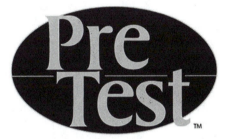

Clinical Vignettes for the USMLE Step 1

PreTest™ Self-Assessment and Review

Notice

Medicine is an ever-changing science. As new research and clinical experience broaden our knowledge, changes in treatment and drug therapy are required. The authors and the publisher of this work have checked with sources believed to be reliable in their efforts to provide information that is complete and generally in accord with the standards accepted at the time of publication. However, in view of the possibility of human error or changes in medical sciences, neither the authors nor the publisher nor any other party who has been involved in the preparation or publication of this work warrants that the information contained herein is in every respect accurate or complete, and they disclaim all responsibility for any errors or omissions or for the results obtained from use of the information contained in this work. Readers are encouraged to confirm the information contained herein with other sources. For example and in particular, readers are advised to check the product information sheet included in the package of each drug they plan to administer to be certain that the i nformation contained in this work is accurate and that changes have not been made in the recommended dose or in the contraindications for administration. This recommendation is of particular importance in connection with new or infrequently used drugs.

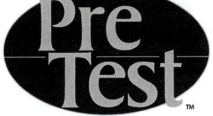

Clinical Vignettes for the USMLE Step 1

PreTest™ Self-Assessment and Review

Fourth Edition

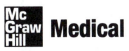

New York   Chicago   San Francisco   Lisbon   London   Madrid   Mexico City
Milan   New Delhi   San Juan   Seoul   Singapore   Sydney   Toronto

Clinical Vignettes for the USMLE Step 1: PreTest™ Self-Assessment and Review, Fourth Edition

Copyright © 2008 by The McGraw-Hill Companies, Inc. All rights reserved. Printed in the United States of America. Except as permitted under the United States Copyright Act of 1976, no part of this publication may be reproduced or distributed in any form or by any means, or stored in a data base or retrieval system, without the prior written permission of the publisher.

Previous editions copyright © 2005, 2004, and 2001 by The McGraw-Hill Companies, Inc.

PreTest™ is a trademark of The McGraw-Hill Companies, Inc.

1 2 3 4 5 6 7 8 9 0   DOC/DOC   0 9 8 7

ISBN: 978-0-07-147184-8
MHID: 0-07-147184-7

This book was set in Berkeley by International Typesetting and Composition.
The editors were Catherine A. Johnson and Regina Y. Brown.
The production supervisor was Sherri Souffrance.
Project management was provided by International Typesetting and Composition.
The cover designer was Maria Scharf.
RR Donnelley was printer and binder.

This book is printed on acid-free paper.

Library of Congress Cataloging-in-Publication Data

Clinical vignettes for the USMLE step 1 : pretest self-assessment and review.—4th ed.
    p. ; cm.
  Includes bibliographical references.
  ISBN-13: 978-0-07-147184-8 (pbk. : alk. paper)
  ISBN-10: 0-07-147184-7 (pbk. : alk. paper)
    1. Medicine—Examinations, questions, etc.   2. Medical sciences—Examinations, questions, etc.   3. Physicians—Licenses—United States—Examinations—Study guides. [DNLM: 1. Medicine—Examination Questions. W 18.2 C6412   2008]
  R834.5.C563   2008
  610.76—dc22

                                        2007026595

Contents

Introduction

The current format of the United States Medical Licensing Examination Step 1 (USMLE Step 1) exam emphasizes clinical vignettes—in single-best-answer multiple-choice format—as the only test question. The examination is 350 questions broken into seven blocks of 50 questions each. Examinees have one hour to complete each block.

Clinical Vignettes for the USMLE Step 1: Fourth Edition parallels this format. The book contains 350 clinical vignette-style questions covering the core basic sciences and was assembled based on the published content outline for the USMLE Step 1. The questions are divided into 7 blocks of 50 questions. As on the Step 1 exam, each block tests the examinee on all core basic science areas. Answers are in the second half of the book. Each answer is accompanied by a concise but comprehensive explanation and is referenced to a key textbook or journal article for further reading.

The questions in this book were culled from the seven *PreTest Basic Science* books. The publisher acknowledges and thanks the following authors for their contributions to this book:

Anatomy, Histology, and Cell Biology: Robert M. Klein, PhD and George C. Enders, PhD
Biochemistry and Genetics: Golder Wilson, MD
Microbiology: James D. Kettering, PhD and Hansel M. Fletcher, PhD
Neuroscience: Allan Siegel, PhD
Pathology: Earl J. Brown, MD
Pharmacology: Marshal Shlafer, PhD
Physiology: Patricia Metting, PhD

McGraw-Hill
November 2007

Block I

Questions

1-1. A patient has been referred to your academic medical center because of recent-onset ventricular ectopy, second degree AV nodal block, chromatopsia, and other extracardiac signs and symptoms of digoxin intoxication. His family doctor, who has been treating him for a host of common medical problems over the last 30 years, had prescribed furosemide and digoxin for this gentleman's heart failure. Blood tests show that serum digoxin levels are well within a normal range. We believe the problems are diuretic-induced. Which of the following does the diuretic most likely do to account for the digoxin toxicity?

a. Caused hypercalcemia
b. Caused hypokalemia
c. Caused hyponatremia
d. Displaced digoxin from tissue binding sites
e. Inhibited digoxin's metabolic elimination

1-2. A 62-year-old male who was diagnosed with lung cancer also displays weakness in his arms and legs. A battery of tests are administered to the patient, including those involving nerve conduction. The nerve conduction test reveals a reduction in the compound motor action potential relating to muscles of the hand. However, the amplitude of this potential improves significantly following exercise involving the relevant muscles. Which of the following is the most likely diagnosis?

a. MS
b. ALS
c. Myasthenia gravis
d. Lambert-Eaton syndrome
e. MD

1-3. A 29-year-old woman (gravida 3, para 2) gave birth to a healthy baby after 38 weeks of gestation and delivered the intact placenta spontaneously. The pregnancy was complicated by preeclampsia, but fetal monitoring and ultrasound were normal throughout gestation. The predominant structures shown in the accompanying photomicrograph of the placenta are derived from which of the following?

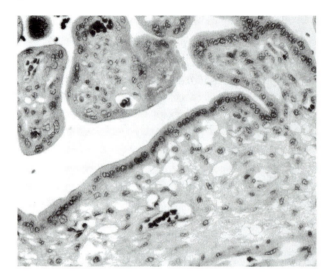

a. A combination of fetal and maternal tissues
b. Endometrial glands
c. Endometrial stroma
d. Fetal tissues
e. Maternal blood vessels

1-4. A 48-year old woman suffering from a severe tension headache is brought to the Emergency Department after her husband discovered her unresponsive and barely breathing when he stopped at home from work during his lunch hour. A bottle of Vicodin was found next to the bathroom sink. Which of the following arterial blood gases are most consistent with her clinical presentation?

a. pH = 7.27; Paco$_2$ = 60 mmHg, [HCO$_3^-$] = 26 mEq/L, Anion Gap = 12 mEq/L
b. pH = 7.02; Paco$_2$ = 60 mmHg, [HCO$_3^-$] = 15 mEq/L, Anion Gap = 12 mEq/L

c. pH = 7.10; $Paco_2$ = 20 mmHg, $[HCO_3^-]$ = 6 mEq/L, Anion Gap = 30 mEq/L
d. pH = 7.51; $Paco_2$ = 49 mmHg, $[HCO_3^-]$ = 38 mEq/L, Anion Gap = 14 mEq/L
e. pH = 7.40; $Paco_2$ = 20 mmHg, $[HCO_3^-]$ = 10 mEq/L, Anion Gap = 26 mEq/L

I-5. A 6-month old infant is admitted to the hospital with acute meningitis. The Gram stain reveals gram-positive, short rods, and the mother indicates that the child has received "all" of the meningitis vaccinations. Which of the following is the most likely cause of the disease?

a. *H. influenzae*
b. *L. monocytogenes*
c. *N. meningitidis,* group A
d. *N. meningitidis,* group C
e. *S. pneumoniae*

I-6. An AIDS patient complains of headaches and disorientation. A clinical diagnosis of *Toxoplasma encephalitis* is made, and *Toxoplasma* cysts are observed in a brain section (see figure below). Which of the following antibody results would be most likely in this patient?

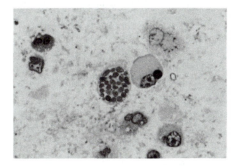

a. IgM nonreactive, IgG nonreactive
b. IgM nonreactive, IgG reactive (low titer)
c. IgM reactive (low titer), IgG reactive (high titer)
d. IgM reactive (high titer), IgG reactive (high titer)
e. IgM reactive (high titer), IgG nonreactive

I-7. A 14-month-old boy presents with a fever of 102°F. The child has a longstanding history of recurrent lower respiratory tract infections including bronchitis and pneumonia. Chronic diarrhea is a longstanding problem. His mother reports that she had numerous upper respiratory infections and chronic diarrhea as a young child. A complete blood count, lung function tests, and urinalysis values are all within normal range. Serum immunoglobulin levels are normal for IgG and IgM, but IgA was 25 mg/dL (normal = 40–60 mg/dL). There are numerous neutrophils and other white cells in the stool sample and the stool is cultured for specific bacteria. IgA coats pathogens facilitating repulsion of the negative charge on the cell membrane. That negative charge on the cell membrane is primarily caused by which of the following?

a. Free saccharide groups
b. Glycoprotein
c. Cholesterol
d. Peripheral membrane protein
e. Integrins

I-8. A 47-year-old man presents with headaches, muscle weakness, and leg cramps. He is not currently taking any medications. Physical examination finds a thin adult man with mild hypertension. Laboratory examination reveals slightly increased sodium, decreased serum potassium level, and decreased hydrogen ion concentration. Serum glucose levels are within normal limits. A CT scan reveals a large tumor involving the cortex of his left adrenal gland. Which of the following combinations of serum laboratory findings is most likely to be present in this individual?

a. Decreased aldosterone with increased renin
b. Decreased cortisol with decreased ACTH
c. Increased aldosterone with decreased renin
d. Increased cortisol with increased ACTH
e. Increased deoxycorticosterone with increased cortisol

I-9. Following hemisection of the spinal cord at the level of approximately T3, a patient experiences loss of pain and temperature on the left side of the leg. Which of the following tracts was affected by the hemisection of the cord that could account for this deficit?

a. Right fasciculus cuneatus
b. Right fasciculus gracilis
c. Right spinothalamic tract
d. Left spinothalamic tract
e. Left corticospinal tract

1-10. A 27-year-old patient with insulin-dependent diabetes mellitus told his roommate that he could not afford to refill his insulin prescription until he got a paycheck. The roommate offered to get it for him, but the patient assured him he could wait until after the weekend. When the roommate returned from a weekend trip on Sunday evening, he found the man unresponsive on the couch, and called 9-1-1. Which of the following arterial blood gases taken in the Emergency Department would be expected in diabetic coma?

a. pH = 7.22; $Paco_2$ = 60 mmHg, [HCO_3^-] = 26 mEq/L, Anion Gap = 12 mEq/L
b. pH = 7.02; $Paco_2$ = 60 mmHg, [HCO_3^-] = 15 mEq/L, Anion Gap = 12 mEq/L
c. pH = 7.10; $Paco_2$ = 20 mmHg, [HCO_3^-] = 6 mEq/L, Anion Gap = 30 mEq/L
d. pH = 7.51; $Paco_2$ = 49 mmHg, [HCO_3^-] = 38 mEq/L, Anion Gap = 14 mEq/L
e. pH = 7.40; $Paco_2$ = 20 mmHg, [HCO_3^-] = 10 mEq/L, Anion Gap = 26 mEq/L

1-11. A 63-year-old man presents with signs of congestive heart failure, including shortness of breath, cough, and paroxysmal nocturnal dyspnea. Physical examination reveals a hyperdynamic, bounding, "water-hammer" pulse and a decrescendo diastolic murmur. His hyperdynamic pulse causes "bobbing" of his head. Which of the following is the most frequent cause of the cardiac valvular abnormality present in this individual?

a. Aortic dissection
b. Infective endocarditis
c. Latent syphilis
d. Marfan syndrome
e. Rheumatic fever

1-12. An elderly female suffering from an infection complained that she could not salivate and was unable to display lacrimation on the right side of her face. Following a neurological examination, it was determined that a peripheral component of a cranial nerve was affected by this disorder. Which of the following cell bodies of origin form the origin of the affected cranial nerve?

a. Dorsal motor nucleus of the vagus
b. Nucleus ambiguus
c. Inferior salivatory nucleus
d. Superior salivatory nucleus
e. Edinger-Westphal nucleus of cranial nerve III

1-13. An immunocompromised person with a history of seizures has an MRI that reveals a temporal lobe lesion. Brain biopsy results show multinucleated giant cells with intranuclear inclusions. Which of the following is the most probable cause of the lesion?

a. Coxsackievirus
b. Hepatitis C virus
c. Herpes simplex virus
d. *Listeria monocytogenes*
e. Parvovirus

1-14. Soon after returning from a trip to Costa Rica, a 41-year-old woman develops recurrent chills and high fever that recur every 48 h. Examination of her peripheral blood reveals red granules (*Schüffner's dots*) in enlarged, young erythrocytes. Which of the following organisms is most likely to have produced her signs and symptoms?

a. *Afipia felis*
b. *Ancyclostoma duodenale*
c. *B. microti*
d. *P. ovale*
e. *Toxoplasma gondii*

1-15. A 22-year-old woman presents at the ophthalmology clinic. She describes an initial inability to drive at night because of what she describes as "night blindness." She says that the deterioration of her vision has continued and she is having difficulty seeing objects on the periphery of her vision. Visual acuity, color, visual field, dark adaptation, and ERG testing is completed. The tests show rod degeneration with limited peripheral vision. She has pigment deposits in the mid-peripheral retina known as "bone spicules." She also has attenuated vessels in the retina and paleness of the optic nerves. An electroretinogram (ERG) is reduced in amplitude. The cause may be related to a failure of opsin and other protein vesicle transport. This transport would occur along which of the following?

a. Microfilaments (thin filaments)
b. Thick filaments
c. Microtubules
d. Intermediate filaments
e. Spectrin heterodimers

1-16. A 57-year-old woman is undergoing a femoral popliteal bypass for her peripheral vascular disease. The vascular surgeon wishes to induce a localized arteriolar constriction to help control hemostasis. An increase in the local concentration of which of the following agents will cause systemic vasoconstriction?

a. Nitric oxide
b. Angiotensin II
c. Atrial natriuretic peptide
d. A β_2-adrenergic agonist
e. Adenosine

I-17. We administer a drug with the intent of lowering a patient's elevated LDL and total cholesterol levels, and raising HDL levels. The drug we choose inhibits cholesterol synthesis by inhibiting 3-hydroxy-3-methylglutaryl-coenzyme A (better known as [HMG CoA] reductase). Which of the following drugs best fits this description and works by the stated mechanism of action?

a. Clofibrate
b. Gemfibrozil
c. Lovastatin
d. Nicotinic acid (niacin)
e. Probucol

I-18. A parent is correcting his child's photograph for red eye and notes one of the child's pupils reflects the flash as white rather than red. An ophthalmologist confirms the presence of a tumor in the back of the white-reflecting eye, telling the parents about the possibility of retinoblastoma (180200). The parents return to their pediatrician, confused about the relation of retinoblastoma (Rb) and B-cell lymphoma (bcl) genes they saw on the Internet and the possibility their child's tumor is inherited. Which of the following is the most appropriate response?

a. Rb and bcl proteins are polymerases that prevent oncogenesis by stringent DNA repair; the parents are therefore carriers for autosomal recessive Rb deficiency with a 1 in 4 recurrence risk.
b. Rb protein binds transcription factors needed for cell division and bcl protein (cyclin D1) stimulates it; Rb is a tumor suppressor gene requiring homozygous mutations (two hits) that are likely sporadic in a child with unilateral tumor.
c. Rb and bcl proteins are DNA-binding factors that suppress promoters near oncogenes and act as tumor suppressors; the child represents a new, dominant-acting mutation and the parents have a minimal recurrence risk.
d. Rb protein stimulates cyclins specific for retinal tissue and bcl does the same for lymphatic cyclins; the child represents a new mutation with excess Rb activity.
e. Rb protein forms complexes with bcl protein that promotes cell division in rapidly proliferating tissues; the child represents a new mutation with excess Rb-bcl complex activity.

1-19. A 48-year-old woman presents with a 1.5-cm firm mass in the upper outer quadrant of her left breast. A biopsy from this mass reveals many of the ducts to be filled with atypical cells. In the center of these ducts there is extensive necrosis. No invasion into the surrounding fibrous tissue is seen. Which of the following is the most likely diagnosis?

a. Colloid carcinoma
b. Comedocarcinoma
c. Infiltrating ductal carcinoma
d. Infiltrating lobular carcinoma
e. Lobular carcinoma in situ

1-20. A forest worker experiences a sudden onset of fever, headache, myalgias, and prostration. A macular rash develops several days later, with it appearing first on the hands and feet before moving onto his trunk. Which of the following treatments is most appropriate?

a. Amphoteracin B
b. Cephalosporin
c. Erythromycin
d. Sulfonamides
e. Tetracycline

1-21. A 29-year-old woman presents with nervousness, heat intolerance, and weight loss. Physical examination reveals the presence of exophthalmus, pretibial myxedema, and diffuse enlargement of the thyroid. Laboratory examination reveals elevated serum thyroxine (T4) and triiodothyronine (T3) levels, while the level of serum thyroid-stimulating hormone (TSH) is decreased. Histologic sections from her thyroid gland reveal increased cellularity with scalloping of the colloid at the margins of the follicles. Which of the following types of autoantibodies is most specific for this individual disease?

a. Antimicrosomal antibodies
b. Antithyroglobulin antibodies
c. Antithyroid peroxidase antibodies
d. TSH-receptor-blocking antibodies
e. TSH-receptor-stimulating antibodies

1-22. A 27-year-old woman presents with tender cervical lymphadenopathy. A biopsy of one of the enlarged lymph nodes in this area is diagnosed by the pathologist as being a "reactive lymph node with follicular hyperplasia." The associated schematic depicts the morphology of this reactive change. The majority of the proliferating cells in the area marked by the arrow labeled with an "*" are in the process of transforming into cells that eventually will secrete which substance?

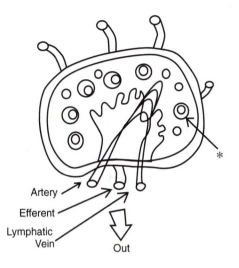

a. Erythropoietin
b. Gamma-interferon
c. Immunoglobulin
d. Interleukin-2
e. Interleukin-3

I-23. A 65-year-old man presents to the neurology clinic with a several year history in which he has less and less energy and spontaneity, memory loss (especially recent events), and mood swings. He is described by his wife as uncharacteristically slow to learn and react and shying away from anything new, preferring the familiar, confused, getting lost easily, and exercising poor judgment. He scores poorly on the mini-mental status examination (MMSE). This disease is believed to be caused by protein misfolding. Chaperonins regulate protein folding in which of the following ways?

a. Stimulating aggregation of proteins
b. Contributing folding information to the native protein
c. Controlling the docking of the signal peptide with its receptor on the rough endoplasmic reticulum
d. Inhibiting proteolytic activity of misfolded proteins
e. Using their ATPase activity to bind and release themselves from hydrophobic regions of the protein

1-24. A 17-year-old boy is admitted to the hospital with a traumatic brain injury, sustained when he fell off his motorcycle. He develops a fever of 39°C, which is unrelated to an infection or inflammation. The fever is most likely due to a lesion of which of the following?

a. The lateral hypothalamus
b. The arcuate nucleus
c. The posterior nucleus
d. The paraventricular nucleus
e. The anterior hypothalamus

1-25. A 3-year-old girl, with no history of vaccination, is brought to the hospital with a sore throat, fever, malaise, and difficulty breathing. Physical examination reveals a gray membrane covering the pharynx. Growth of the etiologic agent on cysteine-tellurite agar forms gray to black colonies with a brown halo. The major virulence factor of this organism is only produced by those strains that will most likely have which of the following characteristics?

a. Encapsulated
b. Glucose fermenters
c. Lysogenic for β-prophage
d. Of the mitis strain
e. Sucrose fermenters

1-26. A patient with epilepsy is started on oral therapy with an appropriate anticonvulsant. Not long after treatment starts he manifests psychotic behaviors that were not present before antiepileptic drug therapy started. Of the following antiepileptic agents, which is associated with the highest risk of causing psychosis?

a. Ethosuximide
b. Phenobarbital
c. Phenytoin
d. Valproic acid
e. Vigabatrin

1-27. A newborn boy is born with first arch congenital malformations classified as Treacher-Collins syndrome, which is an autosomal dominant inherited disorder. The Treacher Collins-Franceschetti syndrome 1 (TCOF) gene encodes the protein treacle. Treacle is localized to the structure labeled with the arrows in the accompanying transmission electron micrograph. Treacle is most likely involved in which of the following?

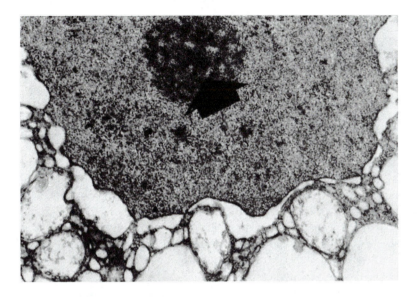

a. Assembly of ribosomal subunits into mature ribosomes
b. Translation of cytosolic proteins
c. Transcription of nuclear proteins
d. Transcription of ribosomal proteins
e. Organelle degradation

I-28. A 34-year-old man with mild anxiety and depression symptoms has heard about buspirone on television and asks whether it might be suitable for him. According to the latest diagnostic criteria, the drug would be appropriate, particularly for short-term symptom control. Which of the following best describes an important property of this drug?

a. Associated with a withdrawal syndrome that, if unsupervised, is frequently lethal
b. Has a significant potential for abuse
c. Is likely to potentiate the CNS depressant effects of alcohol, benzodiazepines, and sedative antihistamines (e.g., diphenhydramine), so such interactants must be avoided at all cost
d. Requires almost daily dosage titrations in order to optimize the response
e. Seldom causes drowsiness

1-29. A 47-year-old female is brought to the Emergency Department because she fainted at the gym during her daily aerobic workout. A prominent systolic murmur is heard and a presumptive diagnosis of aortic stenosis is made. Which of the following is consistent with that diagnosis?

a. A decreased pulse pressure
b. An increased arterial pressure
c. A decreased left ventricular diastolic pressure
d. An increased ejection fraction
e. A decreased cardiac oxygen consumption

1-30. A 5-year-old Egyptian boy receives a sulfonamide antibiotic as prophylaxis for recurrent urinary tract infections. Although he was previously healthy and well-nourished, he becomes progressively ill and presents to your office with pallor and irritability. A blood count shows that he is severely anemic with jaundice due to hemolysis of red blood cells. Which of the following is the simplest test for diagnosis?

a. Northern blotting of red blood cell mRNA
b. Enzyme assay of red blood cell hemolysate
c. Western blotting of red blood cell hemolysates
d. Amplification of red blood cell DNA and hybridization with allele-specific oligonucleotides (PCR-ASOs)
e. Southern blot analysis for gene deletions

1-31. An 11-year-old boy presents with ciliary dyskinesia, sinusitis, and bronchiectasis. He has had persistent infections and otitis media since birth. A PA radiograph shows dextrocardia, and he has a negative saccharin test. In the cross-section of the cilium shown below, which of the following is primarily affected in this disorder?

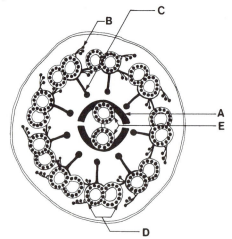

a. Structure A
b. Structure B
c. Structure C
d. Structure D
e. Structure E

I-32. Two weeks after contact with an individual with an acute disease presentation, a 12-year-old girl has fever and malaise, followed by a rash composed of crops of vesicles which lasts 5 days. This common childhood disease is caused by which of the following viruses?

a. Adenovirus
b. Cytomegalovirus
c. Papillomavirus
d. Rubeola
e. Varicella virus

I-33. A 2-day-old neonate becomes lethargic and uninterested in breast-feeding. Physical examination reveals hypotonia (low muscle tone), muscle twitching that suggests seizures, and tachypnea (rapid breathing). The child has a normal heartbeat and breath sounds with no indication of car-diorespiratory disease. Initial blood chemistry values include normal glucose, sodium, potassium, chloride, and bicarbonate (HCO_3^-) levels; initial blood gas values reveal a pH of 7.53, partial pressure of oxygen (Po_2) normal at 103 mmHg, and partial pressure of carbon dioxide (Pco_2) decreased at 27 mmHg. Which of the following treatment strategies is most appropriate?

a. Administer alkali to treat metabolic acidosis
b. Administer alkali to treat respiratory acidosis
c. Decrease the respiratory rate to treat metabolic acidosis
d. Decrease the respiratory rate to treat respiratory alkalosis
e. Administer acid to treat metabolic alkalosis

1-34. A patient is sent to be examined by an endocrinologist after complaining of excessive thirst and increased excretion of urine. The patient is then referred to a neurologist and neuroradiologist, who detect the presence of a secondary brain lesion after viewing an MRI of the patient's brain. Where is the most likely locus of the lesion that could account for these deficits?

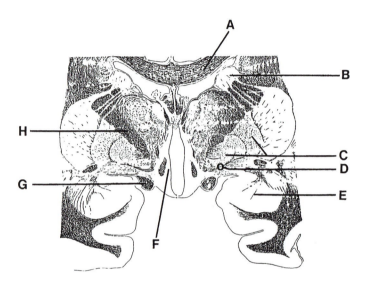

a. A
b. B
c. C
d. D
e. E
f. F
g. G
h. H

I-35. A 32-year-old woman presents at her physician's office complaining of nausea and vomiting. The history reveals that her symptoms have been present for over a month and that they seem to be worse in the morning. A urine sample is taken and shows that the woman is pregnant. Physiological changes that occur during pregnancy include which of the following?

a. Decreased production of cortisol and corticosterone
b. Increased conversion of glucose to glycogen
c. Hypercapnia
d. Increased hematocrit
e. Reduced circulating gonadotropin levels

I-36. After a term uncomplicated gestation, normal delivery, and unremarkable nursery stay, a 10-day-old female is readmitted to the hospital because of poor feeding, weight loss, and rapid heart rate. Antibiotics are started as a precaution against sepsis, and initial testing indicates an unusual echocardiogram with a very short PR interval and a large heart on x-ray. Initial concern about a cardiac arrhythmia changes when a large tongue is noted, causing concern about glycogen storage disease type II (Pompe disease—232300—Table 3). Which of the following best explains why Pompe disease is more severe and lethal compared to other glycogen storage diseases?

a. The deficiency is a degradative rather than synthetic enzyme
b. The deficiency involves a liver enzyme
c. The deficiency involves a lysosomal enzyme
d. The deficiency causes associated neutropenia
e. The deficiency involves a serum enzyme

I-37. A 45-year-old woman presents with increasing fatigue, weakness, and tingling of her arms and legs. Physical examination finds numbness and loss of balance, position, and vibratory sense in both of her lower extremities. Histologic examination of a smear made from a bone marrow aspiration reveals asynchrony in red blood cell precursors between the maturation of their nuclei and their cytoplasm. Additional workup discovers achlorhydria, and a biopsy of the antrum of her stomach reveals chronic atrophic gastritis. Which of the following is the most likely diagnosis?

a. Fanconi anemia
b. Leukoerythroblastic anemia
c. Megaloblastic anemia
d. Myelophthisic anemia
e. Sideroblastic anemia

1-38. An individual was admitted to the emergency room following loss of consciousness. After the patient regained consciousness, he was examined by a neurologist and presented with a right side hemiplegia, loss of sensation on the left side of the face, and his ability to chew. Which of the following arteries was most likely subjected to an infarct that could account for the deficits described in this individual?

a. Posterior inferior cerebellar artery
b. Anterior inferior cerebellar artery
c. Circumferential branches of basilar artery
d. Paramedian branches of basilar artery
e. Anterior spinal artery

1-39. A 34-year-old woman, who has been immobilized with a sprained ankle for the past 4 days, develops a throbbing pain that has spread to her entire left leg. History reveals that she has been taking oral contraceptives for 15 years. Compared to localized pain, such as one might experience from a needle stick, which of the following is true of ischemic pain?

a. Ischemic pain sensory fibers are classified as A delta (Aδ) sensory fibers.
b. Ischemic pain is produced by overstimulating somatic touch receptors.
c. Ischemic pain is transmitted to the brain through the neospinothalamic tract.
d. Ischemic pain receptors quickly adapt to a painful stimulus.
e. Ischemic pain sensory fibers terminate within the substantia gelatinosa of the spinal cord.

1-40. A 40-year-old female reports chronic gastritis. She tests positive for *H. pylori*. After a course of the appropiate antibiotic theraphy her symptoms subside. Which of the following is the most effective noninvasive test for the diagnosis of *Helicobacter*-associated gastric ulcers?

a. Culture of stomach contents for *H. pylori*
b. Detection of *H. pylori* antigen in stool
c. Growth of *H. pylori* from a stomach biopsy
d. Growth of *H. pylori* in the stool
e. IgM antibodies to *H. pylori*

1-41. A 26-year-old woman has rhinorrhea, excessive lacrimation, and ocular congestion from a bout with the common cold. Diphenhydramine provides symptomatic relief. Which of the following is the most likely mechanism by which this drug gave symptom relief in the presence of this rhinovirus?

a. α-Adrenergic activation (agonist)
b. β-Adrenergic blockade
c. Calcium channel blockade

d. Histamine (H_1) receptor blockade
e. Muscarinic receptor blockade

I-42. A pregnant 29-year-old woman diagnosed with type I diabetes 2 decades ago, taking Humulin three times per day, is referred to the ophthalmology clinic. She is complaining of "floaters" and difficulty with night-time driving. Dilated indirect ophthalmoscopy coupled with biomicroscopy and fundus photography detect the presence of proliferative diabetic retinopathy with leaky retinal vessels indicative of increased vascular permeability, growth of new, fragile vessels on the retina and posterior surface of the vitreous and macular edema. Overexpression of fibronectin is a histological marker of diabetic microangiopathy. Which of the following is the primary function of fibronectin in the basement membrane?

a. Elasticity
b. Cell attachment and adhesion
c. Binding to selectins
d. Binding to cadherins
e. Binding to actin filaments

I-43. A 55-year-old male alcoholic presents with symptoms of liver disease and is found to have mildly elevated liver enzymes. A liver biopsy examined with a routine hematoxylin and eosin (H&E) stain reveals abnormal clear spaces in the cytoplasm of most of the hepatocytes. Which of the following materials is most likely forming these cytoplasmic spaces?

a. Calcium
b. Cholesterol
c. Hemosiderin
d. Lipofuscin
e. Triglyceride

I-44. A teenage girl is brought to the medical center complaining of fatigue that prevents participation in gym class. A consulting neurologist finds muscle weakness in the girl's arms and legs. Laboratory testing demonstrates elevated serum triacylglycerides esterified with long-chain fatty acids and borderline low glucose. Muscle biopsy shows increased numbers of lipid vacuoles. Which of the following is the most likely diagnosis?

a. Fatty acid synthase deficiency
b. Tay-Sachs disease
c. Carnitine deficiency
d. Biotin deficiency
e. Lipoprotein lipase deficiency

1-45. A 2-week-old baby is hospitalized for inadequate feeding and poor growth. The parents are concerned by the child's weak cry. An experienced grandmother accompanies them, saying she thought the cry sounded like a cat's meow. The grandmother also states that the baby doesn't look much like either parent. The physician orders a karyotype after noting a small head size (microcephaly) and subtle abnormalities of the face. Which of the results pictured below is most likely?

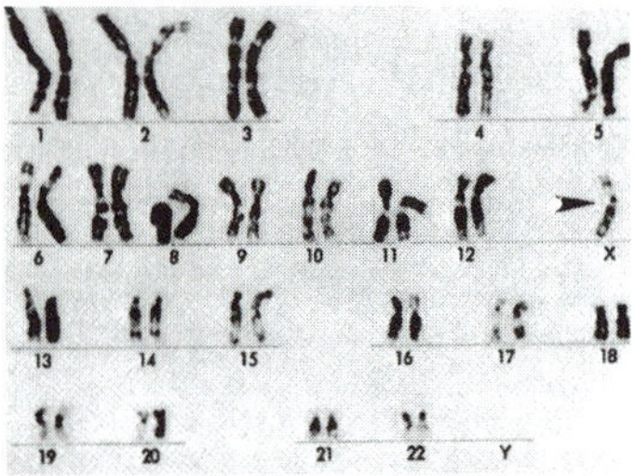

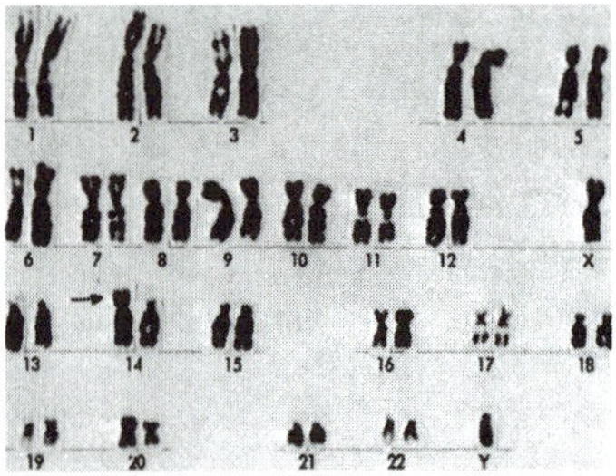

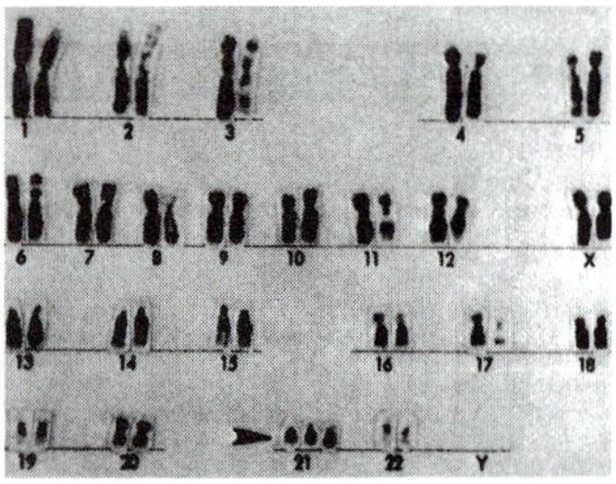

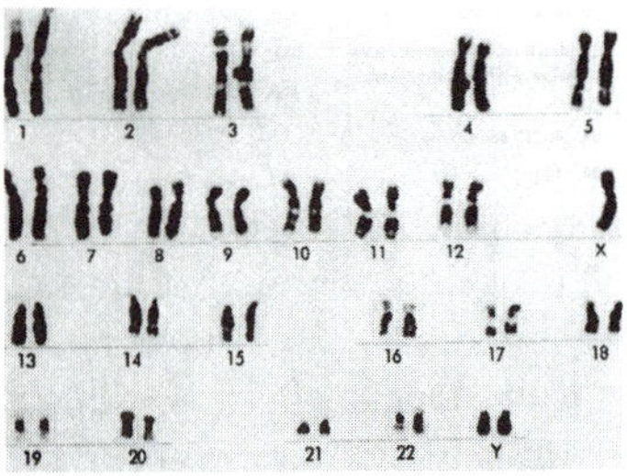

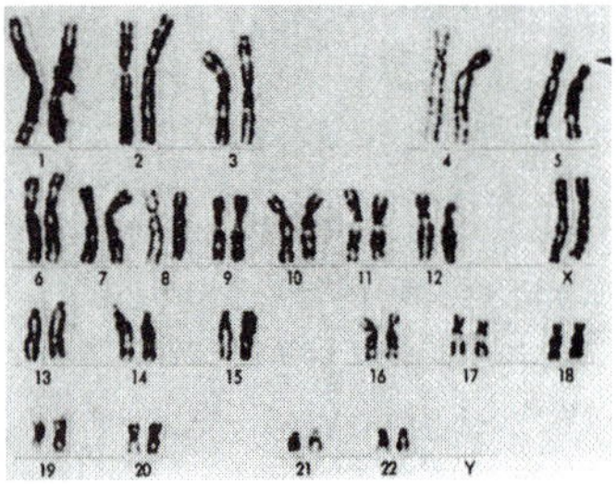

a. Result A
b. Result B
c. Result C
d. Result D
e. Result E

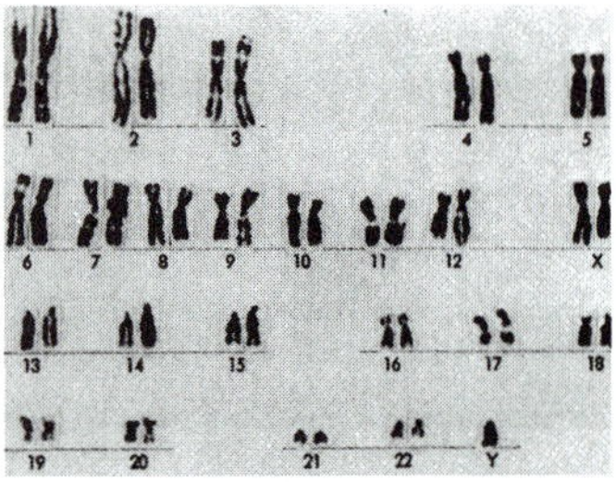

1-46. A woman has severe irritable bowel syndrome characterized by frequent, profuse, and symptomatic diarrhea. She has not responded to first-line therapies and is started on alosetron. Which of the following is the most worrisome adverse effect associated with this drug?

a. Cardiac arrhythmias (serious, e.g., ventricular fibrillation)
b. Constipation, bowel impaction, ischemic colitis
c. Parkinsonian extrapyramidal reactions
d. Pulmonary fibrosis
e. Renal failure

1-47. A patient with renal failure is undergoing periodic hemodialysis while awaiting a transplant. Between dialysis sessions we want to reduce the body's phosphate load by reducing dietary phosphate absorption and removing some phosphate already in the blood. Which of the following drugs would be most suitable for this purpose?

a. Aluminum hydroxide
b. Bismuth subsalicylate
c. Magnesium hydroxide/oxide
d. Sodium bicarbonate
e. Sucralfate

1-48. Histologic sections from a 3-cm mass found in the mandible of a 55-year-old woman reveal a tumor consisting of nests of tumor cells that appear dark and crowded at the periphery of the nests and loose in the center (similar to the stellate reticulum of a developing tooth). Grossly, the lesions consist of multiple cysts filled with a thick, "motor oil"–like fluid. Which of the following is the most likely diagnosis?

a. Pleomorphic adenoma
b. Ameloblastoma
c. Mucoepidermoid carcinoma
d. Adenoid cystic carcinoma
e. Acinic cell carcinoma

1-49. A 24-year-old woman presents after having several "attacks" that last for about 24 h. She states that during these attacks she develops nausea, vomiting, vertigo, and ringing in her ears. Physical examination reveals a sensorineural hearing loss. Which of the following is the most likely cause of this woman's signs and symptoms?

a. Acute suppurative inflammation of the middle ear
b. Dilation of the cochlear duct and saccule
c. Obstruction of the middle ear by a cyst filled with keratin
d. Destruction of the tympanic membrane by a benign neoplasm
e. New bone formation around the stapes and the oval window

1-50. A 2-month-old male infant, who was born at term without any pre-natal abnormalities, is being evaluated for possible visual problems. He is noted to have an abnormal white light reflex involving his right eye, and examination finds a large mass that has almost completely filled the poste-rior chamber of this eye. Which of the following cells are most likely to be seen proliferating in histologic sections from this mass?

a. Benign fibroblasts and endothelial cells
b. Foamy macrophages with cytoplasmic clear vacuoles
c. Plasmacytoid cells within a dense Congo red–positive stroma
d. Small cells forming occasional rosette structures
e. Spindle-shaped cells with cytoplasmic melanin

Block 2

Questions

2-1. Parents bring in their 2-week-old child fearful that he has ingested a poison. They had delayed disposing one of the child's diapers, and noted a black discoloration where the urine had collected. Later, they realized that all of the child's diapers would turn black if stored as waste for a day or so. Knowing that phenol groups can complex to form colors, which of the following amino acid pathways are implicated in this phenomenon?

a. The phenylalanine, tyrosine, and homogentisate pathway
b. The histidine pathway
c. The leucine, isoleucine, and valine pathway
d. The methionine and homocystine pathway
e. The arginine and citrulline pathway (urea cycle)

2-2. A 6-month-old boy is being evaluated for a lesion on his chin. Physical examination finds a raised, nontender, bright red strawberry-colored vascular lesion measuring approximately 4 mm in greatest dimension. At this time, which of the following is the best therapy for this infant?

a. Leave alone and follow up on a routine basis
b. Photocoagulation with yellow-green laser light
c. Repeated injections with steroids
d. Shave biopsy with frozen section diagnosis
e. Wide local excision with sentinel node sampling

2-3. A 52-year-old male develops an abscess following surgery to repair an abdominal gunshot wound. Gram stain of the exudates from his foul-smelling abscess reveals numerous polymorphonuclear neutrophils (PMNs) and several gram-negative rods that did not grow on blood plates in the presence of O_2. Metabolism of O_2 results in toxic reactive oxygen species. Which of the following enzymes is most likely involved in the following reaction?

$$2O^{2-} + 2H^+ \rightarrow H_2O_2 + O_2$$

a. ATPase
b. Catalase
c. Oxygen permease
d. Peroxidase
e. Superoxide dismutase

2-4. A 49-year-old male in end-stage renal failure is able to perform peritoneal dialysis at home. The osmolality of the solution chosen for peritoneal dialysis will determine the rate of ultrafiltration. Which of the following statements best characterizes a molecule whose osmolality is zero?

a. It will not permeate the membrane
b. It can only cross the membrane through the lipid bilayer
c. It causes water to flow across the membrane
d. It is as diffusible through the membrane as water
e. It is transported across the membrane by a carrier

2-5. A 26-year-old African American woman presents with nonspecific symptoms including fever, malaise, and increasing respiratory problems. A chest x-ray reveals enlarged hilar lymph nodes, while laboratory tests find her serum calcium level to be elevated. A transbronchial biopsy reveals scattered chronic inflammatory cells, reactive epithelial changes, and several noncaseating granulomas. The pathomechanism involved in the formation of these noncaseating granulomas involves the activation of macrophages to form epithelial cells by the action of which substance?

a. Gamma-interferon
b. Leukotriene C4
c. Interleukin-2
d. Interleukin-5
e. Interleukin-12

2-6. A nurse develops clinical symptoms consistent with hepatitis. She recalls sticking herself with a needle approximately 4 months before, after drawing blood from a patient. Serologic tests for HBsAg, antibodies to HBsAg, and hepatitis A virus (HAV) are all negative; however, she is positive for IgM core antibody. Which of the following characterizes the current health state of the nurse?

a. Does not have hepatitis B
b. Has hepatitis A
c. Has hepatitis C
d. Is in the late stages of hepatitis B infection
e. Is in the "window" (after the disappearance of HBsAg and before the appearance of anti–HBsAg)

2-7. A 10-year-old boy is brought into your office by his mother. The boy is supporting his left arm at the elbow by using his right hand because he thinks he has "broken his arm." The 10-year-old had been playing tag and tripped over the curb and landed on the grass, catching himself with his hands. Upon physical examination you note a slight drooping of the left shoulder when unsupported, and tenderness over the midclavicular region but *no* palpable fracture or displacement. The jugular notch appears symmetrical. The shoulder has normal movement, but the boy is unwilling to lift his hand above his head because it hurts. Otherwise, hand and arm movements are relatively normal with normal sensation. You order an AP and lateral x-rays of the thorax and upper arm because you suspect which of the following?

a. Colles' fracture
b. Scaphoid fracture
c. Fracture of the surgical head of the humerus
d. Dislocated sternoclavicular joint
e. Greenstick fracture of the clavicle

2-8. A 65-year-old obese male presents with pain radiating down the left arm and shortness of breath. A serum lactate dehydrogenase (LDH) level is obtained to evaluate possible myocardial infarction, and its activity is only slightly elevated. Shortly thereafter the laboratory calls, saying that a more detailed analysis of LDH does suggest myocardial damage. The managing physician knows that lactate dehydrogenase is composed of two different polypeptide chains arranged in the form of a tetramer. Which of the following is the likely correlation between LDH measures and the likelihood of myocardial infarction?

a. LDH is an enzyme specific to the endocardium
b. LDH is mainly localized in liver, and its elevation in cardiac disease occurs because of heart failure
c. LDH isozymes are composed of different subunit combinations, some released during inflammation following heart attacks
d. LDH isozymes are composed of different subunit combinations, some specific for heart and released with myocardial damage
e. LDH isozymes are composed of different subunit combinations, some specific for vascular endothelium and released with infarction

2-9. A patient with a family history of peripheral neuropathy is found to have a decrease in nerve conduction velocity and an X-linked mutation of connexin 32, consistent with Charcot-Marie-Tooth Disease. Connexin is an important component of which of the following?

a. Gap junction
b. Sarcoplasmic reticulum
c. Microtubule
d. Synaptic vesicle
e. Sodium channel

2-10. A 67-year-old female was admitted to a hospital after she reported to her primary care physician that she had been having very painful headaches. Further examination revealed the presence of significant increases in intracranial pressure. After viewing a magnetic resonance imaging (MRI), the neurologist concluded that the woman's condition was due to the presence of a developing tumor along the rostral aspect of the medial wall of the lateral ventricle. Which of the structures in the illustration would be most likely to contain this tumor?

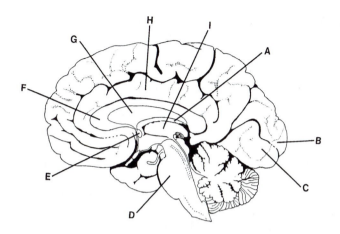

a. A   f. F
b. B   g. G
c. C   h. H
d. D   i. I
e. E

2-11. Your patient has bipolar illness, hypercholesterolemia, chronic-stable angina, and Stage I essential hypertension. He has been taking lithium and an SSRI for the bipolar illness. Cardiovascular drugs include atorvastatin, diltiazem, sublingual nitroglycerin, captopril, and hydrochlorothiazide. Which of the following outcomes, due to interactions involving these drugs, would you most likely expect?

a. Development of acute psychosis from an ACE inhibitor-antipsychotic interaction
b. Development of a hypomanic state from antagonism of lithium's action by the nitroglycerin
c. Lithium toxicity because of hyponatremia caused by the hydrochlorothiazide
d. Loss of cholesterol control from antagonism of the HMG CoA reductase inhibitor by the antipsychotic
e. Worsening of angina because the antipsychotic counteracts the effects of the calcium channel blocker
f. Worsening of angina because the lithium antagonizes the effects of the nitroglycerin

2-12. A hospital worker is found to have hepatitis B surface antigen. Subsequent tests reveal the presence of e antigen as well. Which of the following best describes the worker?

a. Is infective and has active hepatitis
b. Is infective but does not have active hepatitis
c. Is not infective
d. Is evincing a biologic false-positive test for hepatitis
e. Has both hepatitis B and hepatitis C

2-13. A 59-year-old woman presents with headaches and decreasing vision over the past several months. Her children state that she has been bumping into things recently and does not seem to see them when they are not directly in front of her. Physical examination is unremarkable except for the visual field abnormality illustrated in the picture. Her visual problems are most likely to be caused by a tumor originating in which one of the following anatomic areas?

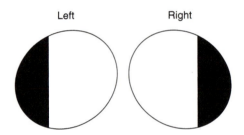

a. Parietal lobe
b. Pineal gland
c. Pituitary gland
d. Posterior orbit
e. Temporal lobe

2-14. A 23-year-old female presents with fatigue and is found to have a systolic murmur and higher than normal cardiac output. The differential diagnosis based on these findings includes which of the following?

a. Hypertension
b. Mitral valve prolapse
c. Anemia
d. Aortic regurgitation
e. Cardiac tamponade

2-15. On November 6, a patient had the onset of an illness characterized by fever, chills, headache, cough, and chest pain. The illness lasted 1 week. On December 5, she had another illness very similar to the first, which lasted 6 days. She had no flu immunization during this period. Her hemagglutination inhibition (HI) antibody titer to swine flu virus was as follows:

November 6   10
November 30   10
December 20   160
(There was no laboratory error)

Which of the following is the best conclusion from these data?

a. The patient was ill with swine flu on November 6
b. The patient was ill with swine flu later, and the November 6 illness was due to another pathogen
c. The patient was ill with swine flu on December 20
d. It is impossible to relate either illness with the specific virus

2-16. A 6-month-old male becomes ill after fruits and vegetables are added to his diet of breast milk. Mother feels that he used to become colicky when she ate fruit, although her pediatrician did not think this was significant. After 1 month of these new foods, the child has stopped gaining weight and the pediatrician feels an enlarged liver. Initial blood tests show a mild acidosis (pH 7.2) with increased lactic acid and low blood glucose. The Clinitest reaction is positive for reducing substances in the urine, but the glucose oxidase test is negative for glucosuria. A glycogen storage disease is suspected, and a liver biopsy dose shows mildly increased glycogen with marked cellular damage suggestive of early cirrhosis. Assays for type IV glycogen storage disease are negative (Table 3), and the initial frozen urine sample is reanalyzed and found to contain fructose. The most likely diagnosis and the reasons for hypoglycemia and glycogen accumulation is which of the following?

a. Hereditary fructose intolerance with inhibition of liver phosphorylase
b. Hereditary fructose intolerance with inhibition of glycogen synthase
c. Essential fructosuria with inhibition of glycogen synthase
d. Essential pentosuria with inhibition of liver phosphorylase
e. Essential fructosuria with allosteric stimulation of glycogen synthase

2-17. A pregnant woman is found to have elevated blood pressure on her check-up at 8 months gestation, and testing by her obstetrician demonstrates anemia with Hemolysis, Elevated Liver enzymes, and Low Platelets that are characteristic of disease represented by the acronym HELLP syndrome. The woman is hospitalized and fetal maturity tests are performed that allow elective premature delivery. The woman quickly recovers but the premature newborn has a dilated heart and elevated liver enzymes that are characteristic of a defect in long chain fatty acid oxidation. The potential enzyme deficiencies are those responsible for sequential oxidation of fatty acids, which include which of the following?

a. Dehydrogenase, hydratase, dehydrogenase, thiolase
b. Transacylase, synthase, reductase
c. Hydratase, reductase, thioesterase
d. Thioesterase, dehydrogenase, thiolase
e. Dehydrogenase, thiolase, thioesterase

2-18. A patient with elevated heart rate and blood pressure is examined by a battery of physicians and they conclude that his condition is due to a deficiency or loss of the carotid sinus reflex. Which of the following is a component of this reflex?

a. Baroreceptor afferent fibers from cranial nerve XI
b. Glossopharyngeal efferent fibers
c. Interneurons within the nucleus ambiguus of the medulla
d. Efferent fibers contained in the intermediate component of the facial nerve
e. Vagal efferent fibers

2-19. A young couple comes to your urology office because of inability to conceive a wanted child after 1 year of unprotected sex. The wife had already undergone a gynecological workup, including testing for 3 months showing a normal ovulation profile as confirmed by an ovulatory kit. The primary care physician describes the husband's physical exam as normal and had already ordered a semen analysis and had forwarded the results to you. The semen volume was 0.5 mL, pH 6.8, and azospermic without any fructose. The husband has a brother, who has two children, one of whom has confirmed cystic fibrosis. You order a pelvic MRI of the husband to determine whether which of the following exist(s)?

a. Bilateral abdominal testicles
b. Hypospadias
c. Congenital absence of ejaculatory ducts and vas deferens
d. Congenital hydrocele
e. Congenital absence of the prostate gland

2-20. A 37-year-old obese man presents with signs and symptoms of hyperglycemia. After appropriate workup, he is diagnosed as having type II diabetes mellitus, which is due in part to insulin resistance. Laboratory evaluation of his serum also finds hypertriglyceridemia, which is due to his diabetes. The most common type of secondary hyperlipidemia associated with diabetes mellitus is characterized by elevated serum levels of which one of the following substances?

a. Chylomicrons
b. High-density lipoproteins
c. Intermediate-density lipoproteins
d. Low-density lipoproteins
e. Very-low-density lipoproteins

2-21. A newborn girl is born with a small mouth, rather widely spaced eyes and low-set ears. Genetic analysis shows a microdeletion on chromosome 22q11.2 leading to a diagnosis of an anomaly which results from failure of the normal development of the third and fourth branchial pouches during embryonic development. Which of the following would be expected to occur in a child with this anomaly?

a. Absence of the parafollicular cells
b. Increased numbers of cells in the deep cortex of the lymph nodes
c. Tetany
d. Excess activity of osteoclasts
e. Increased Ca^{2+} levels in the blood

2-22. A 64-year-old male was admitted to the hospital with edema and congestive heart failure. He was found to have diastolic dysfunction characterized by inadequate filling of the heart during diastole. The decrease in ventricular filling is due to a decrease in ventricular muscle compliance. Which of the following proteins determines the normal stiffness of ventricular muscle?

a. Calmodulin
b. Troponin
c. Tropomyosin
d. Titin
e. Myosin light chain kinase

2-23. A family routinely consumed unpasteurized milk, claiming "better taste." Several members experienced a sudden onset of crampy abdominal pain, fever, and bloody, profuse diarrhea. *C. jejuni* was isolated and identified from all patients. Which of the following is the treatment of choice for this type of enterocolitis?

a. Ampicillin
b. *Campylobacter* antitoxin
c. Ciprofloxacin
d. Erythromycin
e. Pepto-Bismol

2-24. A family is seen for routine prenatal counseling because the mother of two normal children is age 35, the arbitrary "advanced maternal age" when the approximate 1 in 100 risk for fetal chromosome disorders is deemed significant. Family history reveals that the mother's parents and her husband all have had onset of high blood pressure (hypertension) at early ages, and two of mother's grandparents died of strokes that may be hypertension-related. The mother also had some hypertension in the third trimester of her last pregnancy. Recognizing that hypertension is a multifactorial trait, which of the following is the most appropriate explanation and counseling for the couple?

a. Multifactorial determination indicates an interaction between the environment and a single gene, implying a 50% risk for eventual hypertension in mother and offspring
b. Multifactorial determination indicates an interaction between the environment and multiple genes, implying a 5–10% risk for eventual hypertension in mother and offspring
c. Multifactorial determination results from multiple postnatal environmental factors, implying a 75–100% risk for eventual hypertension in mother and a 5–10% risk to offspring
d. Multifactorial determination results from multiple pre- and postnatal environmental factors, implying a 75–100% risk for eventual hypertension in mother and a 5–10% risk to offspring
e. Multifactorial determination implies action of multiple genes independent of environmental factors, implying low risks for hypertension in mother's next pregnancy but a 5–10% risk for eventual hypertension in offspring

2-25. A 23-year-old woman develops the sudden onset of congestive heart failure. Her condition rapidly deteriorates and she dies in heart failure. At autopsy, patchy interstitial infiltrates composed mainly of lymphocytes are found, some of which surround individual myocytes. Which of the following is the most likely cause of this patient's heart failure?

a. Autoimmune reaction (to group A β-hemolytic streptococci)
b. Bacterial myocarditis (due to *S. aureus* infection)
c. Hypersensitivity myocarditis (due to an allergic reaction)
d. Nutritional deficiency (due to thiamine deficiency)
e. Viral myocarditis (due to coxsackievirus infection)

2-26. An apathetic male infant in an underdeveloped country is found to have peripheral edema, a "moon" face, and an enlarged, fatty liver. Which of the following is the basic defect causing this change in the liver?

a. Decreased protein intake leads to decreased lipoproteins
b. Decreased caloric intake leads to hypoalbuminemia
c. Decreased carbohydrate intake leads to hypoglycemia
d. Decreased fluid intake leads to hypernatremia
e. Decreased fat absorption leads to hypovitaminosis

2-27. An 18-year-old girl with a 9-year history of wheezing on exertion is referred for pulmonary function tests. The diagram below represents the spirometry tracing of a forced vital capacity. Her total lung capacity was 110% of predicted. Which of the following values will most likely be above normal?

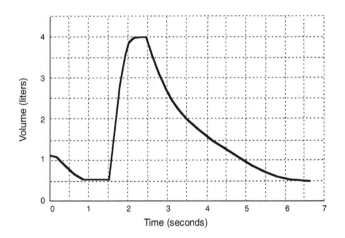

a. Vital capacity
b. Residual volume
c. Expiratory reserve volume
d. $FEV_{1.0}/FVC$
e. Maximum voluntary ventilation

2-28. A 5-year-old boy sustains a tear in his gastrocnemius muscle when he is involved in a bicycle accident. Regeneration of the muscle will occur through which of the following?

a. Differentiation of satellite cells
b. Dedifferentiation of myocytes into myoblasts
c. Fusion of damaged myofibers to form new myotubes
d. Hyperplasia of existing myofibers
e. Differentiation of fibroblasts to form myocytes

2-29. A 45-year-old male is hospitalized for treatment of myocardial infarction. His father and a paternal uncle also had heart attacks at an early age. His cholesterol is elevated, and lipoprotein electrophoresis demonstrates an abnormally high ratio of low- to high-density lipoproteins (LDL to HDL). Which of the following is the most likely explanation for this problem?

a. Mutant HDL is not responding to high cholesterol levels
b. Mutant LDL is not responding to high cholesterol levels
c. Mutant caveolae proteins are not responding to high cholesterol levels
d. Mutant LDL receptors are deficient in cholesterol uptake
e. Intracellular cholesterol is increasing the number of LDL receptors

2-30. A 48-year-old man who has a long history of excessive drinking presents with signs of alcoholic hepatitis. Microscopic examination of a biopsy of this patient's liver reveals irregular eosinophilic hyaline inclusions within the cytoplasm of the hepatocytes. These eosinophilic inclusions are composed of which one of the following substances?

a. Immunoglobulin
b. Excess plasma proteins
c. Prekeratin intermediate filaments
d. Basement membrane material
e. Lipofuscin

2-31. A febrile 52-year-old male patient receiving glucocorticoid treatment presents with vesicular lesions with intense itching, burning, and sharp pain along the back in a specific dermatomal pattern covering his nipple and extending onto the right side of his back. The vesicular lesions do not cross the midline. A Tzanck test is positive. The cause of this illness is the movement of virus from the structures shown in the photomicrograph toward the surface of the skin. This movement occurs in which direction and by which molecular motor?

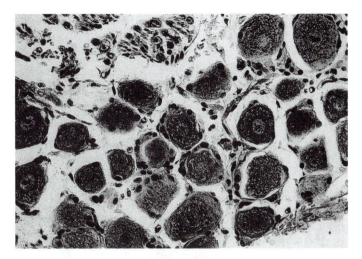

a. Minus end to plus end, dynein
b. Minus end to plus end, kinesin
c. Plus end to minus end, dynein
d. Plus end to minus end, kinesin
e. Minus end to plus end, myosin II

2-32. A 59-year-old male with an ejection fraction of 15%, who is being treated with medications for his heart failure, is asked whether he would like to participate in a trial for an experimental drug. The drug being tested is designed to decrease the expression of phospholamban on ventricular muscle cells. Which of the following would be increased by decreasing phospholamban?

a. The activity of the sodium-potassium pump
b. The diastolic stiffness of the ventricular muscle cells
c. The activity of the L-type calcium channels
d. The duration of the ventricular muscle action potential
e. The concentration of calcium within the SR

2-33. Several employees in a veterinary facility experienced a mild influenza-like infection after working on six sheep with an undiagnosed illness. The etiologic agent causing the human disease is most often transmitted to humans by which of the following methods?

a. Fecal contamination from flea deposits on the skin
b. Inhalation of infected aerosols from animal urine and feces
c. Lice feces scratched into the broken skin during the louse's blood feeding
d. Tick saliva during feeding on human blood
e. Urethral discharge from infected humans

2-34. A 65-year-old man who just retired after having worked for many years as a shipyard worker presents with increasing shortness of breath. Pertinent medical history is that he has been a long time smoker. A CT scan of his chest reveals thick, pleural plaques on the surface of his lungs. The associated picture is from a bronchial washing specimen from this patient. The dumbbell-shaped structures in this picture were found to stain blue with a Prussian blue stain. What are these structures?

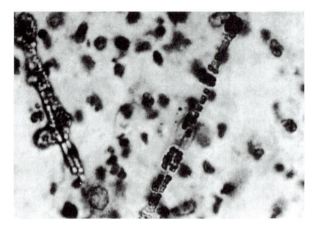

a. *Candida* species
b. Cholesterol crystals
c. Ferruginous bodies
d. Schaumann bodies
e. Silica particles

2-35. Emma is a 64-year-old woman who has had heart disease for many years. While carrying chemicals down the stairs of the dry-cleaning shop where she works, she suddenly lost control of her right leg and arm. She fell down the stairs and was able to stand up with some assistance from a coworker. When attempting to walk on her own, she had a very unsteady gait, with a tendency to fall to the right side. Her supervisor asked her if she was all right, and noticed that her speech was very slurred when she tried to answer. He called an ambulance to take her to the nearest hospital. Upon admission, her face appears symmetric, but when asked to protrude her tongue, it deviates toward the left. She is unable to tell if her right toe is moved up or down by the physician when she closes her eyes, and she can't feel the buzz of a tuning fork on her right arm and leg. In addition, her right arm and leg are markedly weak. The physician can find no other abnormalities in the remainder of Emma's general medical examination.

Where in the nervous system could a lesion occur that would cause arm and leg weakness but spare the face?

a. Right corticospinal tract in the cervical spinal cord
b. Left inferior frontal lobe
c. Right medullary pyramids
d. Occipital lobe
e. Right side of basilar pons

2-36. A 43-year-old anatomy professor is working in her garden, pruning rose bushes without gloves. She has a thorn enter the skin of her forefinger. The area later becomes infected and she removes the thorn, but there is still pus remaining at the wound site. Which of the following cells functions in the formation of pus?

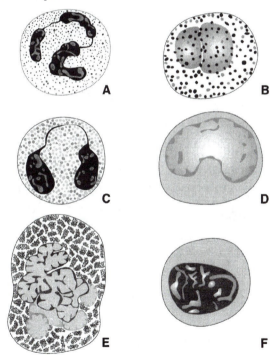

a. A
b. B
c. C
d. D
e. E
f. F

2-37. Valley fever or desert rheumatism is asymptomatic in 60% of individuals, while 40% present with a self limited influenza-like illness with fever, malaise, cough, arthralgia, and headache. Less than 1% develop life-threatening CNS complications. The highly infectious asexual conidia of the etiologic agent are called which of the following?

a. Arthroconidia
b. Blastoconidia
c. Chlamydospores
d. Sporangiospores

2-38. A morbidly obese person visits the local bariatric (weight loss) clinic seeking a pill that will help shed weight. The physician prescribes dextroamphetamine. In addition to causing its expected centrally mediated anorexigenic (appetite-suppressant) effects it causes a host of peripheral adrenergic effects that, for some patients, can prove fatal. Which of the following best summarizes the main mechanism by which dextroamphetamine, or amphetamines in general, cause their peripheral autonomic effects?

a. Activates MAO
b. Blocks NE reuptake via the amine pump/transporter
c. Displaces, releases, intraneuronal NE
d. Enhances NE synthesis, leading to massive neurotransmitter overproduction
e. Stabilizes the adrenergic nerve ending by directly activating α_2 receptors

2-39. A 1-year-old child recently emigrated from Africa exhibits intermittent diarrhea, pallor (pale skin), extreme tenderness of the bones, "rosary" of lumps along the ribs, nose bleeds, bruising over the eyelids, and blood in the urine. Which of the following is the most likely cause?

a. Deficiency of vitamin C due to a citrus-poor diet during pregnancy
b. Hypervitaminosis A due to ingestion of beef liver during pregnancy
c. Deficiency of vitamin C because of reliance on a milk only diet
d. Deficiency of vitamin K because of neonatal deficiency and continued poor nutrition
e. Deficiency of vitamin D due to darker skin pigmentation and poor sun exposure

2-40. An experiment was performed by a physiologist who was interested in identifying a specific kind of neuron within the visual cortex. The type of neuron sought by the investigator was one that responds to an image in a specific position, has discrete excitatory and inhibitory zones, and is associated with a specific axis of orientation. Which of the following cells would respond to such an image?

a. M cells of the lateral geniculate nucleus
b. P cells of the lateral geniculate nucleus
c. Simple cells of the visual cortex
d. Complex cells of the visual cortex
e. Hypercomplex cells of the visual cortex

2-41. A patient stung by a bee is rushed into the emergency room with a variety of symptoms including increasing difficulty in breathing due to nasal and bronchial constriction. Although your subsequent treatment is to block the effects of histamine and other acute-phase reactants released by most cells, you must also block the slow-reacting substance of anaphylaxis (SRS-A), which is the most potent constrictor of the muscles enveloping the bronchial passages. An SRS-A is composed of which of the following?

a. Thromboxanes
b. Interleukins
c. Complement
d. Leukotrienes
e. Prostaglandins

2-42. A 56-year-old man presents to his family medicine physician. He is a 41 year pack/day smoker. He reports that he has had a "typical smoker's cough" for years; however, the morning cough has turned into a chronic productive cough with hemoptysis. He has dyspnea, chest pain, cachexia, increasing dysphonia. He has been treated for 4 respiratory infections in the past 18 months. Examination of the sputum reveals the presence of malignant cells confirmed by fine needle aspiration. Imaging reveals a tumor that is 3 cm in greatest dimension, surrounded by lung parenchyma. Bronchoscopic evaluation reveals a cavitary lesion of a proximal bronchus. Surgical resection is completed and the pathologist classifies the tumor as a T1, N2, MO nonsmall cell lung cancer (NSCLC), specifically a squamous cell carcinoma. Tumor vascularity assessed by bronchial arteriography (BAG) and immunocytochemistry indicates a highly vascular tumor with many microvessels. Vascularity of the tumor is inhibited by upregulation of which of the following?

a. Vascular endothelial growth factor (VEGF)
b. Platelet-derived growth factor (PDGF)
c. Extracellular matrix synthesis
d. Endostatin
e. Periendothelial cell recruitment and proliferation

2-43. A couple has three girls, the last of whom is affected with cystic fibrosis. The first-born daughter marries her first cousin—that is, the son of her
mother's sister—and they have a son with cystic fibrosis. The father has a
female cousin with cystic fibrosis on his mother's side. Which of the
following pedigrees represents this family history?

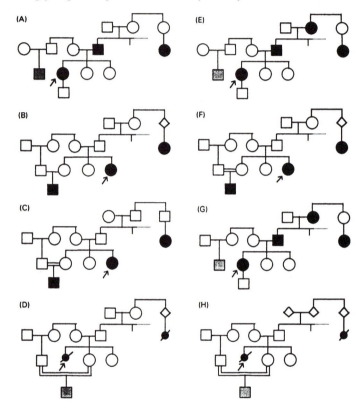

a.   Diagram A
b.   Diagram B
c.   Diagram C
d.   Diagram D
e.   Diagram E
f.   Diagram F
g.   Diagram G
h.   Diagram H

2-44. A 65-year-old man with uncontrolled Type II diabetes and sustained hyperglycemia (serum glucose = 550 mg/dL) and polyuria (5 L/day) is evaluated in the hospital's clinical laboratory because his urine glucose concentration (<100 mM) was much lower than expected. The graph below illustrates the relationship between plasma glucose concentration and renal glucose reabsorption for this patient. The glomerular filtration rate (GFR) is 100 mL/min. Which of the following is the T_{max} for glucose?

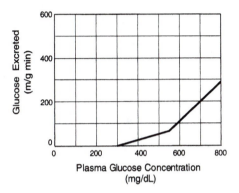

a. 100 mg/min
b. 200 mg/min
c. 300 mg/min
d. 400 mg/min
e. 500 mg/min

2-45. A 3-year-old girl, who has missed several scheduled immunizations, presents to the emergency room with a fever trouble breathing. A sputum sample is brought to the laboratory for analysis. Gram stain reveals the following: rare epithelial cells, 8–10 polymorphonuclear leukocytes per high-power field, and pleomorphic gram-negative rods. As a laboratory consultant, which of the following interpretations is correct?

a. The appearance of the sputum is suggestive of *H. influenzae*
b. The patient has pneumococcal pneumonia
c. The patient has Vincent's disease
d. The sputum specimen is too contaminated by saliva to be useful
e. There is no evidence of an inflammatory response

2-46. A child with developmental delay and unusual features has had routine chromosome analysis that was normal. The physician then considers a "telomere FISH"—analysis of the child's chromosomes using fluorescent DNA probes specific for repetitive DNA sequences near telomeres. The laboratory provides a summary of abnormal FISH results. Which of the following would be the best conclusion from that summary?

a. Longer telomeres in older patients and those with subtle chromosome change
b. Shorter telomeres in cancer tissue and longer telomeres in patients with subtle chromosome change
c. Shorter telomeres in aging patients and a single, specific telomere rearrangement in patients with subtle chromosome change
d. Longer telomeres in cancer tissue and a single, specific telomere rearrangement in patients with subtle chromosome change
e. Shorter telomeres in cancer tissue and a single, specific telomere rearrangement in patients with subtle chromosome change

2-47. An 18-year-old college freshman presents with fever of 103°F, headache, right flank pain, nausea and vomiting, and urinary frequency with hematuria and dysuria. Renal ultrasound demonstrates a right urinary stone with right hydronephrosis. Which of the following antibiotics binds to PBP-2 and is the most appropriate treatment option?

a. Amdinocillin
b. Amphotericin
c. Chloramphenicol
d. Penicillin
e. Trimethoprim

2-48. A 75-year-old African American male with neurogenic bladder presents to the emergency room with hypertension, fever up to 104.6°F, and nausea and vomiting. The urine from his foley catheter gives a positive culture for *Enterococcus faecalis*. Which of the following antibiotics inhibits the final peptide bond between d-alanine and glycine and is the most appropriate treatment for this patient?

a. Amdinocillin
b. Amphotericin
c. Chloramphenicol
d. Penicillin
e. Trimethoprim

2-49. A patient with leukemia has a chest CT finding that suggests aspergillosis. Which of the following antimicrobial binds sterols and alters membrane permeability, and would most likely be used in this patient's treatment?

a. Amdinocillin
b. Amphotericin
c. Chloramphenicol
d. Penicillin
e. Trimethoprim

2-50. A 10-week-old infant is diagnosed with meningitis. A lumbar puncture reveals numerous neutrophils and gram-positive rods. She is admitted to the hospital and is thought to be allergic to β-lactams. Which of the following antibiotics attaches to 50S ribosome, inhibits peptidyl transferase, and would most likely be used to treat this patient?

a. Amdinocillin
b. Amphotericin
c. Chloramphenicol
d. Penicillin
e. Trimethoprim

Block 3

Questions

3-1. A 28-year-old man was exposed to very cold temperatures for several days and noted sometime afterward that he was unable to smile and display other aspects of facial expression on one side of his face. Which of the following is the affected cranial nerve shown on the illustration below?

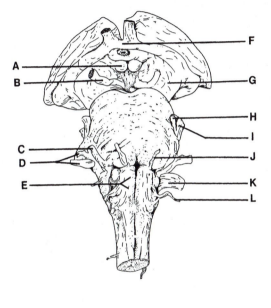

a. A
b. B
c. C
d. D
e. E
f. F
g. G
h. H
i. I
j. J
k. K
l. L

3-2. A 45-year-old male had been receiving drug therapy for the treatment of complex partial seizures when he suffered a deterioration of his condition. One day he fell to the ground with a further loss of consciousness in which all of his extremities were extended and rigid, and jerks of these limbs were displayed as well. Which of the following best characterizes his new condition?

a.   Generalized seizure
b.   Absence seizure
c.   Simple partial seizure
d.   Complex partial seizure
e.   Petit mal epilepsy

3-3. A patient with Alzheimer's disease is taking an acetylcholinesterase inhibitor specifically approved for that indication, primarily because it is quite lipophilic and so enters the CNS well. Which of the following drugs is the patient most likely receiving?

a.   Tacrine
b.   Edrophonium
c.   Neostigmine
d.   Pyridostigmine
e.   Ambenonium

3-4. A 9-year-old schoolchild developed malaise, a low-grade fever, and a morbilliform rash that appeared on the same day. The rash started on the face and spread to the extremities. Which of the following statements best describes the etiologic agent causing this disease?

a.   Incubation time is approximately 3–4 weeks
b.   Measles (rubeola) and German measles (rubella) are caused by the same virus
c.   Onset is abrupt, with cough, coryza, and fever lasts 3 days
d.   Specific antibody in the serum does not prevent disease
e.   Vesicular rashes are characteristic

3-5. A patient presents with Whipple's triad, including plasma glucose <60 mg/dL, symptomatic hypoglycemia, and improvement of symptoms with administration of glucose. CT of the abdomen shows enlargement of the islet cells suggestive of islet cell carcinoma. Which of the following is true regarding the islets of Langerhans?

a. They are found primarily in the head of the pancreas.
b. They constitute approximately 30% of the pancreatic weight.
c. They contain six distinct endocrine cell types.
d. They have a meager blood supply.
e. They secrete insulin and glucagon.

3-6. A 43-year-old woman presents with a cyst on her labia majora with foul-smelling drainage. She says the drainage occurs spontaneously and recently the cyst has enlarged and has become painful. The cyst is associated with the structure in the photomicrograph delineated by the arrow. The mechanism of secretion normally used by this structure is which of the following?

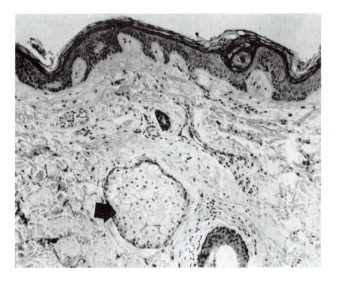

a. Holocrine
b. Merocrine
c. Apocrine
d. Endocrine
e. Autocrine

3-7. A child presents to a pediatrician after being removed from his parents because of severe neglect. The pediatrician notes the child is undersized with sparse hair, boggy subcutaneous tissue, and a hopeless, depressed look. Marasmus is suspected, and supported with laboratory studies that include a low serum protein concentration. The pediatrician institutes a gradual regimen of increased calories and nutrition, gradual because rapid feeding will produce diarrhea and further protein loss. This is because long-term starvation leads to low protein concentrations, reduced osmotic pressure, and acidosis in the tissues, producing the extra tissue fluid (edema) and catabolic state of marasmus. Marasmus and related starvation conditions (like the swollen abdomen and reddish hair of kwashiorkor) demonstrate the importance of proteins in maintaining tissue hydration and pH. The greatest buffering capacity at physiologic pH would be provided by a protein rich in which of the following amino acids?

a. Lysine
b. Histidine
c. Aspartic acid
d. Valine
e. Leucine

3-8. A 59-year-old man has a history of emphysema from 20 years of cigarette smoking; hypercholesterolemia that is being managed with atorvastatin; and Stage 2 essential hypertension for which he is taking metolazone. He presents in clinic today with his main new complaints: nocturia, urinary frequency, and an inability to urinate forcefully and empty his bladder. Following a complete workup, the MD arrives at a diagnosis of benign prostatic hypertrophy (BPH). We start daily therapy with tamsulosin. Which of the following is the most likely side effect the patient may experience from the tamsulosin, and about which he should be forewarned?

a. Bradycardia
b. Increased risk of statin-induced skeletal muscle pathology
c. Orthostatic hypotension
d. Photophobia and other painful responses to bright lights
e. Wheezing or other exacerbations of the emphysema

3-9. A 52-year-old woman with a provisional diagnosis of celiac disease presents with bouts of diarrhea and extreme fatigue. Verification was sought through performance of esophagogastroduodenoscopy to obtain small bowel biopsies. Biopsies of the region shown in the accompanying light micrograph disclose hyperplasia of the structures labeled with the asterisks. The labeled structures produce which of the following?

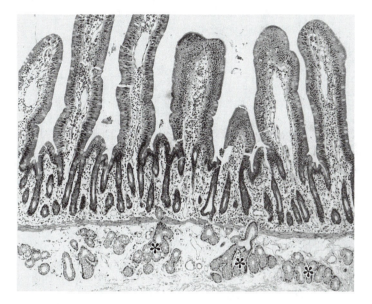

a. Acid
b. Mucus and HCO_3^-
c. Pepsinogen
d. Lysozyme
e. Enterokinase

3-10. A neurological examination of a 75-year-old male revealed that when the abdominal wall was stroked, the muscles of the abdominal wall of the side of the body stimulated failed to contract. Other neurological tests appeared normal. Which of the following is the most likely region of the injury?

a. C1–C5 spinal segments
b. C6–T1 spinal segments
c. T2–T7 spinal segments
d. T8–T12 spinal segments
e. L1–L5 spinal segments

3-11. A 39-year-old man presents with severe writhing back pain, hematuria, and nausea. An intravenous pyelogram (IVP) confirms a diagnosis of renal calculi. The presence of strongly opaque stones on the plain film is suggestive of calcium oxalate stones, which have an increased incidence with hypophosphatemia. The renal clearance of phosphate is increased by which of the following hormones?

a. Aldosterone
b. Parathyroid hormone
c. Norepinephrine
d. Vasopressin
e. Angiotensin

3-12. A 35-year-old man who had been in good health noticed that his right leg was weak. As the day progressed, he found that he was dragging the leg behind him when he walked, and finally asked a friend to drive him home from work because he was unable to lift his right foot up enough to place it on the gas pedal. He also noticed that his left leg felt a little bit numb. Finally, his wife convinced him to go to the emergency room of his local hospital.

In the emergency room, he had a great deal of difficulty walking. He informed the physician that it started slowly several days before but he had ignored the symptoms. His language function, cranial nerves, and motor and sensory examinations of his arms were within normal limits. When the physician examined his right leg, it was markedly weak, with very brisk reflexes in the knee and ankle. Vibration and position sense in the right leg were absent. Pain and temperature testing were normal in the right leg, but these sensations were absent on the left leg and abdomen to the level of his umbilicus. Reflexes in the left leg were normal, but when the physician scratched the lateral portion of the plantar surface on the bottom side of his right foot, the great toe moved up. The remainder of the patient's examination was normal. Which of the following is the primary site of the lesion?

a. Lower brainstem
b. Cervical spinal cord
c. Thoracic spinal cord
d. Lumbar spinal cord
e. Peripheral nerves

3-13. A 45-year-old woman, who works as a corporate executive, presents with the primary complaint of "always being tired." She comments that she has been tired for 4 months even though she is sleeping more. She complains of being unable to finish household chores and "dragging at work." She indicates that she is often constipated and is intolerant to cold. She is continuously turning the thermostats in the house and work to higher temperatures, to the dismay of family members and coworkers, respectively. She also complains that her skin is very dry; use of lotions and creams have not helped the dryness. A biopsy of the thyroid indicates dense lymphocytic infiltration with germinal centers throughout the parenchyma. A battery of tests is carried out. You would expect which of the following?

a. Elevated TSH levels in the serum
b. Elevated T3 and T4 levels in the serum
c. Autoantibodies to the thyroid hormone receptor
d. Elevated calcitonin levels
e. Elevated glucocorticoid levels

3-14. The pediatrician writes a prescription for a combination (of several drugs) product that contains dextromethorphan, which is an isomer of a codeine analog. The patient is a 12-year-old boy. Which of the following is the most likely purpose for which the drug was prescribed?

a. Control mild-moderate pain after the lad broke his wrist playing soccer
b. Manage diarrhea caused by food-borne bacteria
c. Provide sedation because the child has ADD/ADHD
d. Suppress severe cough associated with a bout of influenza
e. Treat nocturnal bed-wetting

3-15. A teenager is brought in by his parents after his physical education teacher gives him a failing grade. The teacher has scolded him for malingering because he drops out of activities after a few minutes of exercise, complaining of leg cramps and fatigue. A stress test is arranged with sampling of blood metabolites and monitoring of exercise performance. Which of the following results after exercise would support a diagnosis of glycogen storage disease in this teenager?

a. Increased oxaloacetate, decreased glucose
b. Increased glycerol and glucose
c. Increased lactate and glucose
d. Increased pyruvate and stable glucose
e. Stable lactate and glucose

3-16. A 30-year-old woman with partial seizures is treated with vigabatrin. Which of the following is the principal mechanism of action of vigabatrin?

a. Sodium channel blockade
b. Increase in frequency of chloride channel opening
c. Increase in GABA
d. Calcium channel blockade
e. Increased potassium channel permeability
f. NMDA receptor blockade

3-17. A previously well 12-year-old boy is brought to the Emergency Department with vomiting and severe abdominal cramps after a prolonged period of exercise. Elevated levels of serum creatinine and blood urea nitrogen suggest acute renal failure. Following treatment and recovery, his serum uric acid concentration (0.6 mg/dL) remains consistently below normal. To determine if his low serum uric acid level is related to renal dysfunction, uric acid clearance studies are conducted and the following data are obtained:

Urine volume = 1 mL/min
Urine uric acid = 36 mg/dL

Which of the following is the patient's uric acid clearance?

a. 6 mL/min
b. 12 mL/min
c. 24 mL/min
d. 48 mL/min
e. 60 mL/min

3-18. A 36-year-old woman presents with increased trouble swallowing. Physical examination finds hypertension and sclerodactyly, while laboratory examination finds an autoantibody against DNA topoisomerase (anti-Scl-70). Which of the following biopsies is most characteristic of this disorder?

a. A conjunctival biopsy that reveals noncaseating granulomas
b. A peripheral nerve biopsy that reveals rare acid-fast bacteria
c. A skin biopsy that reveals dermal fibrosis with an absence of adnexal structures
d. A subcutaneous fat biopsy that reveals an infiltrate of plasma cells and eosinophils
e. A temporal artery biopsy that reveals fragmentation of the internal elastic lamina

3-19. A healthy middle-aged construction worker who engaged in a demolition task 10 days earlier complains of respiratory symptoms similar to those of pneumonia. No causative agent has been isolated from his sputa. The patient does not respond to any antibacterial antibiotics and dies before a definitive diagnosis was established. Microscopic examination of specimens taken of granulomatous and suppurative lesions of the lung obtained during necropsy reveal the presence of large budding yeast cells. The bud is attached to the parent cell by a broad base. Based on this information, which of the following is the most likely diagnosis?

a. Blastomycosis
b. Coccidioidomycosis
c. Cryptococcosis
d. Histoplasmosis
e. Sporotrichosis

3-20. A patient was diagnosed with a form of motor neuron disease that initially affected neurons situated in the dorsolateral aspect of the ventral horn at L1–L4. Which of the following arrangements best describes the deficit likely to be present?

a. LMN paralysis involving the hand
b. UMN paralysis of the upper limb
c. LMN paralysis of the back muscles
d. LMN paralysis of the leg
e. UMN paralysis of the leg

3-21. A 14-year-old girl presents in the pediatric nephrology clinic with fatigue, malaise, anorexia, abdominal pain, and fever. She reports a loss of 6 lb in the last 2 months. Serum gamma globulin as well as the immunoglobulins: IgG, IgA, and IgM are all elevated. She is diagnosed with bilateral photophobia as a result of nongranulomatous uveitis. Her serum creatinine is 1.4 mg/dL (normal: 0.6 to 1.2 mg/dL) and urinalysis of glucose and protein are 2$^+$ on dipstick test and are confirmed by the laboratory at 8.0 g/dL and 0.95 g/dL, respectively. A renal biopsy is prepared for light and electron microscopy. Lymphocytes, plasma cells, and eosinophils are found within infiltrates with pathological change in the tubular basement membrane. The cell most affected is shown in the accompanying transmission electron micrograph. Which of the following is a correct statement about this cell?

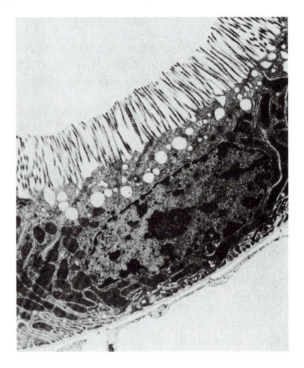

a.   Impermeable to water despite the presence of ADH
b.   The site of the countercurrent multiplier
c.   The site of action of aldosterone
d.   The source of renin
e.   The primary site for the reduction of the tubular fluid volume

3-22. A teenage boy presents to clinic complaining of muscle cramps on exercise. Past history indicates he had some coordination problems in childhood and received occupational therapy. Blood tests show an increased amount of lactic acid at rest, with dramatic increases on exercise testing. Simultaneous measures of capillary oxygenation by a surface probe were normal. The abnormality most likely involves which of the following?

a. Glycolysis in the lysosomes
b. Glycolysis in the cytosol
c. Respiratory chain in the mitochondria
d. Glycogen breakdown in the mitochondria

3-23. A 29-year-old woman is trying to become pregnant. She presents with irregular menstrual cycles and heavy, prolonged, irregular uterine bleeding and undergoes an endometrial biopsy. The biopsy has the appearance shown in the photomicrograph below. Which of the following is characteristic of this stage of the menstrual cycle?

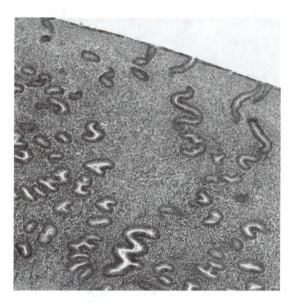

a. It precedes ovulation
b. It depends on progesterone secretion by the corpus luteum
c. It coincides with the development of ovarian follicles
d. It coincides with a rapid drop in estrogen levels
e. It produces ischemia and necrosis of the stratum functionale

3-24. A 64-year-old male complains of difficulty in swallowing and salivating. The patient also fails to elicit a gag reflex following stroking of the pharynx. Further examination reveals a tumor impinging upon a cranial nerve just beyond its exit from the brain. Which cranial nerve in the figure is affected?

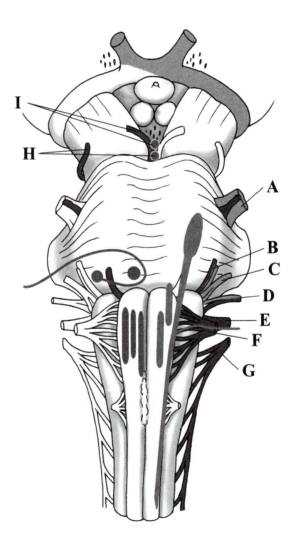

a. A
b. B
c. C
d. D
e. E
f. F
g. G
h. H
i. I

3-25. A patient has Stage III essential hypertension. After evaluating the responses to several other antihypertensive drugs, alone and in combination, the physician places the patient on oral hydralazine. Which of the following adjunct(s) is/are likely to be needed to manage the expected and unwanted cardiovascular side effects of the hydralazine?

a. Captopril plus nifedipine
b. Digoxin plus spironolactone
c. Digoxin plus vitamin K
d. Hydrochlorothiazide and a β blocker
e. Nitroglycerin
f. Triamterene plus amiloride

3-26. An elderly male suffered a stroke that appeared to involve the left internal capsule rather than the cerebral cortex. It resulted in paralysis of the right arm and leg, the tongue deviated to the right side when he was asked to protrude it; lower (jaw) facial expression on the right side was lost, and his speech was slurred, but fluent and grammatically correct. Which of the following best describes the speech deficit in this patient?

a. Wernicke's aphasia
b. Broca's aphasia
c. Anomia
d. Dysarthria
e. Conduction aphasia

3-27. A 57-year-old obese white female is referred to your clinic due to a sore throat characterized by a white pseudomembranous lesion of epithelial cells and organisms. The patient's history reveals type 1 diabetes mellitus and recent penicillin use for a severe bacterial infection in her right foot. Which of the following will most likely be present on microscopic examination?

a. Abundance of septate rhizoids
b. Asci containing 2–8 ascospores
c. Metachromatic granules
d. Spherules containing endospores
e. Yeasts and pseudohyphae

3-28. A man has an aneurysm in the aortic root, a consequence of Marfan's syndrome. He experiences a hypertensive crisis that requires prompt blood pressure control. Nitroprusside will be infused for its immediate antihypertensive effects. Which of the following drugs must we administer along with the nitroprusside to minimize the risk of aneurysm rupture as blood pressure falls?

a. Atropine
b. Diazoxide
c. Furosemide
d. Phentolamine
e. Propranolol

3-29. A second-year medical student was asked to see a nursing home patient as a requirement for a physical diagnosis course. The patient was a 79-year-old man who was apparently in a coma. The student wasn't certain how to approach this case, so he asked the patient's wife, who was sitting at the bedside, why this patient was in a coma. The wife replied, "Oh, Paul isn't in a coma. But he did have a stroke." Slightly confused, the student leaned over and asked Paul to open his eyes. He opened his eyes immediately. However, when asked to lift his arm or speak, Paul did nothing. The student then asked Paul's wife whether she was certain that his eye opening was not simply a coincidence and whether he really was in a coma, since he was unable to follow any commands. Paul's wife explained that he was unable to move or speak as a result of his stroke. However, she knew that he was awake because he could communicate with her by blinking his eyes. The student appeared rather skeptical, so Paul's wife asked her husband to blink once for "yes" and twice for "no." She then asked him if he was at home, and he blinked twice. When asked if he was in a nursing home, he blinked once. The student then asked him to move his eyes, and he was able to look in his direction. However, when the student asked him if he could move his arms or legs, he blinked twice. He also blinked twice when asked if he could smile. He did the same when asked if he could feel someone moving his arm. The student thanked Paul and his wife for their time, made notes of his findings, and returned to class. Where in the nervous system could a lesion occur that can cause paralysis of the extremities bilaterally, as well as in the face, but not of the eyes?

a. High cervical spinal cord bilaterally
b. Bilateral thalamus
c. Bilateral basal ganglia
d. Bilateral basilar pons
e. Bilateral frontal lobe

3-30. A 75-year-old man was rushed to the hospital from his retirement community when he suddenly became confused and could not speak but could grunt and moan. The patient could follow simple commands and did recognize his wife and children although he could *not* name them or speak to them. Additional immediate examination revealed weakness of the right upper extremity. Several days later, a more comprehensive examination revealed weakness and paralysis of the right hand and arm with increased biceps and triceps reflexes. Paralysis and weakness were also present on the lower right side of the face. Pain, temperature, and touch modalities were mildly decreased over the right arm, hand, and face, and proprioception was reduced in the right hand. The patient had regained the ability to articulate a few simple words with great difficulty, but could *not* repeat even simple two or three word phrases. Which artery or major branch of a large artery suffered the occlusion that produced the observed symptoms?

a. Anterior choroidal artery
b. Middle cerebral artery
c. Posterior communicating artery
d. Ophthalmic artery
e. Anterior cerebral artery

3-31. A 61-year-old male presents to his family physician with the chief complaint of frequent diarrhea accompanied by weight loss. He reports a tendency to bruise easily and laboratory data reveal a prothrombin time of 19 seconds (normal = 11–14 seconds). The bruising and prolonged prothrombin time can be explained by a decrease in which of the following vitamins?

a. Vitamin A
b. Vitamin C
c. Vitamin D
d. Vitamin E
e. Vitamin K

3-32. Several young adults camped in a wilderness area and received multiple mosquito bites. Ten days later, one had a sudden onset of headache, chills, and fever, and became stuporous 48 hours later. He was diagnosed with Saint Louis encephalitis (SLE) and recovered completely. Which of the following best describes SLE?

a. It is transmitted to humans by the bite of an infected tick
b. It is caused by a togavirus
c. It is the major arboviral cause of central nervous system infection in the United States
d. It may present initially with symptoms similar to influenza
e. Laboratory diagnosis is routinely made by cultural methods

3-33. A 29-year-old highly promiscuous male with a fever, rash, weight loss, general malaise, and a purulent urethral discharge presents to an STD clinic for the first time. Suspecting a gonococcal infection, the physician obtains a specimen and sends it to the lab for an initial enzyme-linked immunosorbent assay (ELISA) test, a widely used method for detecting antigen. The figure below demonstrates an ELISA for detection of antigen. One of the problems with (ELISA) is nonspecific reactivity due to nonspecific antibody present in the reaction. Of the four steps depicted, A, B, C, and D, which one may be the major cause of nonspecificity?

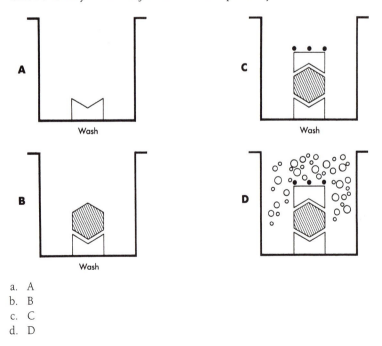

a. A
b. B
c. C
d. D

3-34. A patient with temporal lobe epilepsy is treated with a drug designed to inhibit the principal cell type responsible for the seizures. Which of the following cell types is targeted by this drug?

a. Basket cell
b. Purkinje cell
c. Stellate cell
d. Schwann cell
e. Pyramidal cell

3-35. You are called to the room of a 93-year-old nursing home patient during morning rounds. She is quite upset because she has awoken with double vision and an inability to open her left eye completely. Your presence calms her down somewhat, and you start asking her questions as you perform a complete cranial nerve exam. Her left eye, under her drooping eyelid, is dilated and rotated down and out. It lacks the normal light reflex when you shine light in either eye. There is no evidence of papilledema in either eye. The rest of the cranial nerve exam is normal. Which of the following is the most likely explanation for this condition?

a. An aneurysm of the left posterior cerebral artery compressing cranial nerve III
b. An aneurysm of the right anterior cerebral artery compressing cranial nerve III
c. A tumor at the left optic canal
d. Glaucoma
e. A left parotid gland tumor compressing cranial nerve VII

3-36. A patient suffers badly from a variety of upper respiratory responses during "hay fever" (seasonal allergy) seasons, and his asthma is provoked. We prescribe orally inhaled nedocromil for prophylaxis. Which of the following is the main mechanism by which nedocromil causes its desired effects?

a. Competitively blocks histamine H_1 receptors, thereby blocking bronchoconstriction
b. Decongests mucous membranes via a local vasoconstrictor action
c. Directly binds antigens, preventing them from interacting with mast cell antibodies
d. Inhibits mediator release from immunologically sensitized mast cells
e. Inhibits synthesis of histamine and leukotrienes

3-37. A 2-year-old girl has been healthy until the past weekend when she contracted a viral illness at day care with vomiting, diarrhea, and progressive lethargy. She presents to the office on Monday with disorientation, a barely rousable sensorium, cracked lips, sunken eyes, lack of tears, flaccid skin with "tenting" on pinching, weak pulse with low blood pressure, and increased deep tendon reflexes. Laboratory tests show low blood glucose, normal electrolytes, elevated liver enzymes, and (on chest x-ray) a dilated heart. Urinalysis reveals no infection and no ketones. The child is hospitalized and stabilized with 10% glucose infusion, and certain admission laboratories come back 1 week later showing elevated medium chain fatty acyl carnitines in blood and 6–8 carbon dicarboxylic acids in the urine. The most likely disorder in this child involves which of the following?

a. Defect of medium chain coenzyme A dehydrogenase
b. Defect of medium chain fatty acyl synthetase
c. Mitochondrial defect in the electron transport chain
d. Mitochondrial defect in fatty acid transport
e. Carnitine deficiency

3-38. A 35-year-old man presents to the emergency room with an acute abdomen (severe abdominal pain with tightness of muscles, decreased bowel sounds, and vomiting and/or diarrhea). He has been drinking, and a urine sample is unusual because it has a port-wine color. Past history indicates several prior evaluations for abdominal pain, including an appendectomy. The physician notes unusual neurologic symptoms with partial paralysis of his arms and legs. At first concerned about food poisons like botulism, the physician recalls that acute intermittent porphyria may cause these symptoms (176000) and consults a gastroenterologist. Elevation of which of the following urinary metabolites would support a diagnosis of porphyria?

a. Urobilinogen and bilirubin
b. Delta-aminolevulinic acid and porphobilinogen
c. Biliverdin and stercobilin
d. Urobilin and urobilinogen
e. Delta-aminolevulinic acid and urobilinogen

3-39. A very concerned mother brings her teenager into your pediatric office. The teenager awoke in the morning with a large swollen mass that filled part of his upper eyelid and medial forehead just above his left eye. His eyelid was so swollen he could barely keep it open. His history reveals that he suffers from indoor allergies and a head cold of about a week's length. During your physical examination you note purulent nasal discharge and extreme tenderness to percussion over his paranasal sinuses. The large swollen mass in his eyelid and forehead is quite pliable. You prescribe intravenous antibiotics and give which of the following explanations to the very concerned mother and the teenager?

a. He suffers from trigeminal neuralgia that affects the ophthalmic portion of cranial nerve V
b. He suffers from tic douloureux that affects the ophthalmic portion of cranial nerve V
c. He suffers from sinusitis, which has eroded through the wall on the frontal sinus, and since the frontalis muscle is not attached to bone, allowed pus to leak into the upper eyelid
d. He has Bell's palsy, which is generally caused by herpes simplex virus infection of the facial nerve within the facial canal that caused the loss of ability to raise the upper eyelid and thus allow fluid to accumulate within it
e. He suffers from a sty, which is an inflammation of Meibomian or tarsal glands, which lies on the inner surface of the eyelid

3-40. A 9-year-old child is brought to the emergency room with the chief complaint of enlarged, painful axillary lymph nodes. The resident physician also notes a small, inflamed, dime-sized lesion surrounding what appears to be a small scratch on the forearm. The lymph node is aspirated and some pus is sent to the laboratory for examination. A Warthin-Starry silver impregnation stain reveals many highly pleomorphic, rod-shaped bacteria. Which of the following is the most likely cause of this infection?

a. *Bartonella henselae*
b. *Brucella canis*
c. *Mycobacterium scrofulaceum*
d. *Y. enterocolitica*
e. *Yersinia pestis*

3-41. A 22-year-old woman presents with fever, weight loss, night sweats, and painless enlargement of several supraclavicular lymph nodes. A biopsy from one of the enlarged lymph nodes is shown in the photomicrograph below. The binucleate giant cell with prominent acidophilic "owl-eye" nucleoli shown stains positively with both CD15 and CD30 immunoperoxidase stains. Also present are atypical mononuclear cells that are surrounded by clear spaces (lacunar cells). Which of the following is the most likely diagnosis?

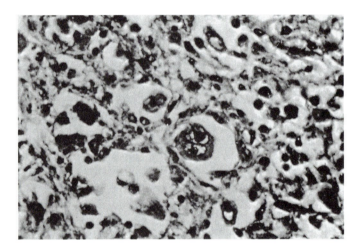

a. Anaplastic large cell lymphoma
b. Diffuse non-Hodgkin's lymphoma
c. Lymphocyte predominate Hodgkin's disease
d. Nodular sclerosis Hodgkin's disease
e. Reactive lymph node hyperplasia

3-42. A 40-year old man presents to the emergency medicine department 1 week following a foot injury. He is experiencing intense pain in the area of injury and the muscles of the jaw. Which of the following is the most common portal of entry for the etiologic organism?

a. Gastrointestinal tract
b. Genital tract
c. Nasal tract
d. Respiratory tract
e. Skin

3-43. A 60-year-old male suffers an upper pontine stroke that selectively damages neuronal pathways mediating auditory signals from the lower brainstem to other relay neurons in higher levels of the brainstem. Which of the following is the principal ascending auditory pathway of the brainstem affected by the stroke?

a. Medial lemniscus
b. Lateral lemniscus
c. Trapezoid body
d. Trigeminal lemniscus
e. Brachium of the superior colliculus

3-44. Your patient reports he spent two weeks on a desert island as part of a television survival show. It rained and was cool the last 5 days, and he developed a cough. He is now in the ER with a productive cough that produces rusty and bloodstained sputum. He also complains of significant pleural pain. You suspect a pneumococcal lobar pneumonia. From this CT scan at the T4 level, which of the following lung lobes (indicated by the asterisk) is involved with the pneumonia?

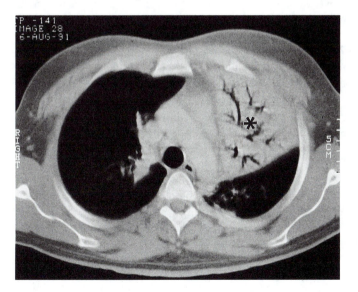

a. Right upper lobe
b. Right middle lobe
c. Right lower lobe
d. Left upper lobe
e. Left lower lobe

3-45. An 83-year-old woman with constipation is prescribed a high-fiber diet, which leads to an increased production of short-chain fatty acids (SCFAs). SCFA absorption occurs almost exclusively from which of the following segments of the GI tract?

a. Stomach
b. Duodenum
c. Jejunum
d. Ileum
e. Colon

3-46. A 47-year-old woman with hypermenorrhea develops an iron-deficiency anemia requiring iron supplements. Which of the following statements is correct regarding iron digestion and absorption?

a. About 100 mg of iron is absorbed per day
b. Iron is absorbed rapidly from the small intestine
c. Iron is transported in the blood bound to transferrin
d. In general, iron must be oxidized from the ferrous to the ferric state for efficient absorption
e. Iron is transported into enterocytes by a ferroportin transporter on the apical membrane

3-47. A patient with alcoholic cirrhosis comes in vomiting blood. After stabilizing him with IV fluids, the next step should be administration of an agonist/analog of which of the following agents to inhibit gastric acid secretion and visceral blood flow?

a. Gastrin
b. Somatostatin
c. Histamine
d. Pepsin
e. Acetylcholine

3-48. A 56-year-old man presents with weight loss, cough, and diffuse chest pain. A chest x-ray reveals normal heart and lungs, but the radiologist detects a "bird's beak" narrowing of the terminal esophagus, which is also seen with a barium swallow. Follow-up history indicates that the patient also has dysphagia and regurgitation. Manometry shows increased lower esophageal sphincter (LES) pressure with no relaxation upon swallowing, indicating a diagnosis of achalasia. Which of the following is the putative inhibitory neurotransmitter responsible for relaxation of gastrointestinal smooth muscle?

a. Dopamine
b. Vasoactive intestinal peptide
c. Somatostatin
d. Substance P
e. Acetylcholine

3-49. A patient has vomiting and severe watery diarrhea after eating spoiled shellfish. Intravenous fluid and electrolyte replacement was started, and a stool specimen was taken, which came back positive for *Vibrio cholerae*. Which of the following statements best describes water and electrolyte absorption in the GI tract?

a. Most water and electrolytes come from ingested fluids
b. The small intestine and colon have similar absorptive capacities
c. Osmotic equilibration of chyme occurs in the stomach
d. The majority of absorption occurs in the jejunum
e. Cholera toxin inhibits sodium-coupled nutrient transport

3-50. An 18-year-old female decides to get a tattoo for her birthday. Two months later she presents with a fever, right upper quadrant pain, nausea, vomiting, and jaundice. Which of the following lab values would most likely be found in a patient with infectious hepatitis?

a. An increase in plasma alkaline phosphatase
b. An increase in plasma bile acids
c. An increase in both direct and indirect plasma bilirubin
d. An increase in direct bilirubin, and a decrease in indirect bilirubin in the plasma
e. An decrease in both direct and indirect plasma bilirubin

Block 4

Questions

4-1. A 3-month-old girl is being evaluated for feeding difficulty and failure to thrive. Physical examination finds pallor, peripheral cyanosis, tachypnea, and fine expiratory wheezing. Chest x-ray shows cardiac enlargement. She is admitted to the hospital, quickly develops severe cardiac failure, and dies 3 days after admission. At the time of autopsy the endocardium is found to have a "cream cheese" gross appearance. Histologic sections from this area reveal thickening of the endocardium due to a proliferation of fibrous and elastic tissue. Which of the following is the most likely diagnosis?

a. Dilated cardiomyopathy
b. Hypertrophic cardiomyopathy
c. Infective endocarditis
d. Libman-Sachs endocarditis
e. Restrictive cardiomyopathy

4-2. A 4-year-old female presents with short stature, web neck, and other features suggestive of Turner syndrome, but also has mild mental disability. Her chromosome studies reveal 90,XX/92,XXXX with about 10% abnormal cells in blood and 20% in skin. These results can be described as which of the following?

a. Aneuploidy
b. Haploidy
c. Triploidy mosaicism
d. Tetraploidy without mosaicism
e. Trisomy with mosaicism

4-3. A 42-year-old patient with a rare blood type is scheduled for surgery that will likely require a transfusion. Because the patient has a rare blood type, an autologous blood transfusion is planned. Prior to surgery, 1500 mL of blood is collected. The collection tubes contain calcium citrate, which prevents coagulation by which of the following actions?

a. Blocking thrombin
b. Binding factor XII
c. Binding vitamin K
d. Chelating calcium
e. Activating plasminogen

4-4. A 25-year-old medical student presented with a ruptured appendix. A peritoneal infection developed, despite prompt removal of the organ and extensive flushing of the peritoneal cavity. An isolate from a pus culture was a gram-negative rod identified as *Bacteroides fragilis*. Anaerobic infection with *B. fragilis* is best characterized by which of the following?

a. A black exudate in the wound
b. A foul-smelling discharge
c. A heme-pigmented colony formation
d. An exquisite susceptibility to penicillin
e. Severe neurologic symptoms

4-5. Dozens of political refugees fleeing from active warfare and living in a dense forest environment with crowded, unsanitary conditions experienced nonspecific symptoms, followed by high fever and severe headache, along with chills, myalgia, and arthralgia. All had body lice. Improved living conditions in a refugee camp and treatment with tetracycline brought resolution to most individuals. Which of the following statements describes the etiological agent responsible for their infection?

a. The disease was caused by an organism with no cell walls
b. The disease was caused by a viral agent
c. The disease was derived from rodents living in the forest area
d. Reoccurrence of milder disease may occur in later years
e. The disease was caused by a tick vector

4-6. A 45-year-old woman was brought to her local hospital's emergency room by her husband because of several days of progressive weakness and numbness in her arms and legs. Her symptoms had begun with tingling in her toes, which she assumed to be her feet "falling asleep." However, this feeling did not disappear, and she began to feel numb, first in her toes on both feet, then ascending to her calves and knees. Two days later, she began to feel numb in her fingertips and had difficulty lifting her legs. When she finally was unable to climb the stairs of her house because of her leg weakness, had difficulty gripping the banister, and experienced shortness of breath, her husband urged her to go to the emergency room. The neurologist who examined the patient in the emergency room noticed that she was short of breath while sitting in bed. He asked the respiratory therapist to measure her vital capacity (the greatest volume of air that can be exhaled from the lungs after a maximal inspiration), and the value for this was far lower than would be expected for her age and weight. Her neurological examination showed that her arms and legs were very weak, so that she had difficulty lifting them against gravity. She was unable to feel a pin or a vibrating tuning fork at all on her legs and below her elbows, but was able to feel the pin on her upper chest. The neurologist could not elicit any reflexes from her ankles or knees. He subsequently advised the emergency room staff that the patient needed to have a spinal tap and be admitted to the intensive care unit immediately. Where in the nervous system was the damage?

a. Frontal lobe
b. Temporal lobe
c. Peripheral nerves and nerve roots
d. Spinal cord
e. Parietal lobe

4-7. A child presents with severe vomiting, dehydration, and fever. Initial blood studies show acidosis with a low bicarbonate and an anion gap (the sum of sodium plus potassium minus chloride plus bicarbonate is 40 and larger than the normal 12 ± 2). Preliminary results from the blood amino acid screen show two elevated amino acids, both with nonpolar side chains. A titration curve performed on one of the elevated species shows two ionizable groups with approximate pKs of 2 and 9.5. Which of the following pairs of elevated amino acids is most likely elevated?

a. Aspartic acid and glutamine
b. Glutamic acid and threonine
c. Histidine and valine
d. Leucine and isoleucine
e. Glutamine and isoleucine

4-8. In a case involving a patient who experienced hoarseness and dysphagia, it was concluded that the patient suffered from a lesion affecting selective brainstem neurons. Which of the following is the most probable nuclei damaged in this case?

a. Solitary nucleus
b. Deep pontine nuclei
c. Nucleus ambiguus
d. Ventral horn cells of cervical cord
e. Inferior salivatory nuclei

4-9. A multiparous mother brings in her second son, an 18-month-old active toddler, because she has noticed blood (sometimes red, one time "currant jelly") in his stools. Although the toddler is trying new foods, she doesn't think the blood is associated with anything in his diet. Your physical exam, including a digital rectal exam, is normal. You order an upper GI barium swallow with small bowel follow through and radiological report describes a 2-inch-long diverticulum, pointing toward the umbilicus, in the ileum, about 2 ft from the ileocecal valve. You explain to the mother that the blood is most likely from which of the following sources?

a. An appendix that must be removed
b. A Meckel's (ileal) diverticulum
c. Active diverticulitis
d. Internal hemorrhoids
e. A duodenal ulcer

4-10. A 71-year-old woman presents with increasing chest pain and occasional syncopal episodes, especially with physical exertion. She has trouble breathing at night and when she lies down. Physical examination reveals a crescendo-decrescendo midsystolic ejection murmur with a paradoxically split second heart sound (S_2). Pressure studies reveal that the left ventricular pressure during systole is markedly greater than the aortic pressure. Which of the following is the most likely diagnosis?

a. Aortic regurgitation
b. Aortic stenosis
c. Constrictive pericarditis
d. Mitral regurgitation
e. Mitral stenosis

4-11. A 63-year-old woman presents with diarrhea, abdominal pain, and flushing. The urinary excretion of the seratonin metabolite,

5-hydroxyindoleacetic acid (5-HIAA) is elevated. Abdominal CT reveals a tumor in the terminal ileum. Surgical resection of the terminal ileum will most likely result in which of the following?

a. A decrease in absorption of amino acids
b. An increase in the water content of the feces
c. An increase in the concentration of bile acid in the enterohepatic circulation
d. A decrease in the fat content of the feces
e. An increase in the absorption of iron

4-12. A box of ham sandwiches with mayonnaise, prepared by a person with a boil on his neck, was left out of the refrigerator for the on-call interns. Three doctors became violently ill approximately 2 hours after eating the sandwiches. Which of the following is the most likely cause?

a. *C. perfringens* toxin
b. Coagulase from *S. aureus* in the ham
c. Penicillinase given to inactivate penicillin in the pork
d. *S. aureus* enterotoxin
e. *S. aureus* leukocidin

4-13. A 35-year-old man who weighs 150 pounds and is 5 feet 10 inches tall is transported to the emergency department in severe distress. He complains of episodes of severe, throbbing headaches, profuse diaphoresis, and palpitations. Eighteen months ago his physician told him he is healthy except for what is assumed to be Stage 2 essential hypertension, but he refused medication and has not seen a health care provider for the last year and a half. He denies use of any drugs, whether prescription or over-the-counter, legal or otherwise.

Assessment now reveals that he is tachycardic and has an irregular pulse (sinus tachycardia, with occasional premature ventricular beats, are noted on his EKG). Heart rate at rest is approximately 130 beats/min, sometimes more. His resting blood pressure is approximately 200/140 mm Hg. These cardiovascular findings are shown in the figure.

The first year house officer who is caring for this patient knows that all the orally effective β-adrenergic blockers are approved for use to treat essential hypertension, and concludes that prompt lowering of blood pressure is essential for this patient. Therefore, he orders intravenous administration of propranolol (at the arrow, in the figure), and a large dose of the drug since the symptoms seem severe.

Unknown to the MD is the fact that the patient's signs and symptoms are due to a pheochromocytoma (epinephrine-secreting tumor of the adrenal/suprarenal medulla).

Which of the following statements best describes the most likely ulti-mate outcome of administering this β blocker (or any other β blocker that lacks α-blocking activity), supplemented with no other medication, to this patient with an undiagnosed pheochromocytoma?

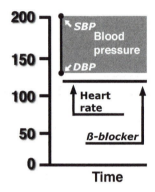

a. Heart failure, cardiogenic shock, death
b. Long-lasting normalization of heart rate, contractility, and blood pressure
c. Normalization of blood pressures but persistence of tachycardia
d. Restoration of normal sinus rate and rhythm, but no change of blood pressure from predrug levels.
e. Sudden and significant rise of systolic blood pressure and heart rate

4-14. An elderly male patient who has just been referred to your practice has been taking a drug for symptomatic relief of benign prostatic hypertrophy. In addition to its effects on smooth muscles of the prostate and urethra, this drug can lower blood pressure in such a way that it reflexly triggers tachy-cardia, positive inotropy, and increased AV nodal conduction. The drug neither dilates nor constricts the bronchi. It causes the pupils of the eyes to constrict and interferes with mydriasis in dim light. Initial oral dosages of this drug have been associated with a high incidence of syncope. Which prototype is most similar to this unnamed drug in terms of the pharmaco-logic profile?

a. Captopril
b. Hydrochlorothiazide (prototype thiazide diuretic)
c. Labetalol
d. Nifedipine
e. Prazosin
f. Propranolol
g. Verapamil

4-15. A 40-year-old woman of fair complexion is admitted for evaluation of acute vomiting with abdominal pain. The episode began the night before after a fatty meal, and she has noted her stools are a peculiar grey white color. Abdominal examination is difficult because she is obese, but she exhibits acute tenderness in the right upper quadrant and has pain just below her left shoulder blade. Interference with which aspect of porphyrin metabolism best accounts for the white stools?

a. Sterile gut syndrome with defective bilirubin oxidation
b. Excess oxidation of bilirubin to urobilinogen
c. Heme synthesis defect causing increased bilirubin clearance
d. Bile duct excretion of bilirubin with oxidation to stercobilin
e. Excess reabsorption of urobilinogen with excess Urobilin

4-16. An adult migrant farm worker in the San Joaquin Valley of California has been hospitalized for 2 weeks with progressive lassitude, fever of unknown origin, and skin nodules on the lower extremities. A biopsy of one of the deep dermal nodules shown in the photomicrograph below reveals the presence of which abnormality?

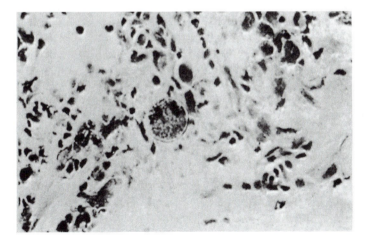

a. Russell bodies
b. Malignant lymphoma
c. Coccidioides spherule
d. Lymphomatoid granulomatosis
e. Erythema nodosum

4-17. A 65-year-old man who is a long-time farmer presents with a small, scaly erythematous lesion on the helix of his left ear. A biopsy from this lesion reveals marked degeneration of the dermal collagen (solar elastosis) along with atypia of the squamous epidermal cells. The atypia, however, does not involve the full thickness of the epidermis, and no invasion into the underlying tissue is seen. Which of the following is the most likely diagnosis?

a. Actinic keratosis
b. Bowen's disease
c. Keratoacanthoma
d. Seborrheic keratosis
e. Squamous cell carcinoma

4-18. A 68-year-old male received a diagnosis of ALS after experiencing weakness in his legs. Over the next year, the disease was progressive and he lost mobility in the use of his arms, legs as well as some cranial nerve functions. Which region or regions of the spinal cord were primarily affected by this disorder?

a. Dorsal horns of the spinal cord
b. Lateral columns of the spinal cord
c. Ventral horns of the spinal cord
d. Dorsal columns and ventral horns of the spinal cord
e. Ventral horns and lateral columns of the spinal cord

4-19. A 12-year-old girl was playing soccer when she began to limp. She has pain in her right leg and upper right thigh. Her temperature is 102°F. X-ray of the femur reveals that the periosteum is eroded. Which of the following is the most likely etiologic agent?

a. *L. monocytogenes*
b. *Salmonella enteritidis*
c. *Staphylococcus saprophyticus*
d. *S. aureus*
e. *Streptococcus pneumoniae*

4-20. A 7-month-old male infant is admitted to the hospital with chronic diarrhea. In his first few months of life this infant has had several episodes of bacterial pneumonia and otitis media along with oral candidiasis and a viral infection. Workup finds that the thymus is small, lymphoid tissues are hypoplastic, and both B and T lymphocytes are decreased in number in the peripheral blood. Serum calcium levels were within normal limits. Which one of the listed defects is associated with the X-linked recessive form for this infant's immunodeficiency disease?

a. Decreased production of NADPH oxidase
b. Decreased synthesis of adenosine deaminase in lymphocytes
c. Mutation in the common gamma chain subunit of cytokine receptors
d. Mutation in the gene coding for the Wiskott-Aldrich syndrome protein (WASP)
e. Mutation in the gene coding for CD40L

4-21. A middle-aged man presents with congestive heart failure with elevated liver enzymes. His skin has a grayish pigmentation. The levels of liver enzymes are higher than those usually seen in congestive heart failure, suggesting an inflammatory process (hepatitis) with scarring (cirrhosis) of the liver. A liver biopsy discloses a marked increase in iron storage. In humans, molecular iron (Fe) is which of the following?

a. Stored primarily in the spleen
b. Stored in combination with ferritin
c. Excreted in the urine as Fe^{2+}
d. Absorbed in the intestine by albumin
e. Absorbed in the ferric (Fe^{3+}) form

4-22. A patient receives a single injection of succinylcholine to facilitate preoperative intubation. The dose is correct for the vast majority of patients, and normally effects of this drug abate spontaneously over a couple of minutes. This gentleman remains apneic for an extraordinarily long time. A genetically based aberrant cholinesterase is eventually determined to be the cause. Which of the following would we administer if we were concerned about this unusually lengthy drug response?

a. Atropine
b. Bethanechol
c. Neostigmine
d. Nothing
e. Physostigmine
f. Tubocurarine

4-23. A 13-year-old boy on the junior high wrestling team experiences attacks of proximal muscle weakness that last from 30 minutes to as long as 4 hours following exercise and fasting. The trainer attributed it to the symptoms of fatigue, but his mother recalled having similar symptoms when she was dieting. Genetic testing revealed an inherited channelopathy. Electrically excitable gates are normally involved in which of the following?

a. The depolarization of the end-plate membrane by acetylcholine
b. Hyperpolarization of rods by light
c. Release of calcium from ventricular muscle sarcoplasmic reticulum
d. Transport of glucose into cells by a sodium-dependent, secondary active transport system
e. Increase in nerve cell potassium conductance caused by membrane depolarization

4-24. A female infant is born approximately 10 weeks prematurely (at 30 weeks) and weighs 1710 g. She has respiratory distress syndrome and is treated with endogenous surfactant. She is intubated endotracheally with mechanical ventilation immediately after birth. Over the first 4 days after birth the ventilator pressure and the fraction of inspired oxygen are reduced. Beginning on the fifth day after birth, she has brief desaturations that become more persistent. She needs increased ventilator and oxygen support on the seventh day after birth. She becomes cyanotic. Further examination, echocardiogram, and x-rays reveal left atrial enlargement, an enlarged pulmonary artery, increased pulmonary vasculature, and a continuous machine-like murmur. Which of the following is the most likely diagnosis?

a. Persistent foramen ovale
b. Patent ductus arteriosus
c. Ventricular septal defect
d. Pulmonary stenosis
e. Coarctation of the aorta

4-25. A young boy is being evaluated for developmental delay, mild autism, and mental retardation. Physical examination reveals the boy to have large, everted ears and a long face with a large mandible. He is also found to have macroorchidism (large testes), and extensive workup reveals multiple tandem repeats of the nucleotide sequence CGG in his DNA. Which of the following is the most likely diagnosis?

a. Fragile X syndrome
b. Huntington's chorea
c. Myotonic dystrophy
d. Spinal-bulbar muscular atrophy
e. Ataxia-telangiectasia

4-26. A mother and newborn are exposed to a pathogen while at the hospital for a routine checkup and breastfeeding clinic. This same pathogen had infected the mother about a year previously, and she had successfully recovered from the subsequent illness. Immunity may be innate or acquired. Which of the following best describes acquired immunity with respect to the newborn?

a. Complement cascade
b. Increase in C-reactive protein (CRP)
c. Inflammatory response
d. Maternal transfer of antibody
e. Presence of natural killer (NK) cells

4-27. A patient presents with a complaint of muscle weakness following exercise. Neurological examination reveals that the muscles supplied by cranial nerves are most affected. You suspect myasthenia gravis. Your diagnosis is confirmed when lab tests indicate antibodies against which of the following in the patient's blood?

a. Acetylcholinesterase
b. Muscle endplates
c. Cranial nerve synaptic membranes
d. Cranial nerve presynaptic membranes
e. Acetylcholine receptors

4-28. A 66-year-old man presents for his annual physical examination. He is asymptomatic and physical examination is unremarkable. Examination of his peripheral smear, however, reveals the presence of small mononuclear cells with little cytoplasm and a mature nucleus with a prominent nuclear cleft. No "smudge cells" are seen. The presence of these "buttock cells" in the peripheral blood warrants further clinical workup to search for which one of the following malignancies?

a. Chronic lymphocytic leukemia
b. Follicular non-Hodgkin's lymphoma
c. Multiple myeloma
d. Nodular sclerosis Hodgkin's disease
e. Small-cell carcinoma of the lung

4-29. A 10-year-old boy is referred to the physician because of learning problems and some behavior changes. His family history is unremarkable. Physical examination reveals tall stature with few anomalies except for single palmar creases of the hands and curved fifth fingers (clinodactyly). The physician decides to order a karyotype. Which of the following indications for obtaining a karyotype best explains the physician's decision in this case?

a. A couple with multiple miscarriages or a person who is at risk for an inherited chromosome rearrangement
b. A child with ambiguous genitalia who needs genetic sex assignment
c. A child with an appearance suggestive of Down syndrome or other chromosomal disorder
d. A child with mental retardation and/or multiple congenital anomalies
e. A child who is at risk for cancer

4-30. A 25-year-old female is treated with a course of broad-spectrum antibiotics for severe pelvic inflammatory disease. She now reports a thick milky white pruritic vaginal discharge. Which of the following is the most prevalent microorganism in the vagina and may also be protective?

a. α-Hemolytic Streptococci
b. *B. fragilis*
c. *E. coli*
d. *Lactobacillus*
e. *S. epidermidis*

4-31. A patient is transported to your emergency department because of a seizure. A review of his history reveals that he has been treated by different physicians for different medical conditions, and there has been no dialog between the two doctors in terms of what they've prescribed. One physician has prescribed a drug for short-term management of depression. Another has prescribed the very same drug to help the patient quit smoking cigarettes. Which of the following was most likely prescribed by both doctors, and was the most likely cause of the seizures?

a. Bupropion
b. Chlordiazepoxide
c. Fluoxetine
d. Imipramine
e. Lithium

4-32. A 12-year-old male with muscular dystrophy is found to have a mutation of the gene that encodes the protein dystrophin. Genetic alterations in dystrophin lead to progressive muscular weakness because dystrophin provides structural support to the sarcolemma by binding which of the followinig?

a. β-Dystroglycan to laminin
b. Actin to β-dystroglycan
c. Actin to the Z lines
d. Z lines to M lines
e. Z lines to the sarcolemma

4-33. A young adult male suffers an injury to the region of the face that affects in part the peripheral nerve innervating the tongue, which results in some loss of ability to identify the taste of foods. Which structure in the brainstem would normally receive these peripheral taste inputs?

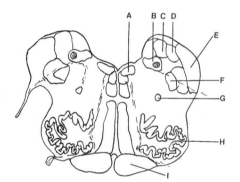

a. A
b. B
c. C
d. D
e. E
f. F
g. G
h. H
i. I

4-34. An 18-year-old male heroin addict, who practices the sharing of needles at a "shooting gallery," is positive in the screening test for AIDS. Since a false positive is possible, the physician orders a confirmatory test. Which of the following best describes the standard confirmatory test, and what this test checks for, respectively?

a. Complement fixation test; antibodies against the virus
b. Enzyme-linked immunosorbent assay; antigens of the virus
c. Radioimmunoassay; specific antibodies against the virus
d. Western blot; antigens of the virus
e. Western blot; specific antibodies against the virus

4-35. A 51-year-old man presents with epigastric pain that is lessened whenever he eats. A gastroscopy is performed to evaluate these gastric symptoms and a solitary gastric ulcer is seen. Which one of the listed gross findings if present would be most suspicious for the lesion being a malignant ulcer?

a. Diameter greater than 2 cm
b. Location on the lesser curvature
c. Outward radiating rugae
d. Perforation into the peritoneal cavity
e. Raised peripheral margins

4-36. A 46-year-old woman who has been a type I diabetic for 35 years visits your family medicine office. She has foot ulcers on both her right and her left feet. You prescribe Beclaperin gel, a prescription drug for the treatment of diabetic foot ulcers. It contains platelet-derived growth factor (PDGF). Which of the following is the most likely mechanism for the action of PDGF in the improvement of wound healing?

a. Acceleration of chemotaxis of monocytes-macrophages
b. Inhibition of vascular smooth-muscle cell proliferation
c. Inhibition of fibroblast proliferation
d. Inhibition of granulation tissue formation
e. Secretion of type II collagen from fibroblasts

4-37. A 2-week-old neonate presents with regurgitation and persistent, severe projectile vomiting. An olive-like epigastric mass is felt during physical examination. A chest x-ray does not reveal the presence of bowel gas in the chest cavity. This infant's mother did not have polyhydramnios during this pregnancy. Which of the following is the most appropriate treatment for this infant's condition?

a. Oral medication with omeprazole and clarithromycin
b. Oral medication with vancomycin or metronidazole
c. Surgery to cut a hypertrophied stenotic band at the pylorus
d. Surgery to remove a mass of the adrenal gland
e. Surgery to resect an aganglionic section of the intestines

4-38. An irritable 18-month-old toddler with fever and blister-like ulcerations on mucous membranes of the oral cavity refuses to eat. The symptoms worsen and then slowly resolve over a period of 2 weeks. Assuming that the etiological agent was HSV type 1, which of the following statements is true?

a. Antivirals do not provide any benefit
b. The virus remains latent in the trigeminal ganglia
c. Recurrence is likely to result in a generalized rash
d. Polyclonal B cell activation is a prominent feature
e. The child is at high risk for developing cancer later in life

4-39. A 16-year-old girl presents to the pediatric genetic and endocrine clinic with short stature, Tanner stage 2 of pubertal development and lack of menstruation. She is 49 in. tall (normal range for age is 59–68 in. mean 64 in.) and weighs 65 lb (normal range for age is 92–158 lb, mean is 126 lb.). She has a short, broad, webbed neck, short fingers and toes, and *cubitus valgus*. Hormonal profile reveals high levels of the gonadotrophins LH and FSH, and very low levels of estrogen. Ultrasound studies show uterine hypoplasia and poorly-defined gonadal streaks. Genetic analysis shows a 45, X0 pattern. The short stature has been linked to reduced protein expression of the short stature homeobox gene (SHOX). That gene working through specific transcription factors would influence the production of which of the following by the cells delineated by the box in the accompanying photomicrograph.

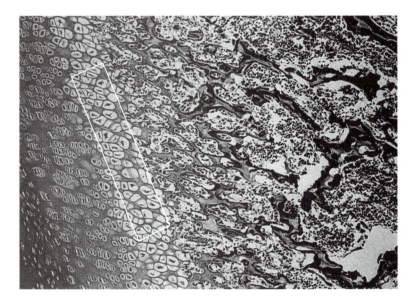

a. Cyclins
b. Acid phosphatase
c. Alkaline phosphatase
d. Type I collagen
e. Osteocalcin

4-40. A 1-year-old child develops fever and vomiting and is unable to keep food down for 2 days. The physical examination discloses no congenital anomalies, and the baby resembles his parents. Which of the following laboratory findings are most likely if the child has a disorder of fatty acid oxidation?

a. Hypoglycemia, acidosis, and elevated urine dicarboxylic acids
b. Alkalosis and elevated serum ammonia
c. Acidosis and elevated urine reducing substances
d. Hypoglycemia, acidosis, and elevated serum leucine, isoleucine, and valine
e. Hepatomegaly, elevated serum liver enzymes, and elevated tyrosine

4-41. While moving furniture, an 18-year-old teenager experiences excruciating pain in his right groin. A few hours later he also develops pain in the umbilical region with accompanying nausea. At this point he seeks medical attention. Examination reveals a bulge midway between the midline and the anterior superior iliac spine, but superior to the inguinal ligament. On coughing or straining, the bulge increases and the inguinal pain intensifies. The bulge courses medially and inferiorly into the upper portion of the scrotum and cannot be reduced with the finger pressure of the examiner. It is decided that a medical emergency exists, and the patient is scheduled for immediate surgery. Nausea and diffuse pain referred to the umbilical region in this patient most probably are due to which of the following?

a. Compression of the genitofemoral nerve
b. Compression of the ilioinguinal nerve
c. Dilation of the inguinal canal
d. Ischemic necrosis of a loop of small bowel
e. Ischemic necrosis of the cremaster muscle

4-42. A 78-year-old man is found on the ground unconscious one morning and taken to the emergency room of a nearby hospital. After regaining consciousness, he is unable to move his right hand or leg. Which of the regions shown on the illustration was most likely directly affected by the stroke?

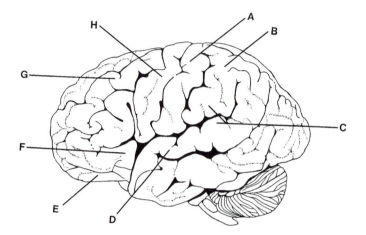

a. A
b. B
c. C
d. D
e. E
f. F
g. G
h. H

4-43. A 36-year-old woman presents because of increasing pain in her hands and knees, which, she says, is worse in the morning. Physical examination finds her fingers to be swollen and stiff, and there is ulnar deviation of her metacarpophalangeal joints. A biopsy from her knee would likely show areas where histiocytes were palisading around irregular areas of necrosis, as seen in the picture. The biopsy would also likely show proliferation and hyperplasia of the synovium with destruction of the articular cartilage. Which one of the following terms best describes these pathologic changes?

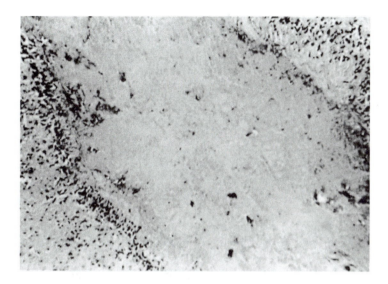

a. Eburnation
b. Gumma
c. Pannus
d. Spondylosis
e. Tophus

4-44. In the operating room, a child receives succinylcholine as a muscle relaxant to facilitate intubation and anesthesia. The operation proceeds until it is time for recovery, when the child does not begin breathing. A hurried discussion with the father discloses no additional problems in the family, but he does say that he and his wife are first cousins. Which of the following is the most likely possibility?

a. An autosomal dominant disorder that interferes with succinylcholine metabolism
b. An autosomal recessive disorder that interferes with succinylcholine metabolism
c. An X-linked disorder that interferes with succinylcholine metabolism
d. A lethal gene transmitted through consanguinity that affects the respiratory system
e. Mismanagement of halothane anesthesia during the operation

4-45. A physician evaluates a 16-year-old boy with a slightly unusual facial appearance and poor school performance. A peripheral blood chromosome study reveals a karyotype of 46,XY/47,XY,+8 mosaicism, with 10% of 100 examined cells showing the extra chromosome 8. Which of the following options is most appropriate for the physician during the counseling session that follows the chromosome result?

a. Recommend karyotyping of the parents
b. Explain that the recurrence risk for such chromosomal aberrations is about 1%
c. Urge that the school receive a copy of the karyotype since these boys often have behavior problems
d. Recommend special education
e. Inform the parents that their child will be sterile

4-46. A young boy is diagnosed with asthma. His primary symptom is frequent cough, not bronchospasm or wheezing. Other asthma medications are started, but until their effects develop fully we wish to suppress the cough without running a risk of suppressing ventilatory drive or causing sedation or other unwanted effects. Which of the following would best meet these needs?

a. Codeine
b. Dextromethorphan
c. Diphenhydramine
d. Hydrocodone
e. Promethazine

4-47. A mother brings her 10-year-old son, who has a long-standing history of poorly controlled asthma, to the emergency department (ED). He is in a relatively early stage of what will prove to be a severe asthma attack. Arterial blood gases have not been analyzed yet, but it is obvious that the lad is in great distress. He is panting with great effort at a rate of about 160/min.

Given the boy's history and the likely diagnosis, the health care team administers all the drugs listed by the stated routes, and with the expected purposes noted. The child's condition quickly improves, and the team leaves the boy with his mother while they go to care for other ED patients. Within a couple of minutes the mother comes out of her son's cubicle frantically screaming "he's stopped breathing!" Which of the listed drugs most likely caused the ventilatory arrest?

a. Albuterol, inhaled, given by nebulizer for prompt bronchodilation
b. Atropine, inhaled, given with the albuterol
c. Midazolam, IV, to normalize ventilatory rate and allay anxiety

d. Methylprednisolone (glucocorticosteroid), IV, for prompt suppression of airway inflammation
e. Normal saline, inhaled, to hydrate the airway mucosae

4-48. We prescribe an orally inhaled corticosteroid for a patient with asthma. Previously they were using only a rapidly acting adrenergic bronchodilator for both prophylaxis and for treatment of acute attacks. They use the steroid as directed for 5 days, then stop taking it. Which of the following is the most likely reason why the patient quit using the drug?

a. Disturbing tachycardia and palpitations occurred
b. Relentless diarrhea developed after just one day of using the steroid
c. She experienced little or no obvious improvement in breathing
d. The drug caused extreme drowsiness that interfered with daytime activities
e. The drug caused him to retain fluid and gain weight

4-49. A patient consumes an excessive dose of theophylline and develops toxicity in response to the drug. Which of the following is the most likely consequence of this?

a. Bradycardia
b. Drowsiness progressing to sleep and then coma
c. Hepatotoxicity
d. Paradoxical bronchospasm
e. Seizures

4-50. A patient suffering status asthmaticus presents in the emergency department. Blood gases reveal severe respiratory acidosis and hypoxia. Even large parenteral doses of a selective β_2 agonist fail to dilate the airways adequately; rather, they cause dangerous degrees of tachycardia. Which of the following pharmacologic interventions or approaches is most likely to control the acute symptoms and restore the bronchodilator efficacy of the adrenergic drug?

a. Add inhaled cromolyn
b. Give a parenteral corticosteroid
c. Give parenteral diphenhydramine
d. Switch to epinephrine
e. Switch to isoproterenol (β_1/β_2 agonist)

Block 5

Questions

5-1. A postoperative patient will require prolonged analgesia. We choose a drug that has the following pharmacokinetic properties:

Half-life: 12 h
Clearance: 0.08 L/min
Volume of distribution: 60 L

The patient has an indwelling venous catheter with a slow drip of 0.9% NaCl, and we will use this to administer intermittent injections of the drug every 4 h. The target blood level of the drug, following each injection, is 8 mcg/mL.

With this plan in mind, which of the following comes closest to the dose that should be administered every 4 h?

a. 0.960 mg (or 1 mg)
b. 6.4 mg (or 6 mg)
c. 25.6 mg (or 25 mg)
d. 150 mg
e. 550 mg

5-2. A 42-year-old woman consults a dermatologist to evaluate and treat her glabellar lines (frown lines on the forehead just above the nose). After her treatment options are explained, the patient asks the dermatologist to administer Botox (botulinum type A). Botox injections smooth out glabellar lines by which of the following methods?

a. Blocking the release of synaptic transmitter from α-motoneurons
b. Preventing the opening of sodium channels on muscle membranes
c. Decreasing the amount of calcium released from the sarcoplasmic reticulum
d. Increasing the flow of blood into the facial muscle
e. Enhancing the enzymatic hydrolysis of acetylcholine at the neuromuscular junction

5-3. A 50-year-old multiparous woman comes to your office to rule out cancer. She reports a growing mass or fullness on the anterior wall of her vagina. Upon physical examination you detect a soft, bulging, and a very compressible mass on the anterior surface of the vagina. When you push on the bulging mass she feels the need to urinate. You order a CT because you suspect which of the following?

a. Rectocele
b. Cystocele
c. Cervical cancer
d. Didelphic uterus
e. Indirect inguinal hernia

5-4. A 55-year-old man discovered that he had pain in the neck and right arm and weakness in extending the fingers of his right hand, with loss of sensation in the right thumb and middle fingers. A neurological examination further revealed a weakness of the right biceps reflex, but other neurological signs could not be detected. Which of the following is the most likely diagnosis?

a. Syringomyelia involving the cervical cord
b. A knife wound of the right arm completely severing nerves innervating the biceps muscle
c. Prolapse of a cervical disk
d. Poliomyelitis involving the cervical cord
e. AIDS

5-5. A young man in his mid-twenties presents with mucosal lesions in his mouth. Based on his CD4 cell count and other signs during the past few months, he is diagnosed as having AIDS. Which of the following is the most likely etiology of the oral lesions?

a. *Aspergillus*
b. *Candida*
c. *Cryptococcus*
d. *Mucor*
e. *Rhizopus*

5-6. A 65-year-old man presents with bone pain and is found to have hypocalcemia and increased parathyroid hormone. Surgical exploration of his neck finds all four of his parathyroid glands to be enlarged. Which of the following disorders is the most likely cause of this patient's enlarged parathyroid glands?

a. Primary hyperplasia
b. Parathyroid adenoma
c. Chronic renal failure
d. Parathyroid carcinoma
e. Lung carcinoma

5-7. A person has a stroke involving the ventral aspect of the diencephalon, resulting in significant damage to the mammillary bodies. As a result, there is considerable loss of input that normally supplies a major target region of the mammillary bodies. Which structure is now deprived of such input?

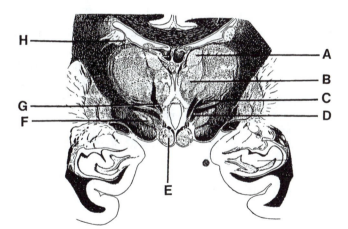

a. A
b. B
c. C
d. D
e. E
f. F
g. G
h. H

5-8. A 67-year-old woman slipped on a scatter rug and fell with her right arm extended in an attempt to ease the impact of the fall. She experienced immediate severe pain in the region of the right clavicle and in the right distal arm. Painful movement of the right arm was minimized by holding the arm close to the body and by supporting the elbow with the left hand. There is marked tenderness and some swelling in the region of the clavicle about one-third of the distance from the sternum. The examining physician can feel the projecting edges of the clavicular fragments. The radiograph confirms the fracture and shows elevation of the proximal fragment with depression and subluxation (underriding) of the distal fragment. Traction by which of the following muscles causes subluxation (the distal fragment underrides the proximal fragment)?

a. Deltoid muscle
b. Pectoralis major muscle
c. Pectoralis minor muscle
d. Sternomastoid muscle
e. Trapezius muscle

5-9. A patient is transported to the emergency department. A friend who accompanies the patient to the ED says "he was experimenting with (PCP phencyclidine)." Which of the following best describes the actions of phencyclidine?

a. Causes its peripheral and central effects via antimuscarinic properties
b. Causes significant withdrawal symptoms
c. Has hallucinogenic properties
d. Has strong opioid receptor-activating activity
e. Overdoses should be treated with flumazenil

5-10. Three weeks after a patient with AIDS traveled to California to study desert flowers, he develops fever, chest pain, and muscle soreness. Two months later, red, tender nodules appear on the shins, and he has pain and tenderness in the right ankle. An x-ray film of the chest shows a left pleural effusion. Which of the following is the most likely diagnosis?

a. Blastomycosis
b. Coccidioidomycosis
c. Histoplasmosis
d. *Mycobacterium marinum* infection
e. *Mycoplasma pneumoniae* infection

5-11. A newspaper correspondent has diarrhea for 2 weeks following a trip to St. Petersburg (Leningrad). She is most likely to have which one of the following?

a. Giardiasis
b. Schistosomiasis
c. Toxoplasmosis
d. Trichinosis
e. Visceral larva migrans

5-12. A patient in the emergency department requires suturing of a deep 2-cm laceration. To reduce discomfort we first infiltrate the surrounding area with lidocaine. Which of the following functions or sensations is most likely to disappear first as the drug's effects build up, and the last to reappear as the drug's effects wear off?

a. Autonomic efferent function
b. Motor nerve activity
c. Pain
d. Pressure (deep or heavy pressure)
e. Temperature

5-13. An 18-month-old boy presents with delayed dentation, short stature, difficulty and painful walking, and bowing of the legs. In vitamin D deficiency, which of the following is defective in bone?

a. Bone formation by osteoblasts
b. The composition of bone collagen
c. Calcification of the bone matrix
d. Bone resorption by osteoclasts
e. The blood supply to the haversian canals

5-14. Martin Causubon weighed 3.5 kg at birth and appeared to be perfectly normal. Through his first 2 years of life, Martin had persistent otitis media, dry cough, and on one occasion bilateral pneumonia. At 5 months, Martin had oral *Candida spp.* and a red rash in the diaper area. He was not gaining weight; Martin was admitted to the hospital with tachypnea. His tonsils were observed to be very small, he had hepatomegaly, and cultures of his nasal fluid grew *Pseudomonas aeruginosa.* He also had coarse, harsh breath sounds from both lungs. Blood work showed a white blood count = 4800 cells μL^{-1} (normal 5000–10,000 cells μL^{-1}), absolute lymphocyte count = 760 cells μL^{-1} (normal 3000 lymphocytes μL^{-1}). None of his lymphocytes reacted with anti-CD3; 99% of his lymphocytes bound antibody against the B-cell molecule CD20 and 1% were natural killer cells reacting with anti-CD16. His serum contained IgG at a concetration of 30 mg dL^{-1}, IgA at 27 mg dL^{-1}, IgM at 42 mg dL^{-1} (IgG levels are normally 400 mg dL^{-1}; the IgA and IgM levels were at the low end of the normal range for Martin's age). His blood mononuclear cells were completely unresponsive to phytohemagglutinin (PHA), concanavalin A (ConA), and pokeweed mitogen (PWM), as well as to specific antigens to which he had been previously exposed by immunization or infection—tetanus and diphtheria toxoids, and *Candida* antigen. His B lymphocytes did not react with an antibody to the γ chain of the interleukin-2 receptor (IL-2Rγ).

The accompanying images are low magnification (A) and high magnification (B) photomicrographs. In Martin's case what would you expect to find immediately surrounding the region labeled with the arrow?

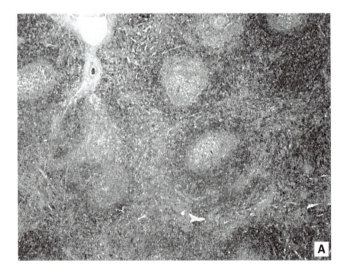

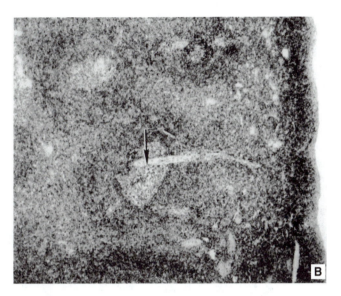

a. Absence of T cells
b. Proliferation of T cells
c. Proliferation of B cells
d. Absence of B cells
e. Absence of antigen-presenting cells (APCs)

5-15. A child presents with deeply pigmented and scarred skin despite her Caucasian heritage, and her growth is delayed. Her dermatologist obtains a skin biopsy, suspecting the xeroderma pigmentosum group of diseases (278730); these have decreased ability to repair thymine-thymine dimers in DNA that are caused by ultraviolet light (sunlight exposure). Which of the following strategies would best measure unscheduled DNA synthesis (DNA repair) in the patient's skin fibroblasts?

a. Cell synchrony, then incubation with labelled iodine in G phase to complex with newly created hydroxyl groups in deoxyribose residues
b. Incubation with labelled purines to replace newly synthesized bases on the outside of the DNA duplex
c. Cell synchrony, then incubation with labelled deoxyribonucleotides in G phase to measure extension of single DNA strands in the 3′ to 5′ direction
d. Incubation with labelled deoxyribonucleotide triphosphates to measure extension of both strands in the 5′ to 3′ direction
e. Incubation with labelled deoxyribonucleotide triphosphates to measure extension of both strands in the 3′ to 5′ direction

5-16. A patient presents with cerebellar ataxia and nystagmus. An MRI later identifies the site of the lesion. To which of the following deep cerebellar nucleus or related structure do the neurons in the damaged region project?

a. Globose nucleus
b. Emboliform nucleus
c. Fastigial nucleus
d. Dentate nucleus
e. Superior cerebellar peduncle

5-17. A 45-year-old man presents with increasing "heartburn," especially after eating or when lying down. Endoscopic examination finds a red velvety plaque located at the distal esophagus. Biopsies from this area, taken approximately 4 cm proximal to the gastroesophageal junction reveal metaplastic columnar epithelium as seen in the associated picture. Which of the following is the most likely diagnosis?

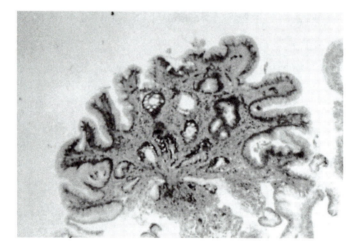

a. Acquired achalasia
b. Barrett's esophagus
c. Hamartomatous polyp
d. Metastatic adenocarcinoma
e. Reflux esophagitis

5-18. A 76-year-old man farmer presents with a 2-cm mass on the left side of his forehead. A biopsy reveals squamous cell carcinoma. Which one of the following causes the formation of pyrimidine dimers in DNA and is associated with the formation of squamous cell carcinoma?

a. Aflatoxin B1
b. Vinyl chloride
c. UVC
d. UVB
e. Epstein-Barr virus

5-19. A 42-year-old female complained about a painful and burning sensation in both hands and arms. Following a neurological examination, it was determined that the patient was suffering from a peripheral neuropathy caused by a virus that selectively attacked sensory fibers in the arms mediating pain and temperature signals. Concerning the distribution and sites of termination of these sensory fibers in the central nervous system (CNS), their sites of termination include which of the following regions?

a. Laminas I and II of the gray matter of the spinal cord ipsilateral to their site of entry into the cord
b. Laminas III and IV of the gray matter of the spinal cord contralateral to their site of entry into the cord
c. Laminas VIII and IX of the gray matter of the spinal cord ipsilateral to their site of entry into the cord
d. Laminas VIII and IX of the gray matter of the spinal cord contralateral to their site of entry into the cord
e. Lower brainstem nuclei ipsilateral to their site of entry into the cord

5-20. A mammogram of a woman, age 48, reveals macrocalcification within the right breast, indicating the need for biopsy. The surgeon visually and manually examines the breast with negative results. The surgeon closely examines the nipple for indications of ductal carcinoma. At surgery for the biopsy, a locator needle is inserted into the region of macrocalcification and the position confirmed by mammography. The surgeon incises the skin and dissects a block of tissue. The pathology report indicates ductal carcinoma with microinvasion necessitating surgery. Both patient and surgeon agree that a modified radical mastectomy offers the best prognosis in her case. At surgery for mastectomy, the surgeon carries the dissection along the major pathway of lymphatic drainage from the mammary gland. The major lymphatic channels parallel which of the following?

a. Subcutaneous venous networks to the contralateral breast and abdominal wall
b. Tributaries of the axillary vessels to the axillary nodes
c. Tributaries of the intercostal vessels to the parasternal nodes
d. Tributaries of the internal thoracic (mammary) vessels to the parasternal nodes
e. Tributaries of the thoracoacromial vessels to the apical (subscapular) nodes

5-21. A 23-year-old woman is being evaluated for the development of polyhydramnios during the 15th week of her first pregnancy. Laboratory testing finds increased α-fetoprotein in her serum, and an ultrasound finds an abnormal shape to the head of the fetus with an absence of the skull. Which of the following therapies would most decrease the probability of this abnormality occurring in subsequent pregnancies for this individual?

a. Completely avoid alcohol
b. Decrease dietary caffeine
c. Vaccinate against rubella
d. Increase dietary folate
e. Increase dietary vitamin A

5-22. A 24-year-old male was hiking in the Rockies on a winter day and became lost. He was discovered a day later and was admitted to a local hospital for a precautionary examination. The patient suffered from overexposure to the cold and, when given a neurological test, had difficulty in closing his eye, displayed a loss of both the eye-blink reflex and increased sensitivity to sounds, and had difficulty displaying his teeth and chewing food, especially on the side of the mouth. In addition, his speech was somewhat slurred and he was unable to whistle upon request. Which of the cranial nerves in the following figure was affected by the cold in this individual?

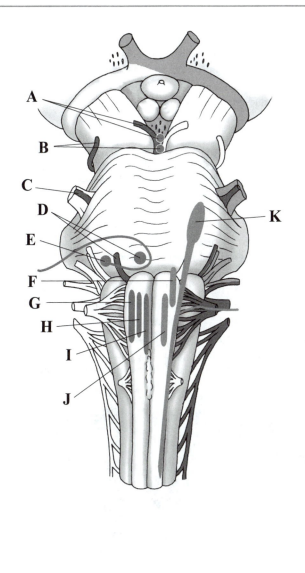

a. A
b. B
c. C
d. D
e. E
f. F
g. G
h. H
i. I
j. J
k. K

5-23. A patient who took a potentially lethal overdose of aspirin was transported by ambulance to the emergency department. Which of the following drugs would be a helpful adjunct to manage this severe aspirin poisoning?

a. Acetaminophen
b. Amphetamines (e.g., dextroamphetamine)
c. N-acetylcysteine
d. Phenobarbital
e. Sodium bicarbonate

5-24. A 23-year-old, semiconscious man is brought to the emergency room following an automobile accident. He is tachypneic and cyanotic. The right lower anterolateral thoracic wall reveals a small laceration and flailing. Air does *not* appear to move into or out of the wound, and it is assumed that the pleura have *not* been penetrated. After the patient is placed on immediate positive pressure endotracheal respiration, his cyanosis clears and the abnormal movement of the chest wall disappears. Radiographic examination confirms fractures of the fourth through eighth ribs in the right anterior axillary line and of the fourth through sixth ribs at the right costochondral junction. There is *no* evidence that bony fragments have penetrated the lungs or of pneumothorax (collapsed lung). The small superficial laceration, once it is ascertained that it has *not* penetrated the pleura, is sutured and the chest bound in bandages; positive pressure endotracheal respiration is maintained. Several hours

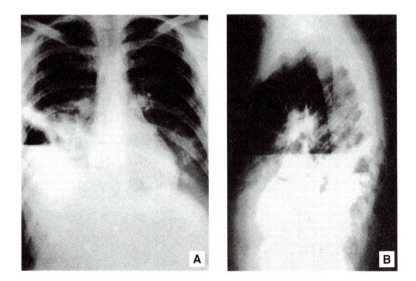

later, the cyanosis returns. The right side of the thorax is found to be more expanded than the left, yet moves less during respiration. Chest x-rays are shown in previous page.

Which of the following is the most obvious abnormal finding in the inspiratory posteroanterior and lateral chest x-ray of this patient (viewed in the anatomic position)?

a. Flail chest
b. Right hemothorax
c. Right pneumothorax
d. Paralysis of the right hemidiaphragm

5-25. A 50-year-old man comes in for a physical so he can attend a boy scout camp with one of his sons. You suggest a colonoscopy after he returns from camp. He agrees, but wants you to describe the procedure and potential risks and complications. You explain that the goal of a colonoscopy is to look at the entire length of the large intestine from the anus to the small intestine (ileocecal junction), observing polyps or diverticuli with a flexible fiber optic colonoscope inserted through the anus. There is a small risk of perforating the bowel especially when the colon takes a sudden turn or twists on itself at regions where it is intraperitoneal rather than attached to the posterior abdominal wall (retroperitoneal). Which of the following regions of the colon generally poses the greatest risk for perforation because the bowel takes either a sudden change in direction or is suspended by a mesentery?

a. Rectum, sigmoid colon and descending colon
b. Sigmoid colon, descending colon and splenic flexure
c. Sigmoid colon, splenic flexure and descending colon
d. Sigmoid colon, splenic flexure and hepatic flexure
e. Descending colon, transverse colon and ascending colon

5-26. Morris is a 79-year-old man who was brought to the emergency room because his family was worried that he suddenly was not using his right arm and leg and seemed to have a simultaneous behavior change. He was unable to write a reminder note to himself, even with his left hand, and he put his shoes on the wrong feet. A neurologist was called to the emergency room to examine the patient. A loud bruit was heard with a stethoscope over the left carotid artery in his neck. When asked to show the neurologist his left hand, he pointed to his right hand, since it could not move. The neurologist asked him to add numbers, and he was unable to do this, despite having spent his life as a bookkeeper. Morris was unable to name the fingers on either hand, and he could not form any semblance of a letter using his left hand. Morris's eyes did not blink when the neurologist waved his hands close to them in the left temporal and right nasal visual fields. The right lower two-thirds of his face drooped. There was some asymmetry of his reflexes between the right and left sides, and there was a positive Babinski's response of his right toe. Where in the CNS is the damage?

a. Right frontal and parietal lobes
b. Left frontal and parietal lobes
c. Right frontal lobe
d. Left frontal lobe
e. Right temporal lobe

5-27. A 25-year-old pregnant woman living in the San Joaquin Valley (California) experienced an influenza-like illness with fever and cough. She was diagnosed with *Coccidioides* infection that disseminated from her lungs to other organs while in the third trimester of pregnancy. Patients who have disseminated coccidioidomycosis usually demonstrate which of the following?

a. Absence of complement-fixing (CF) antibodies
b. A negative coccidioidin skin test and a rising CF titer
c. A negative coccidioidin skin test and a stable CF titer
d. A positive skin test and a mildly elevated CF titer
e. Lack of immunity to reinfection

5-28. In between your M1 and M2 years you are volunteering in a hospital in a very poor part of the world. Their drug selection is limited. A patient presents with acute cardiac failure, for which your preferred drug is dobutamine, given intravenously. However, there is none available. Which of the following other drugs, or combination of drugs, would be a suitable alternative, giving the pharmacologic equivalent of what you want the dobutamine to do? (All these drugs are available in parenteral formulations.)

a. Dopamine (at a very high dose)
b. Ephedrine
c. Ephedrine plus propranolol
d. Norepinephrine plus phentolamine
e. Phenylephrine plus atropine

5-29. A 3-month-old boy presents with poor feeding and growth, low muscle tone (hypotonia), elevation of blood lactic acid (lactic acidemia), and mild acidosis (blood pH 7.3 to 7.35). The ratio of pyruvate to lactate in serum is elevated, and there is decreased conversion of pyruvate to acetyl coenzyme A in fibroblasts. Which of the following compounds should be considered for therapy?

a. Pyridoxine
b. Thiamine
c. Free fatty acids
d. Biotin
e. Ascorbic acid

5-30. A patient taking an oral diuretic for about 6 months presents with elevated fasting and postprandial blood glucose levels. You check the patient's HbA_{1c} and find it is elevated compared with normal baseline values obtained 6 months ago. You suspect the glycemic problems are diuretic-induced. Which of the following was the most likely cause?

a. Acetazolamide
b. Amiloride
c. Chlorothiazide
d. Spironolactone
e. Triamterene

5-31. A child from Nigeria is evaluated for developmental delay. His coloring seems much lighter than that of his family background, and his physician orders a blood amino acid test that demonstrates elevated phenylalanine. A special low phenylalanine formula is begun (Lofenelac) as treatment for phenylketonuria (261600), but the parents refuse to come in for follow-up appointments. A public health evaluation reports that the child is failing to thrive despite apparent adherence to the diet by his parents. The symptoms of decreased skin pigment and later failure to thrive in this child are most likely related to which of the following?

a. Deficiency of alanine
b. Deficiency of tyrosine and melanin
c. Deficiency of tryptophan and niacin
d. Deficiency of leucine and isoleucine
e. Deficiency of phenylalanine

5-32. A tourist who recently returned from a Caribbean cruise suddenly develops arthralgia, a maculopapular rash, and lymphadenopathy with back and bone pain. Which of the following is the most likely diagnosis?

a. Dengue fever
b. Hepatitis
c. HIV infection
d. Infectious mononucleosis
e. Saint Louis encephalitis

5-33. A 55-year-old man with difficulty urinating, blood in the urine, burning during urination and accelerating prostate-specific antigen (PSA) has a radical prostatectomy. The diagnosis is prostate carcinoma with a Gleason score of 7. Rb, p53, and bcl-2 genes are involved in the development of prostate carcinoma. Which of the following mechanisms may be involved in the loss of cell cycle control that occurs in prostate carcinoma?

a. Increased CdkI activity
b. Decreased transcription of G_1/S cyclin
c. Decreased expression of bcl-2
d. Increased transcription of gene regulatory proteins such as E2F
e. Dephosphorylation of Rb

5-34. A 7-year-old boy is referred to the endocrine clinic with short stature, rhizomelic shortening of the arms and legs, a disproportionately long trunk, trident hands, midfacial hypoplasia, prominent forehead (frontal bossing), thoracolumbar gibbus, and megalencephaly. Radiological examination by

MRI reveals caudal narrowing of the interpedicular spaces of T1 and T2 vertebrae and spinal stenosis at L2–L4. Genetic analysis reveals a gain of function mutation, G1138A, in the fibroblast growth factor receptor-3 (FGFR3), band 4p16.3. His parents are requesting the initiation of treatment with growth hormone. The endocrinologist is concerned about harmful growth hormone effects: deposition of abnormally-formed bone and worsening of the patient's kyphoscoliosis. During this child's postnatal development, which of the following is the most likely effect of the FGFR-3 gene mutation?

a. Decreased bone deposition under the periosteum
b. Decreased proliferation of osteoblasts in the primary ossification center
c. Decreased proliferation of osteoblasts in the secondary ossification center
d. Decreased appositional growth of chondroblasts in the primary ossification center
e. Decreased interstitial growth of chondroblasts in the epiphyses

5-35. A 55-year-old woman undergoes surgery. She receives several drugs for preanesthesia care, intubation, and intraoperative skeletal muscle paralysis; and a mixture of inhaled anesthetics to complete the balanced anesthesia. Toward the end of the procedure she develops hyperthermia, hypertension, hyperkalemia, tachycardia, muscle rigidity, and metabolic acidosis. Which of the following drugs is most likely to have participated in this reaction?

a. Fentanyl
b. Halothane
c. Ketamine
d. Midazolam
e. Propofol

5-36. A postoperative patient develops a thready pulse, tachycardia, and hypotension. A decision is made to take the patient back to surgery to check for bleeding. Laboratory analysis shows an increase in plasma angiotensin II accompanied by an increase in glomerular filtration rate (GFR). When GFR increases, proximal tubular reabsorption of salt and water increases by a process called glomerulotubular balance. Contributions to this process include which of the following?

a. An increase in peritubular capillary hydrostatic pressure
b. A decrease in peritubular sodium concentration
c. An increase in peritubular oncotic pressure
d. An increase in proximal tubular flow
e. An increase in peritubular capillary flow

5-37. An elderly man was brought to the emergency room after fainting in his home. A subsequent magnetic resonance imaging (MRI) suggested the presence of a small stroke limited to the medial aspect of the rostral part of the midbrain tegmentum. Which pathway would most likely be affected by the stroke?

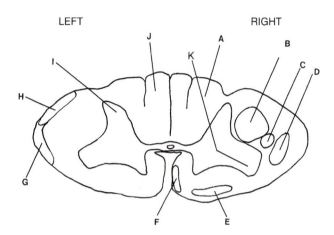

LEFT   RIGHT

a. A
b. B
c. C
d. D
e. E
f. F
g. G
h. H
i. I
j. J
k. K

5-38. An immigrant family from rural Mexico brings their 3-month-old child to the emergency room because of whistling inspiration (stridor) and high fever. The child's physician is perplexed because the throat examination shows a gray membrane almost occluding the larynx. A senior physician recognizes diphtheria, now rare in immunized populations. The child is intubated, antitoxin is administered, and antibiotic therapy is initiated. Diphtheria toxin is often lethal in unimmunized persons because it does which of the following?

a. Inhibits initiation of protein synthesis by preventing the binding of GTP to the 40S ribosomal subunit
b. Binds to the signal recognition particle receptor on the cytoplasmic face of the endoplasmic reticulum receptor
c. Shuts off signal peptidase
d. Blocks elongation of proteins by inactivating elongation factor 2 (EF-2, or translocase)
e. Causes deletions of amino acid by speeding up the movement of peptidyl-tRNA from the A site to the P site

5-39. A 39-year-old man with aortic insufficiency and a history of multiple antibiotic resistance is given a prophylactic intravenous dose of antibiotic before surgery to insert a prosthetic heart valve. As the antibiotic is being infused, the patient becomes flushed over most of his body. Which of the following antibiotics is most likely responsible?

a. Erythromycin
b. Gentamicin
c. Penicillin G
d. Tetracycline
e. Vancomycin

5-40. A 65-year-old female patient is admitted to an intensive care unit because of sudden swelling on the right side of the face and an episode of bleeding from the right nostril. According to her daughter, these signs were not apparent a few days ago. She has a long history of diabetes, high blood pressure, and recently developed clinical signs of ketoacidosis and renal insufficiency. Her blood sugar level at the time of admission is 700 mg/dL. The facial lesion becomes partially necrotic and shows slight protrusion of the right eye and facial paralysis. The patient dies on the second day. Histopathologic examination of the lesions reveals occlusion of the small vessels and the presence of nonseptate hyphae. This is most probably caused by which of the following?

a. Candadiasis
b. Erysipelis
c. Gas gangrene
d. Mucormycosis
e. Nocardiosis

5-41. A 49-year-old male patient with AIDS and declining CD4 counts has an increased frequency of systemic infections and develops sick euthyroid syndrome with a decline in T_4 and T_3 levels. With normal thyroid function, which of the following is correct?

a. TSH initiates thyroid hormone secretion via activation of nuclear receptors in thyroid gland cells.
b. Secretion of TSH is regulated primarily by the pituitary level of T_3
c. TSH is secreted from the posterior pituitary
d. T_4 is the physiologically active hormone
e. T_4 is formed from T_3 by the process of monodeiodination.

5-42. An individual has difficulty adjusting his head, especially after he changes his posture. Which of the following is the most likely pathway affected that might cause this deficit?

a. Lateral vestibulospinal tract
b. Medial vestibulospinal tract
c. Medial reticulospinal tract
d. Lateral reticulospinal tract
e. Rubrospinal tract

5-43. A 58-year-old Caucasian woman is seen in the endocrine clinic. She has been followed for type 1 diabetes for the past decade. She sustained a Colles' fracture last year when she fell over the hose while watering the garden. She took hormone replacement therapy (HRT) for 3 years at the start of menopause, but was taken off HRT 5 years ago because of her concerns about ovarian cancer. She drinks three glasses of milk a day and eats other dairy products frequently. She drinks socially, a drink, a glass of wine, or a beer twice/week. She does not smoke. She once was a "runner," but now walks 2 miles twice/week when weather permits. She is 5 ft 4 in. and she weighs 122 lb. Her height has decreased by an inch over the past 5 years and her weight has increased by 12 lb. CBC and blood chemistries are normal. Her "T" score on dual-energy absorptiometry (DXA) is -2 for spine and -2.5 for hip. Bisphosphonates are prescribed. Which of the following is the most likely mechanism of action for the bisphosphonates?

a. Inhibition of osteoblastic activity
b. Increased RANK-L secretion by osteoblasts
c. Increased M-CSF secretion by osteoblasts
d. Apoptosis of osteoclasts
e. Increased RANK expression by osteoclasts

5-44. A newborn girl presents with a mutation in the erythropoietin receptor gene which leads to primary familial erythrocytosis (familial polycythemia). During the 5th to 9th months of fetal development, the primary effect was on red blood cell production in which of the following?

a. Liver
b. Yolk sac
c. Spleen
d. Thymus
e. Bone marrow

5-45. A 35-year-old man visits his family medicine physician complaining of bloating, a sense of urgency, cramping abdominal pain, meteorism, diarrhea with excessive flatulence several hours after ingestion of milk or dairy products. He says that he has always enjoyed milk and dairy products without any problems, but now eating them causes him abdominal distress. In this disorder, the area shown by the arrows would have a decrease in which of the following?

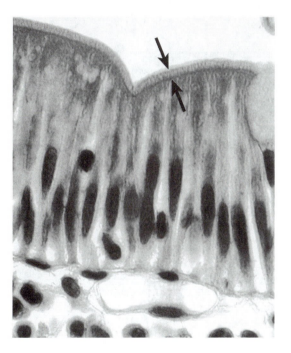

a. Specific disaccharidase activity
b. Glucose/galactose transporter activity
c. Passive diffusion of monosaccharides
d. Uptake of triglycerides by endocytosis
e. Active transport of glycerol

5-46. A 6-month-old boy is brought into the pediatric clinic. He weighs 12 lb, 2 oz and is 22 in. tall. Neither his height nor his weight is on the growth chart for his age; mean weight and height for a 6-month-old are 17 lb, 4 oz and 26.5 in., respectively. Through functional tests, you determine that he is suffering from an inherited condition known as I-cell disease and is missing UDP N-acetylglucosamine: lysosomal enzyme N-acetylglucosamine-1-phosphotransferase, which is more conveniently referred to as phospho-transferase. You recall from your cell biology that the phosphotransferase enzymes phosphorylate mannose to form mannose-6-phosphate. Electron microscopy is performed on a biopsy, and blood tests are completed. Which of the following explains the altered cell biological processes in this patient?

a. Lysosomal enzymes missorted back to the Golgi apparatus
b. Peroxisomal proteins missorted to other organelles
c. Abnormal KDEL sequence on vesicles
d. Absence of SNARE proteins on vesicles
e. Secretion of lysosomal enzymes into the blood

5-47. A woman presents with gallstones and no jaundice. She is prepared for exploratory surgery. The lesser omentum is incised close to its free edge, and the biliary tree is identified and freed by blunt dissection. The liquid contents of the gallbladder are aspirated with a syringe, the fundus incised, and the stones are removed. The entire duct system is carefully probed for stones, one of which is found to be obstructing a duct. In view of her symptoms, where is the most probable location of the obstruction?

a. The bile duct
b. The common hepatic duct
c. The cystic duct
d. Within the duodenal papilla proximal to the juncture with the pancreatic duct
e. Within the duodenal papilla distal to the juncture with the pancreatic duct

5-48. A 72-year-old man presents with increasing fatigue. Physical examination reveals an elderly man in no apparent distress (NAD). He is found to have multiple enlarged, nontender lymph nodes along with an enlarged liver and spleen. Laboratory examination of his peripheral blood reveals a normocytic normochromic anemia, a slightly decreased platelet count, and a leukocyte count of 72,000 cells/μL. An example of his peripheral blood is seen in the picture below. Which of the following is the most likely diagnosis?

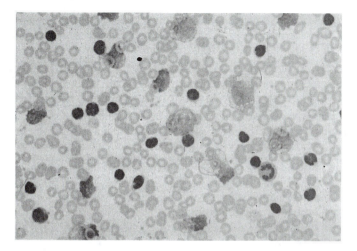

a. Acute lymphoblastic leukemia
b. Atypical lymphocytosis
c. Chronic lymphocytic leukemia
d. Immunoblastic lymphoma
e. Prolymphocytic leukemia

5-49. A 65-year-old man presents with increasing fatigue and shortness of breath. Examination of his peripheral blood finds pancytopenia, and a few (less than 5%) immature cells are present. Some of the neutrophils are bilobed (Pelger-Huët change) and a dimorphic red blood cell population is seen. A bone marrow biopsy reveals a hypercellular marrow with about 15% of the cells being immature cells. Approximately 20% of the red cell precursors have iron deposits that encircled the nucleus. Which of the following is the most likely cause of these clinical findings?

a. Chronic blood loss
b. Iron deficiency
c. Lead poisoning
d. Myelodysplasia
e. Vitamin B_{12} deficiency

5-50. A 30-year-old man presents because of a swelling involving the posterior distal portion of his right leg. Physical examination finds a single tumor nodule in his right Achilles tendon that is consistent with a xanthoma. Pertinent medical history is that his father died of a myocardial infarct before the age of 40. Laboratory evaluation finds elevated serum cholesterol and normal serum triglycerides. His serum HDL levels are found to be decreased in amount. The signs and symptoms in this individual, who has familial hypercholesterolemia, most likely resulted from an abnormality involving the receptor for which one of the following substances?

a. Apoprotein CI
b. Beta-myosin
c. Chylomicron remnants
d. Lipoprotein lipase
e. Low-density lipoproteins

Block 6

Questions

6-1. A 6 feet 3 inches tall, 140-lb, 20-year-old male was watching television when he felt pain in his shoulder blades, shortness of breath, and fatigue. His father noticed how pale he was and took him to the Emergency Department, where a chest X-ray revealed a 55% pneumothorax of the right lung due to rupture of a bleb on the surface of the lung. Which of the following is true?

a. The intrapleural pressure in the affected area is equal to atmospheric pressure
b. The chest wall on the affected side recoils inward
c. There is hyperinflation of the affected lung
d. The $\dot{V}/\dot{Q}$ ratio on the affected side is higher than normal
e. The mediastinum shifts further to the right with each inspiration

6-2. A mountain climber in excellent physical condition suffers shortness of breath and low oxygen (hypoxia) at high altitude in Nepal. After transport to base camp and oxygen treatment, a family history reveals that his mother has sickle cell anemia. With reference to the accompanying figure, laboratory studies of his β-globin gene structure and expression would be expected to show which of the following results? (Note that the same MstII restriction and β-globin probe in the figure is used for Southern blotting).

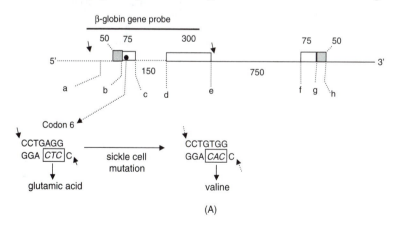

(A)

a. MstII DNA cleavage segment of 515 and 165 bp by Southern blot, RNA segment of ~700 bp by Northern blot, normal and abnormal proteins by hemoglobin electrophoresis
b. MstII DNA cleavage segments of 680, 515, and 165 bp by Southern blot, RNA segment of ~700 bp by Northern blot, normal and abnormal proteins by hemoglobin electrophoresis
c. MstII DNA cleavage segments of 515 and 165 bp by Southern blot, RNA segment of ~1400 bp by Northern blot, single abnormal protein by hemoglobin electrophoresis
d. MstII DNA cleavage segment of 680 bp by Southern blot, RNA segment of ~700 bp by Northern blot, single normal protein band by hemoglobin electrophoresis
e. MstII DNA cleavage segments of 680, 515, and 165 bp by Southern blot, RNA segment of ~700 bp by Northern blot, single abnormal protein by hemoglobin electrophoresis

6-3. A 56-year-old man who drinks a six-pack of beer a day, with higher alcoholic intake on weekends, holidays, and "special days," presents to the internal medicine clinic. He has an abnormal plasma lipoprotein profile. It is known that erythrocyte fluidity is altered in liver disease. Which of the following would increase membrane fluidity in the hepatocytes of this patient's liver?

a. Restriction of rotational movement of proteins and lipids in the membrane
b. Transbilayer movement of phospholipids in the plasma membrane
c. Increased cholesterol/phospholipids ratio in the plasma membrane
d. Binding of integral membrane proteins with cytoskeletal elements
e. Binding of an antibody to a cell-surface receptor

6-4. A 23-year-old HIV-positive man presents with a cough and increasing shortness of breath. A histologic section from a transbronchial biopsy stained with Gomori's methenamine-silver stain is shown in the photomicrograph. Which of the following is the most likely diagnosis?

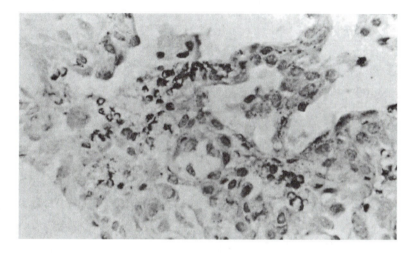

a. *Pseudomonas* pneumonia
b. *Aspergillus* pneumonia
c. *Pneumocystis carinii* pneumonia
d. Cytomegalovirus pneumonia
e. Influenza pneumonia

6-5. A child with an abdominal mass was suspected of having Wilms tumor (194070), supported by blood and unusual cells in the urine sediment. The physicians suspected erosion of surrounding kidney with invasion of the renal pelvis, causing tumor cells to be excreted in urine. Because a version of the p57 gene is known to be silenced preferentially in Wilms tumor, analysis of p57 gene methylation and expression was performed on the urine tumor cells with the results shown below. Which of the following best summarizes these results?

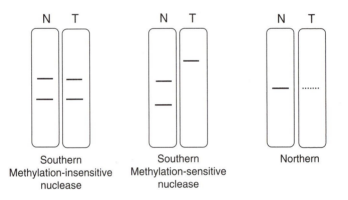

a. Biallelic p57 gene methylation and with normal p57 gene expression making a diagnosis of Wilms tumor unlikely

b. Bi-allelic p57 gene methylation and with increased p57 gene expression making a diagnosis of Wilms tumor unlikely

c. Bi-allelic p57 gene methylation and with decreased p57 gene expression supporting the diagnosis of Wilms tumor

d. Undermethylation of both p57 alleles with increased p57 gene expression supporting the diagnosis of Wilms tumor

e. Methylation of one p57 allele with increased p57 gene expression supporting the diagnosis of Wilms tumor

6-6. An elderly male is admitted to the emergency room after having experienced double vision. Further examination reveals the presence of pressure that is exerted upon the wall of the cavernous sinus. When asked by the neurologist to follow the movement of his fingers when they are directed downward in a medial position, the patient is unable to do so with his right eye. Which of the following cranial nerves is affected in this patient?

a. Cranial nerve VIII
b. Cranial nerve VII
c. Cranial nerve VI
d. Cranial nerve IV
e. Cranial nerve III

6-7. A 14-year-old boy presents with hepatic failure, slurred speech, tremors in the hands and feet, and Kayser-Fleischer rings. A 24 hour urine copper test is 120 micrograms (μg)/24 hours (normal below 100 μg/24 hours) and ceruloplasmin of 15 mg/dL (normal 25 to 50 mg/dL). Liver biopsy reveals 295 μg/g (normal <250 μg/g) dry weight of copper with microscopic changes including glycogen nuclei, microvesicular and macrovesicular fatty changes, steatosis and fibrosis. Genetic studies reveal mutations in the ATP7B gene which has been localized to the late endosome. Such mutations may alter the transport of cargo within late endosomes to which of the following?

a. Lysosome for degradation
b. Clathrin-coated pits and vesicles
c. Multivesicular bodies
d. Cell surface to recycle receptors
e. TGN for further processing

6-8. A 33-year-old woman visits the office of her family medicine physician. Her chief complaint is nervousness. She describes her nervousness as increasing over the past 6 weeks. She says that her children and husband describe her as atypically "easy to anger." She says that she now easily loses her temper and often cries for little or no apparent reason, and she has developed a tremor in her right arm. She has lost 22 lb since her last office visit 9 months ago and indicates that she has not changed her diet. She describes herself as always "hot." You observe that her eyes protrude and appear red and inflamed, and she describes her eyes as feeling "dry." Your examination reveals asthenia, tachycardia, and pretibial myxedema. A biopsy of the organ shown below shows an increase in lymphoid cells. An array of tests is completed. To which of the following would you expect to detect autoantibodies within this organ?

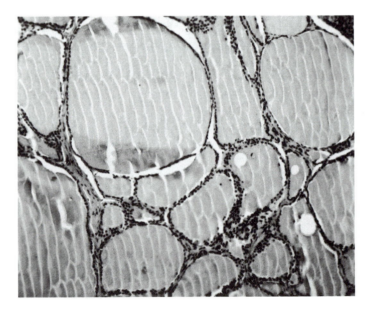

a. C cells
b. Parathyroid principal cells
c. Thyrotropin-releasing factor receptors
d. Thyroglobulin and thyroid peroxidase
e. TSH receptors

6-9. A middle-aged man is brought to the hospital for a neurological examination after displaying uncontrollable movements of his upper limbs. He is diagnosed with a rare genetic disorder affecting dopamine synthesis in brainstem neurons. However, there is some controversy concerning at what step in the biosynthesis of dopamine this failure took place. If the failure lay in the immediate precursor stage in the biosynthesis of dopamine, which of the following is the precursor?

a. Tyrosine
b. Tyrosine hydroxylase
c. Tryptophan
d. L-dihydroxyphenylalanine (L-DOPA)
e. Dopamine β-hydroxylase

6-10. A 30-year-old patient was generally healthy until his impacted wisdom tooth was removed by an oral surgeon. The area where the tooth had been was sore, but what was more alarming was the appearance of eruptions through the skin beneath the area of the jaw where the tooth had been. The exudate draining through the skin eruptions was cultured aerobically, but the results were negative. Which of the following is the most likely etiologic agent responsible for the patient's condition?

a. *Actinomyces bovis*
b. *Actinomyces israelii*
c. *C. albicans*
d. *H. capsulatum*
e. *Nocardia asteroides*

6-11. A child has mononucleosis-like symptoms, yet the tests for mononucleosis and the EBV titers are negative. Which of the following is a cause of heterophile-negative mononucleosis?

a. Adenovirus
b. Coxsackievirus
c. Cytomegalovirus
d. Herpes simplex virus
e. Varicella-zoster virus

6-12. An elderly man, in obvious respiratory distress due to exacerbation of his emphysema and chronic bronchitis, presents in the emergency department. One drug ordered by the physician, to be administered by the respiratory therapist, is N-acetylcysteine. Which of the following is the main action or purpose of this drug?

a. Block receptors for the cysteinyl leukotrienes
b. Inhibit metabolic inactivation of epinephrine or β_2 agonists that were administered
c. Inhibit leukotriene synthesis
d. Promptly suppress airway inflammation
e. Reverse ACh-mediated bronchoconstriction
f. Thin airway mucus secretions for easier removal by suctioning or postural drainage

6-13. A 50-year-old woman has been treated over the past 6 months with lithium for an ongoing emotional disorder. From which of the following disorders is this patient most likely suffering?

a. Panic attacks
b. Schizophrenia
c. Obsessive-compulsive disorder
d. Bipolar disorder
e. Anxiety

6-14. A 45-year-old man was riding a snowmobile and hit a snow-covered rocky outcropping. When standing for the first time after the accident, he slipped and fell on the outcropping and now is experiencing pain in the gluteal region. In this CT scan, the dark linear structure indicated by the arrow is which of the following?

a. A fracture of the sacral body
b. The sacrococcygeal joint
c. A spinal nerve
d. The superior gluteal artery
e. The inferior gluteal artery

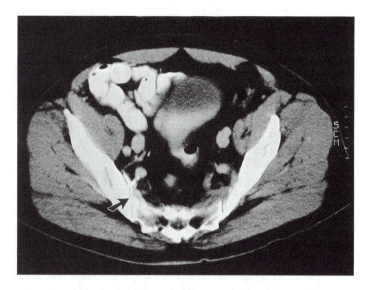

6-15. A 10-year-old female presents with chest pain and unusual skin patches over her elbows and knees. Her father died of a heart attack at age 35 and her mother is known to have high cholesterol. Her physician suspects familial hypercholesterolemia (144010) in the parents with homozygous severe disease in the daughter. This disease results from mutations in the receptor for low-density lipoprotein (LDL) or the ligand portion of its apoprotein coat, which is which of the following?

a. AI
b. B48
c. CII
d. B100
e. E

6-16. A 23-year-old woman complains of abdominal cramps and bloating that are relieved by defecation. Subsequent clinical evaluation reveals an increased maximal acid output, decreased serum calcium and iron concentrations, and microcytic anemia. Inflammation in which area of the GI tract best explains these findings?

a. Stomach
b. Duodenum
c. Jejunum
d. Ileum
e. Colon

6-17. An 82-year-old woman is brought to the emergency room complaining of nausea, vomiting, muscle cramps, and generalized weakness. Laboratory analysis reveals significant hyperkalemia. Elevations of extracellular potassium ion concentration will have which of the following effects on nerve membranes?

a. The membrane potential will become more negative
b. The sodium conductance will increase
c. The potassium conductance will increase
d. The membrane will become more excitable
e. The Na^+-K^+ pump will become inactivated

6-18. A 1-year-old female presents with growth failure and mild elevation of blood urea nitrogen and creatinine (suggesting decreased kidney function). No hormonal or dietary causes of her growth failure are found, and her mother informs her pediatrician that the child seems to avoid light. Referral to an ophthalmologist reveals unusual crystals in her cornea. Measurement of her blood amino acids reveals an unusual peak, which on analysis breaks down into an amino acid with a sulfhydryl group. The derived amino acid furthermore seems to have an ionizable side group with a pK of about 8.3. Which of the following is the most likely amino acid?

a. Lysine
b. Methionine
c. Cysteine
d. Arginine
e. Glutamine

6-19. A patient who has been treated for Parkinson's disease for about a year presents with purplish, mottled changes to her skin. Which of the following drugs is the most likely cause?

a. Amantadine
b. Bromocriptine
c. Levodopa (alone)
d. Levodopa combined with carbidopa
e. Pramipexole

6-20. As a result of a brainstem infarction, an elderly woman was unable to move her right eye to the right in following an object moving from left to right across her visual field. Which of the structures shown in the diagram was affected by this infarction?

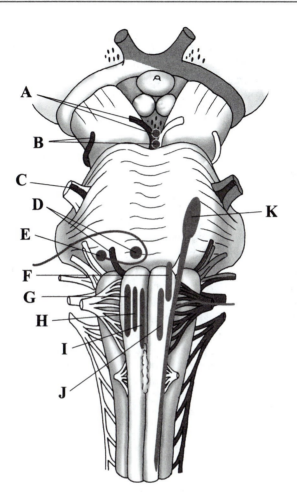

a. A
b. B
c. C
d. D
e. E
f. F
g. G
h. H
i. I
j. J
k. K

6-21. A single, 30-year-old woman presents to her physician with vaginitis. She complains of a slightly increased, malodorous discharge that is gray-white in color, thin, and homogenous. Clue cells are discovered when the discharge is examined microscopically. Which of the following organisms is the most likely cause of her infection?

a. *Candida albicans*
b. *Trichomonas vaginalis*
c. *Escherichia coli*
d. *Gardnerella vaginalis*
e. *Staphylococcus aureus*

6-22. A newborn male is evaluated because of inability to breast feed and found to have severe hypotonia (low muscle tone). The child lays in a frog leg posture with minimal spontaneous movements, and the head and legs dangle to the bed when suspended by his stomach. A large anterior fontanel is noted, and initial laboratory tests indicate elevated liver enzymes. The physician suspects Zellweger syndrome (214100), an end phenotype reflecting peroxisome dysfunction that may be caused by mutations in several different peroxisomal membrane protein genes. The diagnosis is confirmed by demonstrating elevated plasma levels of very long chain fatty acids and of erythrocyte plasmalogens. Which of the following compounds is the starting point of ether lipid and plasmalogen synthesis?

a. Acetyl CoA
b. Pyruvate
c. Dihydroxyacetone phosphate
d. Malonyl CoA
e. Palmitoyl CoA

6-23. An anxious 19-year-old woman presents with perioral numbness and carpopedal spasm. Laboratory examination reveals decreased Pco_2 and decreased bicarbonate. Which of the following is the most likely diagnosis?

a. Metabolic acidosis due to ketoacidosis
b. Metabolic acidosis due to renal tubular acidosis
c. Metabolic alkalosis due to thiazide diuretic
d. Respiratory acidosis due to hypoventilation
e. Respiratory alkalosis due to hyperventilation

6-24. A patient presents in her fifth pregnancy with a history of numbness and tingling in her right thumb and index finger during each of her previous four pregnancies. Currently, the same symptoms are constant, although generally worse in the early morning. Symptoms could be somewhat relieved by vigorous shaking of the wrist. Neurologic examination revealed atrophy and weakness of the abductor pollicis brevis, the opponens pollicis, and the first two lumbrical muscles. Sensation was decreased over the lateral palm and the volar aspect of the first three digits. Numbness and tingling were markedly increased over the first three digits and the lateral palm when the wrist was held in flexion for 30 seconds. The symptoms suggest damage to which of the following?

a. The radial artery
b. The median nerve
c. The ulnar nerve
d. Proper digital nerves
e. The radial nerve

6-25. A middle-aged man presents to his physician because of anxiety attacks accompanied by profuse sweating and heart palpitations. His physician documents a high blood pressure of 175/110 (hypertension) and orders ultrasound studies that show an adrenal tumor called pheochromocytoma. The man has also noted weight loss and fatigue over the past month when the attacks began. Knowing that pheochromocytoma releases epinephrine from the adrenal medulla, alteration of which of the following metabolic processes best explains symptoms of decreased energy and weight loss?

a. Glycolysis
b. Lipolysis
c. Gluconeogenesis
d. Glycogenolysis
e. Ketogenesis

6-26. A 39-year-old man presents with bloody diarrhea. Multiple stool examinations fail to reveal any ova or parasites. A barium examination of the patient's colon reveals a characteristic "string sign." A colonoscopy reveals the rectum and sigmoid portions of the colon to be unremarkable. A biopsy from the terminal ileum reveals numerous acute and chronic inflammatory cells within the lamina propria. Worsening of the patient's symptoms results in emergency resection of the distal small intestines. Gross examination of this resected bowel reveals deep, long mucosal fissures extending deep into the muscle wall. Several transmural fistulas are also found. Which of the following is the most likely diagnosis?

a. Ulcerative colitis
b. Lymphocytic colitis
c. Infectious colitis
d. Eosinophilic colitis
e. Crohn's disease

6-27. A group of students in the Wilderness Medicine Club left for a Spring Break Rocky Mountain hiking trip right after their Organ Systems exam. They arrived at their lodge in Denver by 2 p.m. Mountain time, and then drove to the base camp (10,000 ft), where they camped for the night. The next day, several of the students were experiencing mental and muscle fatigue, and complained of headaches, nausea, and dyspnea, so the guide decided to acclimate at 10,000 ft. for another day. Three of the students grew impatient and announced that they were going to climb to Mt. Elbert, the highest mountain in Colorado (14,400 ft altitude, barometric pressure = 447 mmHg). About 3 hours later (less than 24 hours since they first arrived in Denver), one of the students returned in a panic to get medical help because his friends were disoriented, ataxic, short of breath, and vomiting. The guide called for the search and rescue helicopter, which located the hikers and took them to the nearest Emergency Department. A diagnostic work-up would likely show a decrease in which of the following values?

a. pH
b. Pa_{CO_2}
c. Pulmonary vascular resistance
d. 2,3-Bisphosphoglycerate
e. Erythropoietin

6-28. A patient appears in the emergency room with a submandibular mass. A smear is made of the drainage and a bewildering variety of bacteria are seen, including branched, gram-positive rods. Which of the following is the most clinically appropriate action?

a. Consider vancomycin as an alternative drug
b. Determine if fluorescent microscopy is available for the diagnosis of actinomycosis
c. Do no further clinical workup
d. Suggest to the laboratory that low colony counts may reflect infection
e. Suggest a repeat antibiotic susceptibility test

6-29. A woman who recently traveled through Central Africa now complains of severe chills and fever, abdominal tenderness, and darkening urine. Her febrile periods last for 28 hours and recur regularly. Which of the following blood smears would most likely be associated with the symptoms described?

a. A
b. B
c. C
d. D
e. E

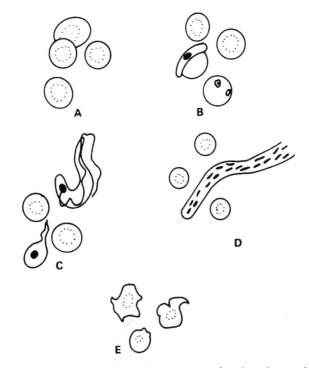

6-30. A patient with tuberculosis becomes confused and complains of muscle cramps and nausea. Lab results show a plasma sodium concentration of 125 mEq/L, serum osmolarity of 200 mOsm/kg, urine osmolarity of 1500 mOsm/kg, urine sodium of 400 mEq/day, and a normal blood volume. These clinical findings are consistent with which of the following?

a. Increased secretion of atrial natriuetic peptide
b. Decreased secretion of aldosterone
c. Increased secretion of aldosterone
d. Decreased secretion of antidiuretic hormone
e. Increased secretion of antidiuretic hormone

6-31. A 67-year-old male with chronic bronchitis is brought to the Emergency Department exhibiting labored breathing and cyanosis. The clinical sign of cyanosis is caused by which of the following?

a. An increase in the affinity of hemoglobin for oxygen
b. A decrease in the percent of red blood cells (hematocrit)
c. An increase in the concentration of carbon monoxide in the venous blood
d. A decrease in the concentration of iron in the red blood cells
e. An increase in the concentration of deoxygenated hemoglobin

6-32. Five days after returning from a trip to mainland China a 25-year-old previously healthy woman acutely develops a cough, shortness of breath, and fever with chills, headaches, diarrhea, nausea, and vomiting. She is found to have a peripheral lymphopenia. After appropriate laboratory tests are performed the diagnosis of severe acute respiratory syndrome (SARS) is made. What type of virus is the cause of this disorder?

a. Alphavirus
b. Coronavirus
c. Filovirus
d. Flavivirus
e. Hantavirus

6-33. A male child is born with an absence of the normal structure labeled between the arrows; inclusions of that structure are found within the cells in the photomicrograph. He presents with refractory diarrhea and is chronically dependent on parenteral nutrition. What is the primary function of the structure labeled between the arrows in the photomicrograph below?

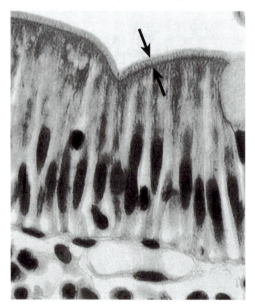

a. Extensive movement of substances over cell surfaces
b. Increase in surface area for absorption
c. Cell motility
d. Transport of intracellular organelles through the cytoplasm
e. Stretch

6-34. A middle-aged man presents with a markedly enlarged tonsil and recurrent infections with serum immunoglobulin deficiency. He has enlarged lymph nodes along his neck. Chromosome analysis demonstrates a translocation between the immunoglobulin heavy-chain locus on chromosome 14 and an unidentified gene on chromosome 8. Which of the following is the most likely cause of his phenotype?

a. The translocation has deleted constant chain exons on chromosome 14 and prevented heavy-chain class switching
b. The translocation has deleted the interval containing diversity (D) and joining (J) regions
c. The translocation has activated a tumor-promoting gene on chromosome 8
d. The translocation has deleted the heavy-chain constant chain Cμ so that virgin B cells cannot produce IgM on their membranes
e. The translocation has deleted an immunoglobulin transcription factor gene on chromosome 8

6-35. An infant is normal at birth but becomes lethargic after several feedings; the medical student describes an unusual smell to the urine but is ignored. Infection (sepsis) is suspected, and blood tests show normal white blood cell counts with a serum pH of 7.0. Electrolytes reveal an anion gap, and evaluation for an inborn error of metabolism shows an abnormal amino acid screen. The report states that branch-chain amino acids are strikingly elevated. Which of the following amino acids does the report refer to?

a. Arginine
b. Aspartic acid
c. Isoleucine
d. Lysine
e. Threonine

6-36. A 20-year-old man presents with low back pain and stiffness. Radiographic examination finds extensive calcification of the vertebral and paravertebral ligaments, producing a "bamboo spine." Rheumatoid factor is not identified in his peripheral blood. This patient's abnormalities are most likely the result of a disorder that is most closely associated with which one of the following HLA types?

a. HLA-A3
b. HLA-B27
c. HLA-BW47
d. HLA-DR3
e. HLA-DR4

6-37. A 30-year-old female with a recent history of serious illness requiring surgery developed fever, nausea, and jaundice. Her condition continued as a clinically mild disease, with AST=552, ALT=712, and the HBV panel was negative. Which one of the following statements best characterizes the illness?

a. Blood products are not tested for antibody to HCV
b. Few cases progress to chronic liver disease
c. HBV but not HCV infections occur in IV drug abusers
d. HCV is a DNA virus
e. HCV is the most common cause of posttransfusion hepatitis

6-38. A patient on the trauma-burn unit receives a drug to ease the pain of debridement and dressing changes. The patient experiences good, prompt analgesia, but despite the absence of pain sensation during the procedure her heart rate and blood pressure rise considerably, consistent with the concept that the sympathetic nervous system was activated by the pain and not affected by the analgesic drug. As the effects of the drug develop, the patient's skeletal muscle tone progressively increases. The patient appears awake at times because the eyes periodically open. As drug effects wear off, the patient hallucinates and behaves in a very agitated fashion. Which of the following drug was most likely given?

a. Fentanyl
b. Ketamine
c. Midazolam
d. Succinylcholine
e. Thiopental

6-39. A 57-year-old female presents with dyspnea on exertion. Pulmonary function studies with plethysmography demonstrate an increase in the work of breathing, and the oxygen consumption is higher-than-normal at rest. Which of the following will decrease the oxygen consumption of the respiratory muscles?

a. A decrease in lung compliance
b. A decrease in airway resistance
c. A decrease in the diffusing capacity of the lung
d. An increase in the rate of respiration
e. An increase in tidal volume

6-40. A 62-year-old African-American man presents with exercise-induced angina. His serum cholesterol is 277 mg/dL (normal <200), LDL is 157 (normal <100), HDL is 43 (normal >35), and triglycerides 170 (normal <150). His BMI is 34 and his coronary risk ratio is 6.84 (normal <5). On cardiac catheterization there is occlusion of the left anterior descending and the origin of the right coronary artery. The disease process is initiated by which of the following?

a. Proliferation of smooth muscle cells
b. Formation of an intimal plaque
c. Attraction of platelets to collagen microfibrils
d. Adventitial proliferation
e. Injury to the endothelium

6-41. Medical evaluation of a 55-year-old man finds the following laboratory data: increased hematocrit, increased RBC count, and increased serum erythropoietin. Which of the following abnormalities is most likely to be present in this individual?

a. Acute gastroenteritis
b. Pancreatic adenocarcinoma
c. Polycythemia rubra vera
d. Porphyria cutanea tarda
e. Renal cell carcinoma

6-42. A 67-year-old female suffers a stroke limited to a region of the superior temporal gyrus. Which of the following structures provides the primary input to the superior temporal gyrus?

a. CM thalamic nucleus
b. Medial geniculate thalamic nucleus
c. Lateral geniculate thalamic nucleus
d. Dorsomedial thalamic nucleus
e. Anterior thalamic nucleus
f. VA thalamic nucleus

6-43. A person presented with a contralateral limb ataxia, together with a weakness of the medial rectus muscle and a fixed dilated pupil. The neurologist concluded that the patient sustained an infarction of the brainstem. Which structure constituted the principal focus of the infarction?

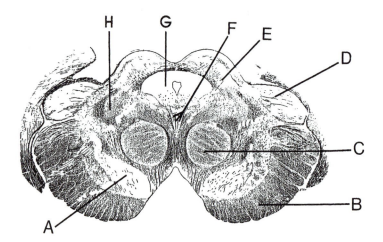

a. A
b. B
c. C
d. D
e. E
f. F
g. G
h. H

6-44. A 47-year-old male who had a reputation as a very friendly and quiet individual suddenly displayed marked changes in his personality. In particular, he became short-tempered, impulsive, and threatening to his colleagues in response to what most people would consider innocuous statements. He was referred to the psychiatric ward of the community hospital, and an MRI revealed a cortical tumor. Which of the structures in the illustration is most likely to contain this tumor?

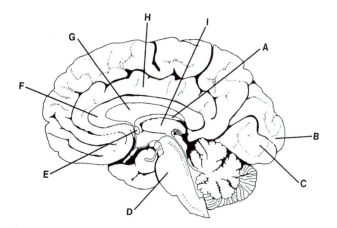

a. A
b. B
c. C
d. D
e. E
f. F
g. G
h. H
i. I

6-45. A 60-year-old male suffered from excruciating pain on the left side of his face. Since drug therapy was found to be ineffective in alleviating the pain, surgery was indicated. Which of the following structures should be surgically cut or destroyed in order to alleviate the pain?

a. First-order descending sensory fibers contained in the ipsilateral spinal tract of cranial nerve V
b. Neurons in the ventral posterolateral nucleus of the thalamus
c. Cells contained in the main sensory nucleus of the trigeminal nerve
d. Substantia gelatinosa
e. Midbrain periaqueductal gray

6-46. A 37-year-old man presents with a cough, fever, night sweats, and weight loss. A chest x-ray reveals irregular densities in the upper lobe of his right lung. Histologic sections from this area reveal groups of epithelioid cells with rare acid-fast bacilli and a few scattered giant cells. At the center of these groups of epithelioid cells are granular areas of necrosis. What is the source of these epithelioid cells?

a. Bronchial cells
b. Fibroblasts
c. Lymphocytes
d. Monocytes
e. Pneumocytes

6-47. A 47-year-old man presents with pain in the midportion of his chest. The pain is associated with eating and swallowing food. Endoscopic examination reveals an ulcerated area in the lower portion of his esophagus. Histologic sections of tissue taken from this area reveal an ulceration of the esophageal mucosa that is filled with blood, fibrin, proliferating blood vessels, and proliferating fibroblasts. Mitoses are easily found, and most of the cells have prominent nucleoli. Which of the following statements best describes this ulcerated area?

a. Caseating granulomatous inflammation
b. Dysplastic epithelium
c. Granulation tissue
d. Squamous cell carcinoma
e. Noncaseating granulomatous inflammation

6-48. A routine H&E histologic section from an irregular white area within the anterior wall of the heart of a 71-year-old man who died secondary to ischemic heart disease reveals the myocytes to be replaced by diffuse red material. This material stains blue with a trichrome stain. Which of the following statements correctly describes this material?

a. It is secreted by endothelial cells and links macromolecules to integrins
b. It is secreted by fibroblasts and has a high content of glycine and hydroxyproline
c. It is secreted by hepatocytes and is mainly responsible for intravascular oncotic pressure
d. It is secreted by monocytes and contains a core protein that is linked to mucopolysaccharides
e. It is secreted by plasma cells and is important in mediating humoral immunity

6-49. A 27-year-old woman presents because of trouble with her vision. Physical examination reveals a very tall, thin woman with long, thin fingers. Examining her eyes reveals the lens of her left eye to be in the anterior chamber. Her blood levels of methionine and cystathionine are within normal levels. Which of the following is the most likely cause of this patient's signs and symptoms?

a. Abnormal copper metabolism
b. Decreased levels of vitamin D
c. Decreased lysyl hydroxylation of collagen
d. Defective synthesis of fibrillin
e. Defective synthesis of type I collagen

6-50. A 50-year-old man presents with headaches, vomiting, and weakness of his left side. Physical examination reveals his right eye to be pointing "down and out" along with ptosis of his right eyelid. His right pupil is fixed and dilated and does not respond to accommodation. Marked weakness is found in his left arm and leg. Swelling of the optic disk (papilledema) is found during examination of his retina. Which of the following is most likely present in this individual?

a. Aneurysm of the vertebrobasilar artery
b. Arteriovenous malformation involving the anterior cerebral artery
c. Subfalcine herniation
d. Tonsillar herniation
e. Uncal herniation

Block 7

Questions

7-1. A 73-year-old male is admitted to a local hospital after he first began complaining of headaches, which were then followed by a significant weakness in his right arm and leg, slurred speech, and lack of expression on the right side of the jaw. An MRI reveals the presence of a well-defined brain tumor (shown in the following figure). Which of the following structures or regions damaged by. the tumor best accounts for the observed deficits?

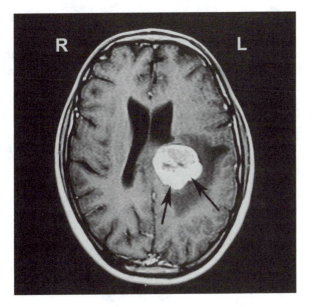

a. Caudate nucleus
b. Globus pallidus
c. Internal capsule
d. Temporal neocortex
e. Dorsal thalamus

7-2. A 48-year-old woman presents to the allergy and rheumatology clinic with itching eyes, dryness of the mouth, difficulty swallowing, loss of sense of taste, hoarseness, fatigue, and swollen parotid glands. She reports increasing joint pain over the past 2 years. She complains of frequent mouth sores. Laboratory tests show a positive antinuclear antibody (ANA) and rheumatoid factor levels of 70U/mL (normal levels less than 60U/mL) by the nephelometric method. A parotid gland biopsy shows inflammatory infiltrates in the interlobular connective tissue with damage to acinar cells and striated ducts. In this case, resorption of which of the following will be most altered by destruction of the striated ducts?

a. Na^+
b. K^+
c. HCO_3^-
d. Cl^-
e. Ca^{2+}

7-3. A 62-year-old woman is referred to a neurologist by her family physician because of a recent loss of initiative, lethargy, memory problems, and a loss of vision. She is diagnosed with primary hypothyroidism and referred to an endocrinologist for treatment of her thyroid problem and to a neuro-ophthalmologist for visual field evaluation. Which of the following visual field defects is most likely to be found?

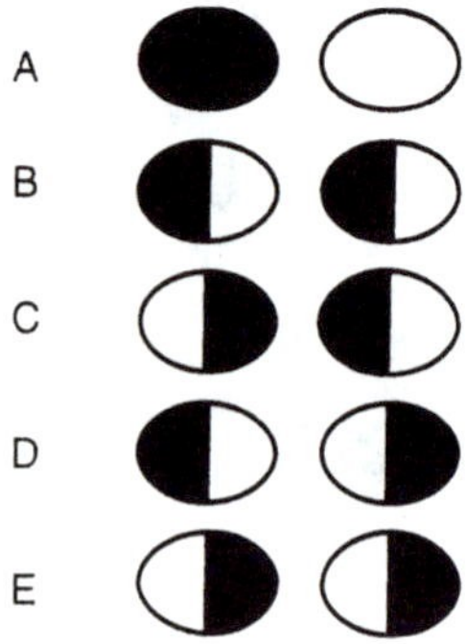

a. A
b. B
c. C
d. D
e. E

7-4. A 44-year-old obese man has extremely high plasma triglyceride levels, but cholesterol levels are within normal limits. Following treatment with a drug specifically indicated for hypertriglyceridemia, triglyceride levels decrease to almost normal. Which of the following agents is most likely to have caused this desired change?

a. Atorvastatin
b. Cholestyramine
c. Colestipol
d. Ezitemibe
e. Gemfibrozil

7-5. A patient is admitted to the emergency room after having lost consciousness. Later on, a neurological examination reveals loss of ability to move his right eye laterally when requested to do so. An MRI further reveals the presence of a brainstem infarction. Which of the following is the most likely locus of the infarction?

a. Ventromedial medulla
b. Ventrolateral medulla
c. Dorsolateral pons
d. Dorsomedial pons
e. Dorsomedial midbrain

7-6. A 35-year-old woman with fever, weight loss, fatigue, and painful joints and muscles presents to her physician's office. The physician notes that she has marked photosensitivity and a rash on the cheeks and over the bridge of her nose. Laboratory tests reveal anemic conditions and the presence of anti-DNA antibodies. Which of the following is the most likely diagnosis?

a. Goodpasture's syndrome
b. Graves' disease
c. Hashimoto's disease
d. Juvenile onset diabetes mellitus
e. Myasthenia gravis
f. Pernicious anemia
g. Rheumatoid arthritis
h. Systemic lupus erythematosus (SLE)

7-7. A patient has supraventricular tachycardia. We inject a drug and heart rate falls to a normal or at least more acceptable level. Although this drug caused the desired response, it did so without any direct effect in or on the heart. Which of the following drugs was most likely used?

a. Edrophonium
b. Esmolol
c. Phenylephrine
d. Propranolol
e. Verapamil

7-8. A 47-year-old male is brought into the emergency room and is diagnosed with a small brainstem stroke. The patient presents with an inability to display reflex movements of the head in response to vestibular stimulation. Which structure is most likely affected by this lesion?

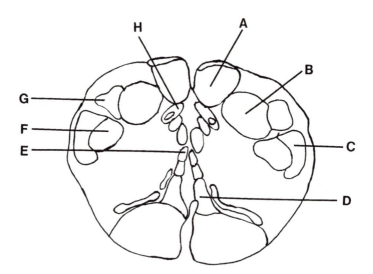

a. A
b. B
c. C
d. D
e. E
f. F
g. G
h. H

7-9. A child is evaluated by an ophthalmologist and is found to have retinitis pigmentosa, a disorder characterized by pigmentary granules in the retina and progressive vision loss. The pedigree below is obtained and the family comes in for counseling. What is the risk for individual II-2 of having an affected child if he mates with an unrelated woman?

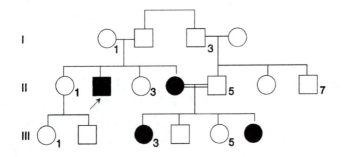

a. 100%
b. 75%
c. 50%
d. 25%
e. Virtually 0

7-10. A routine eye examination reveals the presence of inflammation limited to the left optic disk, probably due to neuritis of this region. Which of the following is the likely visual deficit resulting from this disorder?

a. Total blindness of the left eye
b. Left homonymous hemianopsia
c. Left heteronymous hemianopsia
d. Left enlargement of the blind spot
e. Left upper quadrantanopia

7-11. A 25-year-old man presents with Triple A (Allgrove) syndrome including the clinical triad of adrenal failure, achalasia, and alacrima. The patient shows progressive neurological impairments involving cranial nerves IX, X, XI, and XII, optic atrophy, upper and lower limb muscle weakness, and Horner's syndrome. Causative mutations for the disease have been identified in a gene that encodes the protein ALADIN, a component of the structure labeled with the arrows in the transmission electron micrograph. Which of the following would be directly affected by the mutation?

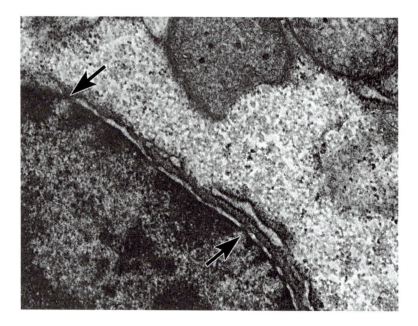

a. Import of macromolecules to the nucleus
b. Reconstitution of the nuclear envelope in telophase
c. Breakdown of the nuclear envelope in prometaphase
d. Condensation of chromatin
e. RNA synthesis

7-12. The parents of a girl with Tay-Sachs disease decide to pursue bone marrow transplantation in an attempt to provide a source for the missing lysosomal enzyme. Preliminary testing of the girl's normal siblings is performed to assess their carrier status and their human leukocyte antigen (HLA) locus compatibility with their affected sister. What is the chance that one of the three siblings is homozygous normal (i.e., has a good supply of enzyme) and HLA-compatible?

a. $\frac{1}{2}$
b. $\frac{1}{3}$
c. $\frac{1}{4}$
d. $\frac{1}{6}$
e. $\frac{1}{12}$

7-13. A 7-month-old male infant presented to the emergency department with severe middle ear and upper respiratory tract infections, which responded promptly to antibiotics. Two months later he was again admitted, this time with *Streptococcus pneumoniae* pneumonia. After several more episodes of bacterial infections, genetic testing was done and the presence of a defective B-cell tyrosine kinase gene (*btk* gene or *X-LA* gene) was revealed. In addition, physical examination detected very small tonsils. Which of the following pathogens presents the most serious threat to this child?

a. *Chlamydia trachomatis*
b. Measles virus
c. *Mycobacterium tuberculosis*
d. Varicella-zoster virus (VZV)

7-14. A patient with AIDS, being treated with multiple antiviral and immunosuppressive drugs, develops an opportunistic infection caused by *P. carinii*. Which of the following drugs are we most likely to use to treat the pulmonary infection caused by this protozoan?

a. Carbenicillin
b. Metronidazole
c. Nifurtimox
d. Penicillin G
e. Pentamidine

7-15. A 60-year-old man with rheumatoid arthritis will be started on a nonsteroidal anti-inflammatory drug to suppress the joint inflammation. Published pharmacokinetic data for this drug include:

Bioavailability (F): 1.0 (100%)
Plasma half-life $(t_{1/2})$: 0.5 h
Volume of distribution (V_d): 45 L

For this drug it is important to maintain an average steady-state concentration 2.0 mcg/mL in order to ensure adequate and continued anti-inflammatory activity.

The drug will be given (taken) every 4 h.

What dose will be needed to obtain an average steady-state drug concentration of 2.0 mcg/mL?

a. 5 mg
b. 100 mg
c. 325 mg
d. 500 mg
e. 625 mg

7-16. A 17-year-old male was diagnosed with epilepsy after developing repeated episodes of generalized tonic-clonic sezures following a motor vehicle accident in which he received a closed head injury. After treating acute seizures with the proper injectable drugs, he is started on a regimen of oral phenytoin, the daily dose titrated upwards until symptom control and a therapeutic plasma concentration were reached. The elimination half-life of the drug during initial treatment was measured to be 24 h, a value that is quite typical for otherwise healthy adults taking no other drugs.

Today he presents in the neurology clinic with nystagmus, ataxia, diplopia, cognitive impairment, and other signs and symptoms consistent with phenytoin toxicity. A blood sample, drawn at noon, has a plasma phenytoin concentration of 30 mcg/mL. That value is 50% higher than typical peak therapeutic serum concentrations and twice the usual minimum effective blood level. These values are summarized in the figure.

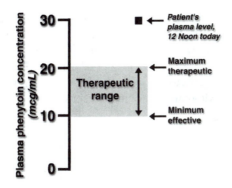

We will withhold further doses of phenytoin until plasma levels fall into the therapeutic range, and the patient is largely free of signs and symptoms of phenytoin toxicity. However, which of the following statements correctly summarizes what we should do, or expect to occur, next?

a. Administer flumazenil, which will quickly reverse signs and symptoms of phenytoin toxicity but may cause seizures to recur
b. Elimination of phenytoin from the plasma will follow zero-order kinetics for several days
c. Give an amphetamine or other CNS stimulant to reverse generalized CNS depression due to the phenytoin excess
d. Give phenobarbital to induce the P450 system, thereby hastening phenytoin's metabolic elimination
e. Plasma phenytoin concentrations will fall to 15 mcg/mL, in the middle of the therapeutic range, by noon the next day (24 h later, per the usual half-life)

7-17. A 55-year-old woman presents with pain in her right hip and thigh. The pain started approximately 6 months ago and is a deep ache that worsens when she stands or walks. Your examination reveals increased warmth over the right thigh. The only laboratory abnormalities are alkaline phosphatase 656 IU/L (normal 23–110 IU/L), elevated 24-hour urine hydroxyproline, and osteocalcin 13 ng/mL (normal 6 ng/mL). X-ray of hips and pelvis shows osteolytic lesions and regions with excessive osteoblastic activity. Bone scan shows significant uptake in the right proximal femur. Which of the following would you include in your differential diagnosis?

a. Paget's disease
b. Multiple myeloma
c. Osteomalacia
d. Osteoporosis
e. Hypoparathyroidism

7-18. An infant with severe muscle weakness is born to a mother with mild muscle weakness and myotonia (sustained muscle contractions manifested clinically by the inability to release a handshake). The mother's father is even less affected, with some frontal baldness and cataracts. Worsening symptoms in affected individuals of successive generations suggest which of the following inheritance mechanisms?

a. Genomic imprinting
b. Heteroplasmy
c. Unstable trinucleotide repeats
d. Multifactorial inheritance
e. Mitochondrial inheritance

7-19. A patient with peptic ulcer disease is taken off their medication because of undesirable side effects. As a result, the patient has rebound gastric acid hypersecretion. Which of the following drugs best accounts for the observed result?

a. An H_1-receptor antagonist
b. A proton pump inhibitor
c. A cholinergic receptor antagonist
d. An antacid
e. A CCKB receptor antagonist

7-20. A 46-year-old man found that, over a period of time, he developed progressive bilateral weakness of both upper and lower limbs beginning with the muscles of the hands. However, testing revealed that sensory functions appeared normal. Eventually, this individual was found to have wasting of muscles, fasciculations, and evidence of upper motor neuron (UMN) dysfunction, together with an increase in tendon reflexes. After a few additional months, the patient developed facial weakness and an inability to swallow (dysphagia). Further analysis revealed abnormalities in the electromyegram (EMG) of the upper and lower extremities, denervation atrophy. However, the cerebrospinal fluid (CSF) remained normal. Which of the following is the most likely diagnosis?

a. MS
b. Amyotrophic lateral sclerosis (ALS)
c. Poliomyelitis
d. Myasthenia gravis
e. A cerebral cortical stroke

7-21. A 2-year-old female presents with mildly enlarged liver, history of low blood sugar (hypoglycemia) on several occasions, and growth just below the third percentile for age (of concern because her parents are tall). Evaluation for glycogen storage disease includes glycogen phosphorylase enzyme assay, which is low-normal and does not increase with addition of cyclic AMP. Which of the following explanations is most likely?

a. Glycogen phosphorylase is activated by a cyclicAMP-regulated enzyme that is deficient in the patient
b. Glycogen phosphorylase is an allosteric enzyme regulated by a cyclic AMP binding site that is mutated in the patient
c. Glycogen phosphorylase gave a false normal value in the patient because it was not properly diluted to give excess substrate
d. Glycogen phosphorylase is subject to feedback inhibition by its product cyclic AMP
e. Glycogen is a complex substrate, so a linear relation of enzyme amount and activity cannot be expected.

7-22. A 12-year-old boy has sudden onset of fever, headache, and stiff neck. Two days eariler, he swam in a lake that is believed to have been contaminated with dog excreta. Leptospirosis is suspected. Which of the following laboratory tests is most appropriate to determine whether he has been infected with leptospira?

a. Agglutination test for leptospiral antigen
b. Counterimmunoelectrophoresis of urine sample
c. Gram stain of urine specimen
d. Spinal fluid for dark-field microscopy and culture in Fletcher's serum medium
e. Urine culture on EMB and Thayer-Martin agar

7-23. A 45-year-old man presents at the neurology clinic with memory loss, mood swings, and clinical depression. Laboratory results reveal a CD4 level of 170/mm^3 (normal range is 500–1200) and a CD4 percentage of 12% (normal approximately 40%). His viral load is 12,000 copies/mL. He has previously been treated for pneumocystis pneumonia. The cells in the accompanying photomicrograph, labeled with anti-GFAP, are involved in the progress of this disease. These cells function to do which of the following?

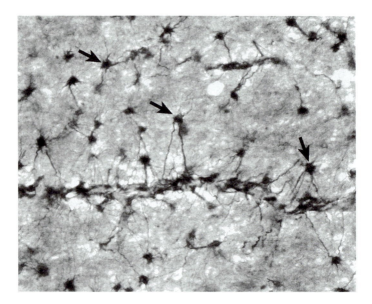

a. Form synaptic contacts with neurons
b. Present antigen
c. Phagocytose dying neurons
d. Form a glial scar following damage
e. Form myelin in the CNS

7-24. A patient is transported to the emergency department shortly after taking a massive overdose of her levothyroxine in an apparent suicide attempt. Which of the following drugs should we administer first for prompt control of the hormone-related effects that are most likely to lead to her death if not correctly managed?

a. Iodine/iodide
b. Liothyronine
c. Propranolol
d. Propylthiouracil
e. Radioiodine (^{131}I)

7-25. A normal female infant begins having jittery spells, vomiting, and falloff in growth when introduced to fruits and vegetables at age 6 months. Serum tests reveal low glucose and increased blood lactate, and her physician suspects hereditary fructose intolerance (229600), which is a deficiency of the enzyme aldolase B. The symptoms and serum abnormalities of this disease are due to which of the following?

a. Accumulation of hexose phosphates, phosphate and ATP depletion, defective electron transport, and glycogen phosphorylase inhibition
b. Accumulation of triose phosphates, phosphate and ATP excess, defective glycolysis, and glycogen synthase inhibition
c. Accumulation of triose phosphates, phosphate and ATP depletion, defective electron transport, and glycogen synthase inhibition
d. Accumulation of hexose phosphates, phosphate and ATP depletion, defective electron transport, and glycogen phosphorylase stimulation
e. Accumulation of hexose phosphates, phosphate and ATP excess, defective electron transport, and glycogen phosphorylase stimulation

7-26. Two siblings, ages 2 and 4, experienced fever, rhinitis, and pharyngitis that resulted in laryngotracheo bronchitis. Both had a harsh cough and hoarseness. Which of the following viruses is the leading cause of their syndrome?

a. Adenovirus
b. Group B coxsackievirus
c. Parainfluenza virus
d. Rhinovirus
e. Rotavirus

7-27. A child is suffering from a developmental abnormality that affects the primary transmitter released from terminals of both neostriatal and paleostriatal neurons. Which neurotransmitter is most likely affected by this abnormality?

a. Glycine
b. Enkephalin
c. Dopamine
d. GABA
e. Glutamate

7-28. An African American infant presents with prominent forehead, bowing of the limbs, broad and tender wrists, swellings at the costochondral junctions of the ribs, and irritability. The head is deformable, able to be depressed like a ping-pong ball, while palpation of the joints is very painful. Which of the following treatments is recommended?

a. Lotions containing retinoic acid
b. Diet of baby food containing leafy vegetables
c. Diet of baby food containing liver and ground beef
d. Milk and sunlight exposure
e. Removal of eggs from diet

7-29. A 27-year-old man develops acute diarrhea consisting of foul-smelling, watery stools, along with severe abdominal cramps and flatulence, after returning from a trip to the Caribbean. The associated photomicrograph is from a duodenal aspiration smear. These signs and symptoms are caused by infection with which one of the following organisms?

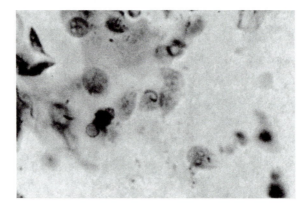

a. Acanthamoeba
b. *Entamoeba histolytica*
c. *E. vermicularis*
d. *Giardia lamblia*
e. Sporothrix

7-30. A patient on long-term warfarin therapy arrives at the clinic for her weekly prothrombin time measurement. Her INR is dangerously prolonged, and the physical exam reveals petechial hemorrhages. She's had episodes of epistaxis over the last 2 days. We are going to stop the warfarin until the INR becomes acceptable (and perhaps admit the patient for follow-up). However, we are concerned with her ongoing bleeding. Which of the following drugs would you most likely administer to counteract the warfarin's excessive effects?

a. Aminocaproic acid
b. Epoetin alfa
c. Ferrous sulfate
d. Phytonadione (vitamin K)
e. Protamine sulfate

7-31. A medical student is admitted to the emergency department with symptoms of hemorrhagic colitis. An aliquot of *Escherichia coli* strain, which is considered the etiologic agent of the infection, is treated with ethylenediaminetetraacetic acid (EDTA). The first wash is analyzed and found to contain alkaline phosphatase, DNase, and penicillinase. Which of the following is the anatomic area of the cell most likely affected by the EDTA?

a. Chromosome
b. Mesosomal space
c. Periplasmic space
d. Plasma membrane
e. Slime layer

7-32. A 5-year-old girl is brought to your office by her mother, who states that the girl has been drinking a lot of water lately. Physical examination reveals a young girl whose eyes protrude slightly. Further workup reveals the presence of multiple lytic bone lesions involving her calvarium and the base of her skull. Which of the following is the most likely diagnosis?

a. Letterer-Siwe disease
b. Hand-Schüller-Christian disease
c. Dermatopathic lymphadenopathy
d. Unifocal Langerhans cell histiocytosis
e. Sarcoidosis

7-33. A male child presents with delayed development and scarring of his lips and hands. His parents have restrained him because he obsessively chews on his lips and fingers. Which of the following is likely to occur in this child?

a. Increased levels of 5-phosphoribosyl-1-pyrophosphate (PRPP)
b. Decreased purine synthesis
c. Decreased levels of uric acid
d. Increased levels of hypoxanthine-guanosine phosphoribosyl transferase (HGPRT)
e. Glycogen storage

7-34. A patient with an inferior MI develops a stable bradycardia of 50/min. The cardiologist orders an ECG to evaluate whether there is sinus node dysfunction or an atrioventricular conduction disturbance. The diagnosis of a first-degree heart block is made in which of the following cases?

a. The PR interval of the ECG is increased
b. The P wave of the ECG is never followed by a QRS complex
c. The P wave of the ECG is sometimes followed by a QRS complex
d. The T wave of the ECG is inverted
e. The ST segment of the ECG is elevated

7-35. A 65-year-old man with severe congestive heart failure (CHF) is unable to climb a flight of stairs without experiencing shortness of breath. After several years of therapy with first-line drugs for heart failure, we empirically try digoxin to improve cardiac muscle contractility. Within 4 weeks, he has a marked improvement in his symptoms. Which of the following best describes the main cellular action of digoxin that accounts for its ability to improve his overall wellness and his cardiovascular function in particular?

a. Activates β_1-adrenergic receptors
b. Facilitates GTP binding to specific G proteins
c. Increases mitochondrial calcium (Ca^{2+}) release
d. Inhibits sarcolemmal Na^+-K^+-ATPase
e. Stimulates cyclic adenosine 5'-monophosphate (cAMP) synthesis

7-36. A 24-year-old man who was sitting in a bar found himself in a fight with another slightly intoxicated individual. During the fight, the young man was stabbed in the back. He was taken to the emergency room and following a thorough neurological examination, it was determined that he received a knife wound that destroyed the right half of the spinal cord at the level of the lower cervical cord. Which of the following deficits would most likely result from the knife wound?

a. Impaired bladder functions only
b. Impaired movements of the lower limb only
c. Impaired movements of the upper limb only
d. Loss of sensory functions of the lower limb only
e. Loss of sensory and motor functions of upper and lower limbs

7-37. A 35-year-old woman presents with a 2.2-cm mass in her left breast. The mass is excised, and histologic sections reveal a tumor composed of a mixture of ducts and cells, as seen in the photomicrograph. The epithelial cells within the ducts are not atypical in appearance. There is a marked increase in the stromal cellularity, but the stromal cells are not atypical in appearance and mitoses are not found. Which of the following is the most likely diagnosis?

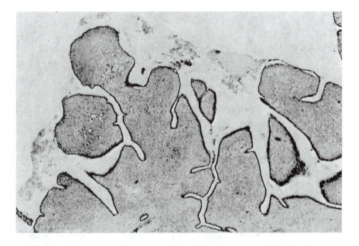

a. Atypical epithelial hyperplasia
b. Benign phyllodes tumor
c. Fibroadenoma
d. Malignant phyllodes tumor
e. Medullary carcinoma

7-38. A 66-year-old man patient who was diagnosed with type II diabetes 10 years ago presents with an aching pain in the muscles of his lower extremity. He says the pain is relieved by rest and worsened by resumed physical activity. His lower limbs appear cold, pale, and discolored, and he has a sore on the skin of his left calf. He has a weak tibial pulse on both sides and poor skin filling from capillaries. In this patient, which of the following functions would be primarily affected in the blood vessel from the lower extremity shown in the accompanying transmission electron micrograph?

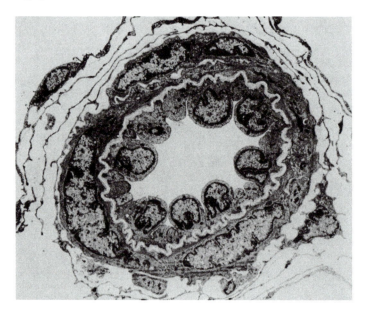

a. Adaptation to systolic pressure
b. Distribution of blood within an organ
c. Blood flow from the aorta to specific organs
d. Return of lymphocytes to the blood
e. Return of venous blood to the heart

7-39. We have a 48-year-old female patient with a history of myasthenia gravis. She has been treated with an oral acetylcholinesterase inhibitor for several years, and has done well till now. She presents with muscle weakness and other signs and symptoms that could reflect either a cholinergic crisis (excess dosages of her maintenance drug) or a myasthenic crisis (insufficient treatment). We will use a rapidly acting parenteral acetyl-cholinesterase inhibitor (AChE) to help make the differential diagnosis. Which of the following drugs would be most appropriate for this use?

a. Edrophonium
b. Malathion
c. Physostigmine
d. Pralidoxime
e. Pyridostigmine

7-40. A newborn with ambiguous genitalia and a 46,XY karyotype develops vomiting, low serum sodium concentration, and high serum potassium. Which of the following proteins is most likely to be abnormal?

a. 21-hydroxylase
b. An ovarian enzyme
c. 5β-reductase
d. An androgen receptor
e. A testicular enzyme

7-41. Eighteen hours after eating undercooked chicken, a 50-year-old farmer presents to the emergency room with abdominal pain, cramping, bloody diarrhea, and nausea. An isolate from the stool is serologically recognized as *Salmonella enteritidis* serovar *newport*. A mutant of this organism has lost region 1 (O-specific polysaccharide) of its LPS. This mutant would be identified as which of the following?

a. *Arizona*
b. *Salmonella typhi*
c. *Salmonella newport*
d. *S. enteritidis*
e. *S. enteritidis* serovar *newport*

7-42. A young woman in her early twenties experiences loss of sensation in her legs and weakness in her limbs. A neurological examination further indicated some spasticity of the limbs as well. The neurologist provided a preliminary diagnosis of onset of multiple sclerosis (MS). Assuming that this diagnosis is correct, which of the following best accounts for the diminution of sensory and motor functions?

a. Loss of Schwann cells in peripheral neurons
b. An overall loss of dopaminergic release throughout the brain and spinal cord
c. Loss of peripheral cholinergic neurons
d. Demyelination of CNS neurons
e. Proliferation of oligodendrocytes

7-43. A 38-year-old woman is admitted to the hospital by her physician because of decreased urine output. Prior to admission, she was rehearsing for a dance performance and had been taking Motrin for pain. Laboratory data reveal: blood urea nitrogen, 49 mg/dL; serum sodium, 135 mmol/L; serum creatinine, 7.5 mg/dL; urine sodium, 33 mmol/L, and urine creatinine, 90 mg/dL. Her fractional sodium excretion is approximately which of the following?

a. 0.5%
b. 1.0%
c. 1.5%
d. 2.0%
e. 3.0%

7-44. A 55-year-old man presents with increasing fatigue, weakness, anorexia, and jaundice over the past several months. Physical examination finds mild ascites and gynecomastia. A liver biopsy reveals regenerative nodules of hepatocytes surrounded by fibrosis, as seen in the picture below. Which of the following is the source of the excess collagen deposited in these fibrotic bands?

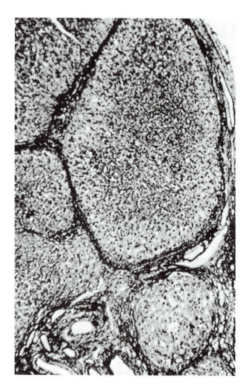

a. Hepatocytes
b. Kupffer cells
c. Ito cells
d. Endothelial cells
e. Bile duct epithelial cells

7-45. A 42-year-old woman with mitral prolapse is admitted to the hospital for evaluation of her cardiac function. Which of the following values is the best index of the preload on her heart?

a. Blood volume
b. Central venous pressure
c. Pulmonary capillary wedge pressure
d. Left ventricular end-diastolic volume
e. Left ventricular end-diastolic pressure

7-46. A patient presents to the Emergency Department with intermittent chest pain. The ECG and blood tests are negative for myocardial infarction, but the echocardiogram shows thickening of the left ventricular muscle and narrowing of the aortic valve. Medications to lower afterload are prescribed. Which of the following values would provide the best measure of the effectiveness of the medication in lowering left ventricular afterload in this patient?

a. Left ventricular end-diastolic pressure
b. Left ventricular mean systolic pressure
c. Pulmonary capillary wedge pressure
d. Total peripheral resistance
e. Mean arterial blood pressure

7-47. A 55-year-old male reports several recent episodes of syncope. An electrocardiogram is performed. Which of the following arrhythmias is most commonly associated with syncope?

a. Sinus arrhythmia
b. First-degree heart block
c. Second-degree heart block
d. Third-degree heart block
e. Tachycardia

7-48. During a routine physical examination, a 32-year-old female is found to have second-degree heart block. Which of the following ECG recordings was obtained from the patient during her physical examination?

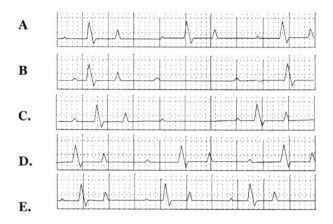

a.   A
b.   B
c.   C
d.   D
e.   E

7-49. A 56-year-old male was admitted to the hospital with angina and diaphoresis. A myocardial infarction is suspected, and a 12-lead electrocardiogram (ECG) is ordered. The ECG is most effective in detecting a decrease in which of the following?

a.   Ventricular contractility
b.   Mean blood pressure
c.   Total peripheral resistance
d.   Ejection fraction
e.   Coronary blood flow

7-50. The spouse of a 58-year-old-man calls 9-1-1 because her husband complains of chest pain radiating down his left arm. He is transported to the Emergency Department, where an electrocardiogram and cardiac enzymes indicate a recent myocardial infarction. The man is sent for a cardiac catheterization, including coronary angiography and hemodynamic recordings throughout the cardiac cycle. No valvular defects were present. During ventricular ejection, the pressure difference smallest in magnitude is between which of the following?

a. Pulmonary artery and left atrium
b. Right ventricle and right atrium
c. Left ventricle and aorta
d. Left ventricle and left atrium
e. Aorta and capillaries

Block I

Answers

1-1. The answer is b. (*Brunton, pp 751, 763, 765–766, 886–889. Craig, pp 249–251, 154–155. Katzung, pp 211–212.*) While many ionic and other factors can predispose a patient to digoxin toxicity, hypokalemia, as can be caused by a loop diuretic (usually used for edema and/or ascites, including that associated with heart failure) or thiazide diuretic (mainly used for treating essential hypertension), is arguably the most important, if not the most common. There is a competition between extracellular K^+ and digoxin for binding to digoxin's cellular receptor, the Na^+, K^+-ATPase on the sarcolemma. When serum K^+ levels are reduced (i.e., when hypokalemia develops), the binding of digoxin is enhanced and so its effects are increased, even without a rise of serum digoxin concentrations, and usually those increased effects are deleterious, as described here. Hypercalcemia can increase the risk or severity of digoxin toxicity. However, loop diuretics increase renal Ca^{2+} loss, and so hypercalcemia (a) is not a likely explanation. Hyponatremia (c) is not likely to have occurred with a loop diuretic, which tends to increase both renal Na^+ and H_2O loss proportionally, such that hyponatremia is not likely to occur as it may with a thiazide. Loop diuretics do not displace digoxin from tissue binding sites (d) or inhibit digoxin's elimination (which involves renal excretion, not metabolism).

Note that in the scenario we described the patient as having been treated by "his family doctor who has been treating him . . . for the last 30 years." This is not at all meant to impugn family doctors or general practitioners. The point is that nowadays, and for a variety of reasons (toxicity being one), digoxin is no longer considered an appropriate drug for managing heart failure, with or without signs or symptoms of congestive failure, until all other reasonable and more suitable options have been tried and the patient's condition has deteriorated to the point that inotropes (digoxin or parenteral agents) are warranted. Recall that our preferred approach for initial therapy of failure involves ACE inhibitors, a β blocker, and perhaps a loop diuretic. Nonetheless, and unfortunately, some physicians still use the "old way," involving digoxin. It is these patients who are likely to be seen in the hospital when the almost inevitable problems due to digoxin develop.

I-2. The answer is d. *(Siegel and Sapru, pp 88, 102).* This disorder is usually associated with small cell carcinoma and results in muscle weakness. There is a reduction in size of the compound action potentials in affected muscles, but such effects can be partially reversed with exercise. (See explanations to Questions 99, 101, and 102 for further details concerning why other possible answers were not correct).

I-3. The answer is d. *(Sadler, pp 95–100. Moore and Persaud, Developing, pp 47–50.)* The placental structures shown in the photomicrograph are chorionic villi that are fetal tissues. The mother's contribution to the placenta **(answers a and e)** is the blood that flows past the chorionic villi. A fertilized ovum reaches the uterus about 4 days after fertilization. At that time, it has developed into a multicellular, hollow sphere referred to as a blastocyst. The blastocyst soon adheres to the secretory endometrium and differentiates into an inner cell mass that will develop into the embryo and a layer of primitive trophoblast. The expanding trophoblast penetrates the surface endometrium **(answers b and c)** and erodes into maternal blood vessels. Eventually, it develops two layers, an inner cytotrophoblast and an outer syncytiotrophoblast. Solid cords of trophoblast form the chorionic villi, which then are invaded by fetal blood vessels.

I-4. The answer is a. *(Ganong, pp 734–738. Stead et al., pp 221, 223–225, 262–263, 321.)* Narcotics used for the treatment of severe headache may depress the medullary respiratory center causing alveolar hypoventilation, as evidenced by an elevation in arterial $Paco_2$. The hypercapnia lowers the ratio of HCO_3^- to dissolved CO_2 in the plasma, and thus lowers the pH according to the Henderson-Hasselbalch equation. Renal compensation for respiratory acidosis takes hours to start and days to be complete, and thus there has not been sufficient time for the body's compensatory mechanisms to take effect and for plasma $[HCO_3^-]$ to rise. Thus, the scenario is most consistent with an acute, uncompensated respiratory acidosis. The slight rise in plasma bicarbonate concentration can be attributed to extracellular buffering of the excess H^+.

I-5. The answer is b. *(Brooks, pp 279–281. Levinson, pp 24, 34, 76, 112–113, 147–148. Murray PR—2005, pp 369–371. Ryan, pp 302–305.)* No vaccine is available for *Listeria*. Except during a meningococcal epidemic, *H. influenzae* is the most common cause of bacterial meningitis in children.

The organism is occasionally found to be associated with respiratory tract infections or otitis media. *H. influenzae, N. meningitidis, S. pneumoniae,* and *Listeria* account for 80–90% of all cases of bacterial meningitis. A purified polysaccharide vaccine conjugated to protein for *H. influenzae* type B is available. A tetravalent vaccine is available for *N. meningitidis* and a 23-serotype vaccine for *S. pneumoniae.*

1-6. The answer is b. *(Brooks, pp 685–687, 759t. Levinson, pp 319, 353–354, 499s. Murray PR—2005, p 882. Ryan, pp 722–727.)* One of the leading causes of death among AIDS patients is central nervous system toxoplasmosis. It is thought that *Toxoplasma* infection is a result of reactivation of old or preexisting toxoplasmosis. Occasionally, the infection may be acquired by needle sharing. Because the disease is a reactivation of old or preexisting toxoplasmosis, routine quantitative tests for IgM antibody are usually negative, and IgG titers are low (≤1:256, IFA). More sophisticated methods, such as IgM capture or IgG avidity, may reveal an acute response.

1-7. The answer is b. *(Alberts, pp 584, 612, 613. Junqueira, pp 23–25. Ross and Pawlina, pp 23–25. Kasper, pp 1943–1944.)* The child in the scenario suffers from IgA deficiency, the most common immunoglobulin deficiency. IgA functions in several ways, one of which is to coat pathogens with a negative charge that repels the polyanionic charge on the cell surface. In IgA deficiency,

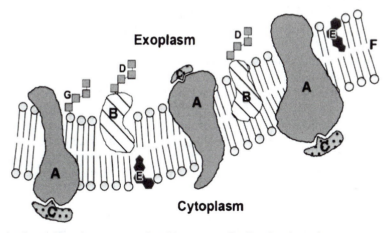

A = Integral membrane protein, B = Glycoprotein, C = Peripheral membrane protein (more abundant on cytosolic surface), D = sugar, E = cholesterol, F = hydrophobic fatty acid chains (hydrophilic polar head groups are not labeled), G = glycolipid

pathogens can more easily attach to the cell surface leading to persistent infections. The carbohydrate of biological membranes is found in the form of glycoproteins and glycolipids rather than as free saccharide groups (answer a). The polyanionic charge of the membrane is produced by the sugar side chains on the glycoproteins and glycolipids. Glycoproteins often terminate in sialic acid side chains, which impart a negative (polyanionic) charge to the membrane. Similarly, the glycolipids (also called glycosphingolipids), particularly the gangliosides, terminate in sialic acid residues with a strong negative charge. Cholesterol (answer c) alters membrane fluidity (see figure on the previous page) and is amphipathic (hydrophilic and hydrophobic properties). It reduces the packing of lipid acyl groups through its steroid ring structure and hydrocarbon tail and cements hydrophilic regions of the membrane through interactions with its hydroxyl (OH⁻) region. Peripheral membrane proteins (answer d) are found primarily on the cytosolic leaflet of the membrane bilayer. Integrins (answer e) are heterodimeric receptors that bind with extracellular matrix (ECM) molecules such as laminin and fibronectin.

1-8. The answer is c. (*Kumar, pp 1207–1210. Rubin, pp 1189–1194.*) Excess aldosterone secretion may be due to an abnormality of the adrenal gland (primary aldosteronism) or an abnormality of excess renin secretion (secondary aldosteronism). Causes of primary hyperaldosteronism (Conn's syndrome), which is independent of the renin-angiotensin-aldosterone (RAA) system, include adrenal cortical adenomas (most commonly), hyperplastic adrenal glands, and adrenal cortical carcinomas. These diseases are associated with decreased levels of renin. The signs of primary hyperaldosteronism include weakness, hypertension, polydipsia, and polyuria. The underlying physiologic abnormalities include increased serum sodium and decreased serum potassium, the latter due to excessive potassium loss by the kidneys, which together with the loss of hydrogen ions produces a hypokalemic alkalosis. The elevated level of serum sodium causes expansion of the intravascular volume. In contrast to Conn's syndrome, secondary hyperaldosteronism results from conditions causing increased levels of renin, such as renal ischemia, edematous states, and Bartter's syndrome. Causes of renal ischemia include renal artery stenosis and malignant nephrosclerosis, while Bartter's syndrome results from renal juxtaglomerular cell hyperplasia.

1-9. The answer is c. (*Afifi, pp 91–103. Siegel and Sapru, pp 147–149.*) The spinothalamic tract carries fibers mediating pain and temperature. The primary pain fibers enter the spinal cord and pass one or two segments in

Lissauer's marginal zone before making a synapse with neurons that form the lateral spinothalamic tract. Fibers of the lateral spinothalamic tract then cross to the contralateral side one or two segments above or before where the primary afferent fibers have entered the cord. Accordingly, pain and temperature are lost below the lesion on the contralateral side. The cuneate and gracile fasciculi mediate proprioception and vibration in association with the same side of the body from which these fibers originate, and the corticospinal tract mediates voluntary motor function.

1-10. The answer is c. (*Ganong, pp 735–736. Kasper et al., pp 266–267, 2590. Stead et al., p 222.*) Diabetic ketoacidosis generates a partially compensated metabolic acidosis. The primary disturbance is a decrease in the plasma [HCO_3^-], which lowers the ratio of HCO_3^- to dissolved CO_2 in the plasma, and thus lowers the pH according to the Henderson-Hasselbalch equation. To compensate for the metabolic acidosis, the lungs increase the rate of alveolar ventilation, which decreases $PaCO_2$ and thus dissolved CO_2 and returns the pH toward the normal range. The differential diagnosis of metabolic acidosis is divided into high anion gap and normal anion gap (hyperchloremic) acidosis. The increased anion gap of 30 mEq/L compared to a normal value of ~12 mEq/L is consistent with an increase in ketoacids, that is, acetoacetic acid and β-hydroxybutyric acid, in the diabetic patient.

1-11. The answer is e. (*Damjanov, pp 1257–1272. McPhee, pp 283–286.*) Clinical manifestations of aortic regurgitation (AR) include exertional dyspnea, angina, and left ventricular failure. Owing to the rapidly falling arterial pressure during late systole and diastole, there is often wide pulse pressure, Corrigan's "water-hammer" pulse, capillary pulsations at the nail beds, and a pistol-shot sound over the femoral arteries. A blowing diastolic murmur is heard along the left sternal border. Volume overload of the heart is the basic defect and results in left ventricular dilation and hypertrophy. AR is rheumatic in origin in approximately 70% of cases. Much less frequently it is due to syphilis, ankylosing spondylitis (rarely), infective endocarditis, aortic dissection, or aortic dilation from cystic medial necrosis. Congenital forms of aortic stenosis occur fairly frequently, but AR is rarely congenital in origin.

1-12. The answer is d. (*Afifi, pp 163–166. Gilroy, pp 588–589. Siegel and Sapru, pp 235–237. Simon et al., pp 347–348.*) The preganglionic parasympathetic neurons associated with lacrimation and which contribute to salivation arise from the superior salivatory nucleus of the lower pons. These preganglionic neurons synapse with postganglionic neurons in the submandibular and pterygopalatine ganglia. Since the disorder affected parts of the facial nerve, other choices are clearly incorrect since they relate to other cranial nerves. The inferior salivatory nucleus governs salivation associated with the parotid gland but has no relationship to lacrimation.

1-13. The answer is c. *(Brooks, pp 433–438. Murray PR—2005, pp 546–547. Ryan, pp 559–560.)* HSV causes primary and recurrent disease. The typical skin lesion is a vesicle that contains virus particles in serous fluid. Giant multinucleated cells are typically found at the base of the herpesvirus lesion. Encephalitis, which usually involves the temporal lobe, has a high mortality rate. Severe neurologic sequelae are seen in surviving patients. PCR amplification of viral DNA from CSF has replaced viral isolation.

1-14. The answer is d. *(Kumar, pp 359, 401–403. Mandell, pp 2824–2825.)* Malaria results from infection with one of four species of plasmodia, namely *P. falciparum, P. vivax, P. ovale, and P. malariae.* Malarial organisms (sporozoites) are released into the blood after the bite of an affected *Anopheles* mosquito. These sporozoites then enter the hepatocyte via a hepatocyte receptor for the serum proteins thrombospondin and properdin. In the liver, they multiply asexually to form numerous merozoites, which are released when the hepatocyte ruptures. These merozoites then infect erythrocytes and form either gametocytes, which are taken up and fertilized in the mosquito, or trophozoites, which become schizonts that develop into merozoites that infect other red cells. In the blood, *P. falciparum* merozoites bind to glycophorin molecules on red blood cells, while *P. vivax* merozoites bind to Duffy antigens on red blood cells. (Note that patients who are Duffy antigen-negative are resistant to *P. vivax* infection.) *P. vivax* infects only young erythrocytes (reticulocytes), while *P. malariae* infects only old erythrocytes. Within the red cells, merozoites mature to form schizonts, which then secrete proteins that form knobs on the surface of the red cells. Sequestrins form on top of these knobs and then bind to endothelial cells via ICAM-1, the thrombospondin receptor, and CD46, causing thrombosis.

Clinically, patients with malaria develop recurrent bouts of chills and high fever (paroxysms) that result from rupture of infected erythrocytes. These symptoms cycle at different time intervals depending upon the type of malaria. For example, infection with *P. malariae* causes symptoms to cycle every 72 h, and thus it is called quartan or malarial malaria. The remaining plasmodia cause symptoms that cycle every 48 h. The disease produced by *P. falciparum*, however, is much more serious and is called malignant tertian malaria. *P. falciparum* malaria is more serious because it alters RBCs, making them more adherent to endothelial cells. This in turn leads to capillary plugging and obstruction. In the brain this is called cerebral malaria, while in the kidney the disease produces acute renal failure (called blackwater fever). In contrast, *P. vivax* malaria is called benign tertian malaria, and the disease caused by *P. ovale* is similar to that caused by *P. vivax.*

Babesiosis is caused by *B. microti.* It is somewhat similar to malaria, except that it is transmitted by the hard-shell tick (ixodid) and it infects individuals living on islands off the New England coast, such as Martha's Vineyard. Patients develop the sudden onset of chills and fever due to destruction of erythrocytes. The disease is usually self-limited, but patients may develop hemoglobinemia, hemoglobinuria, and renal failure.

1-15. The answer is c. *(Alberts, pp 923–927, 952–953, 966–968. Rubin, pp 1518, 1519. Kumar, p 172. Junqueira, pp 464–465.)* The woman in the scenario suffers from retinitis pigmentosa. Vesicles and organelles move unidirectionally along microtubules from the inner segment to the outer segment of the photoreceptor. Opsin, which is needed to sense light, is transported to sites of utilization in the disks of the outer segment. Transport occurs through the connecting, non-motile cilium, driven by the microtubule motor, kinesin, an ATPase. Microtubules are composed of tubulin and are involved in motility as the principal protein in the composition of the axoneme (the core of the cilium or flagellum). Microfilaments (thin filaments) are composed of actin, the most abundant protein in cells of eukaryotes **(answer a)**. They are involved in cell motility and changes in cell shape. Myosin is the main constituent of the thick filament **(answer b)** that binds to actin and functions as an ATPase activated by actin. Intermediate filaments **(answer d)** that are "intermediate" in diameter (8 to 10 nm) between thin and thick filaments are of five different types. Type I and type II are the acidic and basic keratins (cytokeratins) respectively and are found specifically in epithelial cells. Type III intermediate filaments are composed of vimentin, desmin, and glial fibrillary acidic protein (GFAP). Vimentin is found in cells of mesenchymal origin, desmin in muscle cells, and glial fibrillary acidic protein in astrocytes. Type IV intermediate filaments are neurofilament proteins found in neurons. Type V intermediate filaments include the nuclear lamins A, B, and C and are associated with nuclear lamina of all cells. Spectrin heterodimers stabilize the plasma membrane and connect the membrane to actin **(answer e)**.

1-16. The answer is b. *(Ganong, pp 454–457, 601–602. Widmaier et al., pp 422–424.)* Angiotensin II is a powerful vasoconstrictor that is formed when renin is released from the kidney in response to a fall in blood pressure or vascular volume. Renin converts angiotensinogen to angiotensin I. Angiotensin II is formed from angiotensin I by angiotensin-converting enzyme localized within the vasculature of the lung. All the other listed substances cause vasodilation.

1-17.   The answer is c. *(Brunton, pp 948–953. Craig, pp 269–271. Katzung, pp 568–570.)* Simvastatin (and atorvastatin and all the other "statins") decreases cholesterol synthesis in the liver by inhibiting HMG CoA reductase, the rate-limiting enzyme in the synthetic pathway. This results in an increase in LDL receptors in the liver, thus reducing blood levels for cholesterol. These drugs, like other lipid-lowering agents, are best used as adjuncts to exercise and proper diet. They are considered essential components in the primary prevention of coronary heart disease. Some have been shown to lower mortality from cardiovascular causes (MI, stroke, etc.).

1-18. The answer is b. *(Scriver, pp 3–45. Murray RK, pp 333–335. Lewis, pp 171–184.)* DNA synthesis occurs only in the S phase of the cell cycle, a process regulated by numerous proteins called cyclins. A key cyclin (cyclin D) is phosphorylated as the cell commits from gap 1 (G1) quiescent phase to the S phase of DNA synthesis, and a cascade of secondary phosphorylations by cyclin-dependent kinases (CDK) activates cyclins, transcription factors, and the DNA synthesis machinery. The Rb protein, discovered as the product of the gene causing hereditary retinoblastoma, undergoes phosphorylation early in S phase and releases its inhibition (binding) of E2F transcription factor, promoting gene activation and DNA synthesis. Rb, like the genes for neurofibromatosis (neurofibromin) or breast cancer (BRCA1), acts as a tumor supressor gene requiring mutation of both Rb alleles to inactivate Rb protein and foster continuous E2F action and cell proliferation. Individuals with germ-line Rb mutations are more likely to incur a "second hit" in several retinal cells and present with retinoblastomas in both eyes. Individuals without germline Rb mutations are much less likely to incur two Rb mutations in the same retinal cell, having unilateral tumors if they occur at all. The bcl protein, discovered by its excess in B-cell lymphomas, was then identified as a stimulator of cell division called cyclin D1. Bcl is thus an oncogene, requiring one abnormal allele or "one hit" to be genetically activated in a cell and stimulate proliferation (oncogenesis). Several proteins of cancer-causing viruses (v-onc) have been adapted from putative cellular oncogenes (c-onc), while others inactivate the Rb protein and promote cell proliferation. Despite characterization of many tumor suppressor and oncogene proteins, the tissue specificity and variable ages of onset of different tumors speak for multifactorial, polygenic pathways to cancer.

1-19. The answer is b. (*Kumar, pp 1139–1142. Rubin, pp 1040–1041.*) Malignant carcinomas of the breast may be either noninvasive or invasive. Noninvasive carcinomas (carcinoma in situ) may be located within the ducts (intraductal carcinoma) or within the lobules (lobular carcinoma in situ). There are several variants of intraductal carcinoma, including comedocarcinoma, cribriform carcinoma, and intraductal papillary carcinoma. Comedocarcinoma grows as a solid intraductal sheet of cells with a central area of necrosis. It is frequently associated with the erb B2/neu oncogene and a poor prognosis. Cribriform carcinoma is characterized by round, ductlike structures within the solid intraductal sheet of epithelial cells, while intraductal papillary carcinoma has a predominant papillary pattern. In contrast, invasive malignancies are characterized by infiltration of the stroma, which may produce a desmoplastic response within the stroma (scirrhous carcinoma). Infiltrating ductal carcinomas also produce yellow-white chalky streaks that result from the deposition of elastic tissue around ducts (elastosis). Other patterns of invasion that produce specific results include infiltration of cells in a single file in infiltrating lobular carcinoma and mucin production in colloid carcinoma.

1-20. The answer is e. (*Brooks, pp 360–365. Levinson, pp 176–178. Murray PR—2005, pp 469–470. Ryan, p 475.*) Tetracyclines and chloramphenicol are effective, provided treatment is started early for rickettsial diseases, including RMSF, as in this case. Those should be given orally daily and continued for several days after the rash subsides. IV dosage can be used in severely ill patients. Sulfonamides enhance the disease and are contraindicated. The other antibiotics are ineffective. Antibiotics only suppress the bacteria's growth, and the patient's immune system must eradicate them.

1-21. The answer is e. (*Kumar, pp 1172–1173. Rubin, pp 1167–1171.*) Graves' disease, or diffuse toxic goiter, is one of the three most common disorders associated with thyrotoxicosis or hyperthyroidism (the other two are toxic multinodular goiter and toxic adenoma). This hyperfunctioning and hyperplastic diffuse goiter is accompanied by a characteristic triad of clinical findings: signs of hyperthyroidism, exophthalmus, and pretibial myxedema. Graves' disease is an autoimmune form of goiter caused by thyroid-stimulating immunoglobulins or thyroid-stimulating hormone (TSH) receptor antibodies. Autoantibodies to TSH receptor antigens are produced because of a defect in antigen-specific suppressor T cells. The antibodies bind to TSH receptors on thyroid follicular cells and function as TSH, with resultant thyroid growth and hyperfunction. Such antibodies can be identified in almost all cases of Graves' disease. In contrast to these stimulating autoantibodies, Hashimoto's thyroiditis, an autoimmune cause of hypothyroidism, is associated with high titers of circulating blocking autoantibodies, such as antithyroglobulin, anti-TSH receptor, and antimicrosomal antibodies.

I-22. The answer is c. (*Henry, pp 878–886, 915–916, 922. Chandrasoma, pp 59–63.*) Follicular hyperplasia is a reactive process involving lymph nodes in which reactive proliferating B lymphocytes produce hyperplasia of the lymphoid follicles and germinal centers. These B lymphocytes are stimulated to proliferate by binding of foreign antigen to membrane-bound surface immunoglobulin (Ig) on the B cells. Upon activation these B cells will then become either memory cells or plasma cells, the product of which is Ig. Igs are composed of light chains and heavy chains, each of which are composed of a variable region and a constant region. The variable regions of both of these chains form the antigen-binding region of Ig, which is called the Fab portion. The portion of Ig that binds complement is called the Fc portion. There are two types of light chains and five types of heavy chains. The two light chains are the kappa chain, the genes of which are located on chromosome 2, and the gamma chain, the genes of which are located on chromosome 22. The heavy chains are M, D, A, E, and G, the genes of all of these being on chromosome 14. The combination of one type of light chain with a particular heavy-chain forms each of the five types of Ig.

In contrast to Ig, erythropoietin is secreted by the peritubular interstitial cells of the kidney, while interleukin-2 and interleukin-3 are secreted by activated T cells. NK cells and T cells are the only known sources of gamma-interferon.

I-23. The answer is e. (*Alberts, pp 355–357.*) The patient in the scenario suffers from Alzheimer disease which is related to protein misfolding leading to neurofibrillary tangles. Three-dimensional folding is required for functional activity of proteins. Native folding of a protein is encoded in its amino acid sequence; however, protein folding inside cells requires molecular chaperones binding and releasing themselves from hydrophobic regions of the newly synthesized protein and ATP to reach their native folded state. Various chaperones protect nonnative protein chains from misfolding and aggregation (**answer a**), but do not contribute conformational information to the folding process (**answer b**). Many chaperones are also stress- or heat-shock proteins (HSPs) that stabilize preproteins for membrane translocation, present misfolded proteins for proteolysis (**answer d**), and regulate the conformation of signaling molecules. The underlying principle in all these functions is the recognition by chaperones of proteins in their nonnative states. Chaperones also inhibit the formation of partially folded intermediates. Chaperones in conjunction with calreticulin monitor the progress of folding and ensure that only properly folded proteins are secreted from the cell or shipped to lysosomes. It is hypothesized that this level of ER "quality control" is absent in Alzheimer and other neurodegenerative diseases. Chaperones assist with translocation of proteins across internal membranes (e.g., mitochondria) by maintaining precursor proteins in their unfolded state during membrane trafficking. They do *not* function in the docking of the signal peptide (**answer c**).

1-24. The answer is e. *(Ganong, pp 251–255.)* The hypothalamus regulates body temperature. Core body temperature, the temperature of the deep tissues of the body, is detected by thermoreceptors located within the anterior hypothalamus. The anterior hypothalamus also contains neurons responsible for initiating reflexes, such as vasodilation and sweating, which are designed to reduce body temperature. Heat-producing reflexes, such as shivering, and heat-maintenance reflexes, such as vasoconstriction, are initiated by neurons located within the posterior hypothalamus.

1-25. The answer is c. *(Brooks, pp 212–216. Levinson, pp 125–126, 474s. Murray PR—2005, pp 280–282. Ryan, p 170.)* All toxigenic strains of *Corynebacterium diphtheriae* are lysogenic for β-phage carrying the *Tox* gene, which codes for the toxin molecule. The expression of this gene is controlled by the metabolism of the host bacteria. The greatest amount of toxin is produced by bacteria grown on media containing very low amounts of iron. Fragment B of the toxin is required for cell entry, while Fragment A stops protein production by inhibiting elongation factor 2 (EF-2).

1-26. The answer is e. *(Brunton, p 481. Katzung, p 387.)* Vigabatrin can induce psychosis. It is recommended that it not be used in patients with preexisting depression and psychosis. None of the other drugs listed are associated with this phenomenon.

1-27. The answer is d. *(Junqueira, pp 52, 56–57. Ross and Pawlina, pp 71, 74–75.)* The TCOF1 gene encodes treacle. Expression of treacle is critical during early embryonic development in structures that form bones and other facial structures. Treacle is active in the nucleolus, the structure labeled in the transmission electron micrograph. The nucleolus is the site of ribosomal protein transcription and treacle regulates ribosomal DNA transcription and therefore ribosomal RNA (rRNA) synthesis. The nucleolus is a highly organized, heterogeneous structure within the nucleus, with distinct regions visible by electron microscopy: (1) fibrillar centers, which represent the nucleolar organizer regions where DNA is not being actively transcribed; (2) dense fibrillar components (*pars fibrosa*) where RNA molecules are being transcribed; and (3) a granular component (*pars granulosa*) where ribosomal subunits undergo maturation. The nucleolar organizer contains clusters of rRNA genes (DNA). The size and number of nucleoli differ with the metabolic activity of cells.

Ribosomal synthesis occurs in the nucleolus, but the complete assembly and maturation of ribosomes requires transport to the cytoplasm (**answer a**). Ribosomal proteins as well as all proteins that function in the nucleus are synthesized in the cytosol and transported into the nucleus (**answer b**). Nuclear proteins are also translated on ribosomes in the cytoplasm (**answer c**) and targeted to the nucleus (traveling through the nuclear pores) by specific nuclear localization signals (NLSs). Cytosolic proteins are synthesized on isolated ribosomes compared with most protein synthesis that occurs on polyribosomes. Nuclear proteins are transcribed on euchromatin (**answer c**). Lysosomes carry out degradation of organelles (**answer e**).

1-28. The answer is e. (*Brunton, pp 436t, 447–451. Craig, pp 356–357t. Katzung, pp 272, 360.*) Buspirone is an attractive drug for managing mild short-term anxiety. Among the reasons (and especially when compared with more traditional anxiolytics, such as benzodiazepines) are a lack of sedation (buspirone is not a CNS depressant); very little or no potentiation of the effects of other CNS depressants, including alcohol; no known abuse potential (it is not regulated by the Controlled Substances Act); or tendency for development of tolerance; and no major withdrawal syndrome. One major drawback is a slow onset of symptom relief (a week or two), and typically it takes about a month from the onset of therapy for antianxiety effects to stabilize. (Knowing this slow onset, one should resist the temptation to titrate the dosage upward, to hasten or increase the drug's effects, prematurely.)

You should recall that long-term benzodiazepine administration is associated with withdrawal phenomena (and, depending on the use, dose, exact drug, and other patient-related factors, the syndrome can be severe). Thus, one can envisage a switch from a benzodiazepine to buspirone.

Because buspirone lacks CNS depressant effects and its effects take some time to develop, one should start the buspirone several weeks before stopping the benzodiazepine and then taper the benzodiazepine dose once it's time to stop the drug.

I-29 The answer is a. (*Ganong, pp 569–570. Stead et al., pp 37–38.*) In aortic stenosis, the resistance of the aortic valve increases, making it more difficult for blood to be ejected from the heart. Because a pressure drop occurs across the stenotic aortic valve, the ventricular pressure is much larger than the aortic pressure. Although stroke volume typically decreases leading to a decrease in pulse pressure, a normal cardiac output and arterial pressure can still be maintained by increasing heart rate. However, the increased afterload will lead to a decreased ejection fraction and increased cardiac oxygen consumption.

I-30. The answer is b. (*Murray RK, pp 396–414. Scriver, pp 4517–4554. Lewis, pp 234, 296.*) Red cell hemolysis after drug exposure suggests a red cell enzyme defect, most easily confirmed by enzyme assay to demonstrate deficient activity. A likely diagnosis here is glucose-6-phosphate dehydrogenase (G6PD) deficiency (305900), probably the most common genetic disease (it affects 400 million people worldwide). Tropical African and Mediterranean peoples exhibit the highest prevalence because the disease, like sickle cell trait, confers resistance to malaria. DNA analysis is available to demonstrate particular alleles, but simple enzyme assay is sufficient for diagnosis. More than 400 types of abnormal G6PD alleles have been described, meaning that most affected individuals are compound heterozygotes. The phenotype of jaundice and red blood cell hemolysis with anemia is triggered by a variety of infections and drugs, including a dietary substance in fava beans. Sulfonamide and related antibiotics as well as antimalarial drugs are notorious for inducing hemolysis in G6PD-deficient individuals. G6PD deficiency exhibits X-linked recessive inheritance, explaining why male offspring but not the parents become ill when exposed to antimalarials.

I-31. The answer is b. (*Alberts, pp 966–968, 1221. Young, p 90. Junqueira, pp 44, 50, 340, 425. Kierszenbaum, pp 7–8, 28–29.*) The patient in the scenario presents with Kartagener's syndrome, also known as immotile cilia syndrome, and has cilia that do not function normally. This leads to chronic infections (otitis media) and infertility (immotile sperm or suboptimal oviductal ciliary function in females). In that disorder, abnormalities occur in the organization of axonemal (ciliary) dynein arms (**answer b**) that bridge the nine outer doublet microtubules (**answer d**) to each other. Dynein is a high-molecular-weight ATPase. When dynein is activated, it produces the sliding motion of the microtubules as it walks along the adjacent doublet. The protein nexin links the outer microtubular doublets, creating a straplike arrangement of paired microtubules around the central microtubule doublet. The radial spokes (**answer c**) restrain the sliding movement of the outer doublets, so those doublets are held in place and sliding is limited lengthwise. The inner sheath (**answer a**) surrounds the central microtubule doublet (**answer e**). The basal body that anchors the microtubules also plays an essential role in converting the sliding of the outer microtubules into the bending of the cilium.

Bronchiectasis is the irreversible, abnormal dilation of one or more bronchi associated with various lung conditions, commonly accompanied by chronic infection. In Kartagener's syndrome it has been found that uncoordinated dyskinesia is more prevalent than immotile cilia. There is therefore a movement in the literature to call this syndrome primary ciliary dyskinesia (PCD), and Kartagener's syndrome would be a subclassification of that group of disorders. Dextrocardia (cardiac apex to the right) occurs in mild cases and *situs inversus* in more severe cases. In *situs inversus*, the morphologic right atrium is on the left, and the morphologic left atrium is on the right. Pulmonary structures (i.e., right and left lungs) as well as abdominal organs may also be reversed in a mirror image of normal. The development of right-left asymmetry is at least partially regulated by ciliary beat at Hensen's node.

The saccharin test is a test of nasal mucociliary clearance. It is carried out by placing a small amount of saccharin behind the anterior end of the inferior turbinate. In the presence of normal mucociliary action, the saccharin will be swept backward to the nasopharynx and a sweet taste perceived. Failure of sweetness to be detected within about 20 minutes indicates delayed mucociliary clearance.

1-32. The answer is e. (*Brooks, pp 438–440, 420–428, 599–601, 562–566, 442–446. Levinson, pp 248–249, 249–250, 255–256, 256–257, 281. Murray—2005, pp 550–553, 533–539, 523–524, 597, 559–561. Ryan, pp 509–510, 564–565, 568, 579, 619.*) Varicella- zoster virus is a herpesvirus. Chickenpox is a highly contagious disease of childhood that occurs in the late winter and early spring. It is characterized by a generalized vesicular eruption with relatively insignificant systemic manifestations.

Adenovirus has been associated with adult respiratory disease among newly enlisted military troops. Crowded conditions and strenuous exercise may account for the severe infections seen in this otherwise healthy group.

Papillomavirus is one of two members of the family Papovaviridae, which includes viruses that produce human warts. These viruses are host-specific and produce benign epithelial tumors that vary in location and clinical appearance. The warts usually occur in children and young adults and are limited to the skin and mucous membranes.

Rubeola (measles) virus produces a maculopapular rash. No vesicles or pustule forms are developed and no successive crops of lesions are formed.

Infectious mononucleosis caused by CMV is clinically difficult to distinguish from that caused by EBV. Lymphocytosis is usually present, with an abundance of atypical lymphocytes. CMV-induced mononucleosis should be considered in any case of mononucleosis that is heterophil-negative and in patients with fever of unknown origin.

I-33. The answer is d. (*Murray RK, pp 5–13. Scriver, pp 3–45. Lewis, pp 185–204.*) Brain injury or metabolic diseases that irritate the respiratory center may cause tachypnea in term infants, resulting in respiratory alkalosis. The increased respiratory rate removes ("blows off") carbon dioxide from the lung alveoli and lowers blood CO_2, forcing a shift in the indicated equilibrium toward the left:

$$CO_2 + H_2O \rightleftharpoons H_2CO_2 \rightleftharpoons H^+ + HCO_3^-$$

Carbonic acid (H_2CO_2) can be ignored because negligible amounts are present at physiologic pH, leaving the equilibrium:

$$CO_2 + H_2O \rightleftharpoons H^+ + HCO_3^-$$

The leftward shift to replenish the exhaled CO_2 of rapid breathing decreases the hydrogen ion concentration [H$^+$] and increases the pH ($^-\log_{10}$[H$^+$]) to produce alkalosis (blood pH above the physiologic norm of 7.4).

Other answers are eliminated because the newborn does not have acidosis, defined as a blood pH below 7.4, either from excess blood acids (metabolic acidosis) or from slower or ineffective respiration with increased [CO_2] (respiratory acidosis). The baby also does not have metabolic alkalosis, caused by loss of hydrogen ion from the kidney (e.g., with renal tubular disease) or stomach (e.g., with severe vomiting). Respiratory alkalosis is best treated by eliminating the underlying disease which will diminish the respiratory rate, elevate blood [CO_2], force the above equilibrium to the right, elevate the [H$^+$], and decrease the pH. The infant would prove to have a urea cycle disorder such as citrullinemia (215700) with neurologic effects (hypotonia, seizures) of high ammonia concentrations. Withdrawal of milk (protein) and other therapies decreased the ammonia, eliminated the seizures, and restored normal respiration.

I-34. The answer is f. (*Nolte, pp 239–240, 261, 507–515, 517–523, 538–561. Siegel and Sapru, pp 204–220, 288–289, 347–349, 434–436, 450–458. Waxman, p 249.*) This section is taken from rostral levels of the diencephalon. Corticobulbar and corticospinal fibers contained within the internal capsule (H) arise from the deeper layers of the cerebral cortex (i.e., layers V–VI). A lesion of the internal capsule would produce a UMN paralysis of the contralateral side of the body because of disruption of corticospinal fibers as well as damage to some corticobulbar fibers contained within the internal capsule. In this instance, there was damage associated with corticobulbar fibers descending from the motor speech area, resulting in a motor aphasia. Fibers associated with the corpus callosum (A) arise from more superficial layers of the cortex (i.e., layers II–III) and project to the homotypic region of the contralateral cortex. Because this commissure represents the principal means by which one side of the cortex communicates with the other, surgical disruption of these fibers is carried out when all means of drug therapy have been shown to be ineffective and when seizures are shown to have spread to the cortices on both sides of the brain. Fibers of the ansa lenticularis (D) arise from the ventral aspect of the medial pallidal segment and can be visualized at more anterior levels of the pallidum. It represents a major output pathway of the basal ganglia and its axons supply the VL, VA, and CM nuclei of the thalamus. The neostriatum [i.e., caudate nucleus (B) and putamen] receives dopaminergic inputs from the substantia nigra. Loss of dopamine levels in the caudate is associated with Parkinson's disease, and experimental strategies have been applied to treat this disorder through replenishment of dopamine in the caudate nucleus.

Different cells of the paraventricular nucleus of the hypothalamus (F), situated in the dorsomedial region at anterior levels, synthesize oxytocin and vasopressin. These hormones are transported down their axons to the posterior pituitary. Loss of vasopressin would result in excessive thirst and increased urine secretion, since vasopressin acts as an antidiuretic hormone. Although the marked changes in emotionality could be accounted for by damage to either the medial hypothalamus or the amygdala (E), psychomotor seizures are typically associated with temporal lobe structures and not with the hypothalamus. Thus, the correct answer in this case is E. Different fiber groups of the amygdala provide major inputs into the medial and lateral regions of the hypothalamus and thus constitute a significant modulator of hypothalamic functions, including rage and aggression. The optic tract (G) arises from the retina. Each optic tract represents fibers associated with the visual fields of the opposite side. Therefore, a lesion of the optic tract will result in a homonymous hemianopsia.

1-35. The answer is e. (*Ganong, pp 448–451.*) During pregnancy, the maternal hypothalamic-pituitary axis is suppressed due to high circulating levels of sex hormones. This leads to reduced gonadotropin levels, and, thus, ovulation does not occur. Additionally, hyperventilation leads to decreased arterial carbon dioxide levels. Increased water retention leads to decreased hematocrit. Maternal use of glucose declines and, as a result, gluconeogenesis increases. Plasma cortisol levels increase as the result of progesterone-mediated displacement from transcortin and its subsequent binding to globulin.

1-36. The answer is c. (*Murray RK, pp 145–152. Scriver, pp 1521–1552.*) Pompe disease has an early and severe onset compared to other glycogen storage diseases because the defective α-glucosidase is a lysosomal enzyme. Accumulation of substances in the lysosome often leads to a more severe and progressive course, illustrated by the mucopolysaccharidoses like Hurler syndrome (607014) or the neurolipidoses like Tay-Sachs disease (272800). Patients with Pompe disease exhibit lysosomal glycogen accumulation in muscle (muscle weakness or hypotonia), brain (with developmental retardation), and heart (with a short PR interval and heart failure). The other glycogen storage diseases lead to glycogen accumulation in liver or muscle with correspondingly milder symptoms.

1-37. The answer is c. (*Kumar, pp 212, 638–642. Rubin, pp 1073–1076.*) The combination of clinical signs suggesting damage to both the posterior spinal cord (such as loss of vibratory and position sense) and the lateral spinal cord (such as arm and leg dystaxia and spastic paralysis) are suggestive of subacute degeneration of the spinal cord, a disorder that results from a deficiency of vitamin B_{12}. Loss of vibratory sensation in the lower extremities is the first neurologic manifestation of this disease. These neurologic abnormalities of B_{12} deficiency do not occur with folate deficiency. They are thought to be the result of abnormal myelin production due to either excess methionine or abnormal fatty acid production (fatty acids with an odd number of carbons), such as propionate.

There are many different causes of vitamin B_{12} deficiency, which also results in a megaloblastic anemia. Examples include inadequate diet, impaired absorption, bacterial overgrowth, or competitive parasitic infections. Dietary deficiencies will take years to produce deficiency states since liver stores are so great (recall that vitamin B_{12} is the only water soluble vitamin that is stored in the body). Dietary deficiency is seen only in strict vegetarians (diet with no animal proteins, milk, or eggs). Normally dietary B_{12} binds to salivary R-binders, forming a B_{12}-R complex that is broken down by pancreatic proteases. Free B_{12} then binds to intrinsic factor (IF is secreted by gastric parietal cells) and the B_{12}-IF complex is absorbed by ileal mucosal epithelial cells. B_{12} is then transported in blood bound to transcobalamin II. Impaired absorption occurs with deficiency of intrinsic factor (patients with pernicious anemia or gastrectomy) or malabsorptive states that involve the ileum (such as celiac disease, Crohn's disease, or chronic pancreatitis). Pernicious anemia, an autoimmune disease, is the most common cause of vitamin B_{12} deficiency. Chronic pancreatitis is associated with B_{12} deficiency because pancreatic enzymes are necessary to enzymatically cleave the R factor from B_{12} in the duodenum before IF can attach to B_{12}. Bacterial overgrowth occurs in the blind-loop syndrome or with broad-spectrum antibiotic therapy, while a competitive parasitic infection is the giant fish tapeworm, *Diphyllobothrium latum.*

In contrast, Fanconi anemia is an autosomal recessive disorder characterized by bone marrow failure combined with certain birth defects, such as abnormalities of the radius. Leukoerythroblastic anemia refers to any space occupying lesion of the bone marrow (myelophthisic anemia) that causes immature red blood cells and immature white blood cells to appear in the peripheral blood. Finally sideroblastic anemia is characterized by the presence of numerous sideroblasts in the bone marrow and may be caused by a deficiency of pyridoxine or it may be a form of myelodysplasia.

1-38. The answer is d. *(Siegel and Sapru, pp 190, 502–503.)* Damage to the paramedian branches of the basilar artery would affect the corticospinal tracts on one side of the brainstem, thus causing paralysis of the contralateral limbs. The distribution of this artery is such that it would also affect both sensory and motor components of cranial nerve V, thus causing loss of ipsilateral facial sensation and the ability to chew. The other choices include arteries that would either not affect the corticospinal tracts (cerebellar arteries) or would not affect the trigeminal fibers (anterior spinal artery).

1-39. The answer is e. *(Ganong, pp 122, 142–147.)* Activating nociceptors on the free nerve endings of C fibers produces ischemic pain. The C fibers synapse on interneurons located within the substantia gelatinosa (laminas II and III) of the dorsal horn of the spinal cord. The pathway conveying ischemic pain to the brain is called the paleospinothalamic system. In contrast, well-localized pain sensations are carried within the neospinothalamic tract. Ischemic pain does not adapt to prolonged stimulation. Pain is produced by specific nociceptors and not by intense stimulation of other mechanical, thermal, or chemical receptors.

1-40. The answer is b. (*Brooks, pp 275–276. Levinson, pp 141, 477s. Murray PR—2005, pp 353–354. Ryan, pp 383–384.*) *H. pylori* antigen tests from a stool sample using an ELISA format and a monoclonal antibody to *H. pylori* are as sensitive as culture of the control portion of the stomach. Urea breath tests are also widely used. *H. pylori* has an active enzyme (urease) that breaks down radioactive urea. The patient releases radioactive CO_2 if *H. pylori* are present. *H. pylori* antibody tests, IgG and IgA, indicate the presence of *H. pylori* and usually decline after effective treatment. Culture of stomach contents is insensitive and not appropriate as a diagnostic procedure for *H. pylori*. Direct tests such as antigen or culture of gastric mucosa are preferred because they are the most sensitive indication of a cure.

1-41. The answer is e. (*Brunton, pp 631–632, 640–641. Craig, pp 138t, 453–455. Katzung, pp 109, 266.*) You may have chosen d (histamine H_1 receptor blocker) as your answer to this question. However, although diphenhydramine is an "antihistamine," histamine plays a minor role in the symptoms of rhinovirus infections (in contrast with a much more important role in, say, seasonal allergies). As a result, blocking the effects of histamine on its receptors does not cause profound symptom relief in this situation. The drying up of nasal secretions afforded by diphenhydramine (an ethanolamine-type H_1 blocker and the prototype of the first generation agents) in this instance is due to the drug's rather intense muscarinic receptor-blocking (atropine-like) actions.

1-42. The answer is b. (*Alberts, pp 1094–1096, 1102–1105. Junqueira, pp 91, 115–116.*) Fibronectin is an adhesive glycoprotein that is important for cell attachment and adhesion. It is important for modulation of cell migration in the adult and during development. Neural crest and other cells appear to be guided along fibronectin-coated pathways in the embryo. Fibronectin is found in three forms: a plasma form that is involved in blood clotting; a cell-surface form, which binds to the cell surface transiently; and a matrix form, which is fibrillar in arrangement. Fibronectin contains a cell-binding domain (RGD sequence), a collagen-binding domain, and a heparin-binding domain. Elastin and type III collagen are responsible for elasticity seen in large arteries and the pinna of the ear **(answer a)**. Cell-cell interactions involve both transient and more long-term, stable processes. Cell-cell adhesion is mediated by transmembrane proteins called cell adhesion molecules which include the calcium or magnesium-dependent selectins, integrins, and cadherins (**answers c and d**) and the non-calcium-dependent immunoglobulin (Ig) superfamily. The stable adhesion junction, known as the zonula adherens, links the cytoskeleton of adjacent cells through cadherins (transmembrane linker proteins) to actin filaments inside the cell (**answer e**).

I-43. The answer is e. (*Kumar, pp 35–37, 41–42. Chandrasoma, 3/e, pp 8–10.*) Substances that can form clear spaces in the cytoplasm of cells as seen with a routine H&E stain include glycogen, lipid, and water. In the liver, clear spaces within hepatocytes are most likely to be lipid, this change being called fatty change or steatosis. In the normal metabolism of lipid by the liver, free fatty acids are either esterified to triglyceride, converted to cholesterol, oxidized into ketone bodies, or incorporated into phospholipids that can be excreted from the liver as very-low-density lipoproteins (VLDLs). Abnormalities involving any of these normal metabolic pathways may lead to the accumulation of triglycerides (not cholesterol) within the hepatocytes. For example, increased formation of triglycerides can result from alcohol use, as alcohol causes excess NADH formation (high NADH/NAD ratio), increases fatty acid synthesis, and decreases fatty acid oxidation.

In contrast to lipid, calcium appears as a dark blue-purple color with routine H&E stains, while hemosiderin, which is formed from the breakdown of ferritin, appears as yellow-brown granules. Lipofuscin also appears as fine, granular, golden-brown intracytoplasmic pigment. It is an insoluble "wear and tear" (aging) pigment found in residual bodies in the cytoplasm of aging cells, typically neurons, cardiac myocytes, or hepatocytes. Lipofuscin is composed of polymers of lipids and phospholipids derived from lipid peroxidation by free radicals of polyunsaturated lipids of subcellular membranes.

I-44. The answer is c. (*Murray RK, pp 180–189. Scriver, pp 2297–2326.*) The most likely cause of the symptoms observed is carnitine deficiency. Under normal circumstances, long-chain fatty acids coming into muscle cells are activated as acyl-coenzyme A and transported as acyl-carnitine across the inner mitochondrial membrane into the matrix. A deficiency in carnitine, which is normally synthesized in the liver, can be genetic, but it is also observed in preterm babies with liver problems and dialysis patients. Blockage of the transport of long-chain fatty acids into mitochondria not only deprives the patient of energy production, but also disrupts the structure of the muscle cell with the accumulation of lipid droplets. Oral dietary supplementation usually can effect a cure. Deficiencies in the carnitine acyltransferase enzymes I and II can cause similar symptoms.

I-45. The answer is e. (*Lewis, pp 241–266. Scriver, pp 3–45.*) Children with chromosome abnormalities often exhibit poor growth (failure to thrive) and developmental delay with an abnormal facial appearance. This baby is too young for developmental assessment, but the catlike cry should provoke suspicion of cri-du-chat syndrome. Cri-du-chat syndrome is caused by deletion of the terminal short arm of chromosome 5 [46,XX,del(5p), also abbreviated as 5p–] as depicted in panel E. When a partial deletion or duplication like this one is found, the parents must be karyotyped to determine if one carries a balanced reciprocal translocation. The other karyotypes show (a) deletion of the short arm of chromosome 4 [46,XY,del(4p) or 4p–]; (b) XYY syndrome (47,XYY); (c) deletion of the long arm of chromosome 13 [46,XX,del(13q) or 13q–]; (d) Klinefelter syndrome (47,XXY). Most disorders involving excess or deficient chromosome material produce a characteristic and recognizable phenotype (e.g., Down, cri-du-chat, or Turner syndrome). The deletion of 4p– (panel A) produces a pattern of abnormalities (syndrome) known as Wolf-Hirschhorn syndrome; deletion of 13q– produces a 13q– syndrome (no eponym). The mechanism(s) by which imbalanced chromosome material produces a distinctive phenotype is completely unknown.

I-46. The answer is b. (*Brunton, pp 999–1003. Craig, p 473. Katzung, pp 1049–1050.*) Constipation is the most common and most worrisome adverse response to alosetron. This drug's mechanism of desired action involves selective blockade of serotonin receptors (5-HT$_3$) in the gut; the main outcomes include slowing of colonic transport time, increased sodium and water reabsorption from the colon, and reduced secretion of water and electrolytes into the colon.

Although constipation might be viewed as "trivial" or a minor complaint with most drugs, with alosetron it is the most worrisome one. Constipation may (and has) progressed to fecal impaction, bowel perforation or obstruction, and ischemic colitis. Fatalities have occurred.

The risks are such that the drug was pulled from the market in early 2000 and reapproved 2 years later with a limited indication (prolonged, severe diarrhea, predominant IBS in women); abundant warnings in the package insert; and a comprehensive risk-management/avoidance program that includes a requirement for (among other things) a special "sign-off" by both the prescriber and the patient that they understand and acknowledge and can identify the risks and agree to treatment anyway.

1-47. The answer is a. (*Brunton, pp 975, 1656. Craig, pp 478–479. Katzung, p 1035.*) Aluminum hydroxide (and all other clinically useful aluminum salts other than the phosphate) has a high affinity for phosphate. In the gut, the aluminum salts bind phosphate and prevent its absorption quite well. They also induce a blood-to-gut gradient that favors elimination of circulating phosphate. (Used inappropriately, it may cause hypophosphatemia: sustained, high-dose use of aluminum-containing antacids is one of the most common causes of hypophosphatemia.) None of the other drugs listed are effective in or used for reducing phosphate absorption or lowering serum levels.

The main limitation to using an aluminum salt by itself is its tendency to cause constipation. This is usually dealt with, when aluminum salts are used as typical "antacids," by coadministering a magnesium salt, which alone tends to cause laxation. (Giving Mg would be inadvisable for patients with renal failure, such as this dialysis patient, who are often unable to excrete Mg at rates sufficient to avoid hypermagnesemia.)

1-48. The answer is b. (*Kumar, p 782. Rubin, pp 1310–1311.*) A rare tumor of the oral cavity (found most commonly in the mandible) that is similar to the enamel organ of the tooth is the ameloblastoma. This locally aggressive tumor consists of nests of cells that at their periphery are similar to ameloblasts and centrally are similar to the stellate reticulum of the developing tooth. A similar lesion occurs in the sella turcica and is called a craniopharyngioma. In contrast, pleomorphic adenomas, mucoepidermoid carcinomas, adenoid cystic carcinomas, and acinic cell carcinomas are all tumors that originate in salivary glands.

1-49. The answer is b. (*Kumar, pp 787–788. Rubin, pp 1331–1333.*) Ménière's disease is an abnormality that is characterized by periodic episodes of vertigo that are often accompanied by nausea and vomiting, sensorineural hearing loss, and tinnitus (ringing in the ears). These symptoms are related to hydropic dilation of the endolymphatic system of the cochlea. Inflammation of the middle ear (otitis media), which occurs most often in children, may be acute or chronic. If otitis media is caused by viruses, there may be a serous exudate, but if it is produced by bacteria, there may be a suppurative exudate. Acute suppurative otitis media is characterized by acute suppurative inflammation (neutrophils), while chronic otitis media involves chronic inflammation with granulation tissue. Chronic otitis media may cause perforation of the eardrum or may lead to the formation of a cyst within the middle ear that is filled with keratin, called a cholesteatoma. The name is somewhat of a misnomer, as cholesterol deposits are not present. Otosclerosis, a common hereditary cause of bilateral conduction hearing loss, is associated with formation of new spongy bone around the stapes and the oval window. Patients present with progressive deafness. Tumors of the middle ear are quite rare, but a neoplasm that arises from the paraganglia of the middle ear (the glomus jugulare or glomus tympanicum) is called a chemodectoma. Other names for this tumor include nonchromaffin paraganglioma and glomus jugulare tumor. This lesion is characterized histologically by lobules of cells in a highly vascular stroma (zellballen). A similar tumor that occurs in the neck is called a carotid body tumor.

I-50. The answer is d. (*Kumar, pp 299–302, 1442–1443. Rubin, pp 1563–1565.*) Retinoblastoma is the most common malignant tumor of the eye in children. Clinically, retinoblastoma may produce a white pupil (leucoria). This is seen most often in young children in the familial form of retinoblastoma, which is due to a deletion involving chromosome 13. These familial cases of retinoblastoma are frequently multiple and bilateral, although like all the sporadic, nonheritable tumors they can also be unifocal and unilateral. Histologically, rosettes of various types are frequent (similar to neuroblastoma and medulloblastoma). There is a good prognosis with early detection and treatment; spontaneous regression can occur but is rare. Retinoblastoma belongs to a group of cancers (osteosarcoma, Wilms' tumor, meningioma, rhabdomyosarcoma, uveal melanoma) in which the normal cancer suppressor gene (antioncogene) is inactivated or lost, with resultant malignant change. Retinoblastoma and osteosarcoma arise after loss of the same genetic locus— hereditary mutation in the q14 band of chromosome 13.

In contrast to the histologic appearance of retinoblastoma, a proliferation of benign fibroblasts and endothelial cells, which can form a retrolental mass, is seen with retinopathy of prematurity (ROP), a cause of blindness in premature infants that is related to the therapeutic use of high concentrations of oxygen. The presence of foamy macrophages with cytoplasmic clear vacuoles is not a specific histologic finding and can be seen with several disorders. Congo red–positive stroma, however, is characteristic of medullary carcinoma of the thyroid, while spindle-shaped cells with cytoplasmic melanin is characteristic of malignant melanoma, the most common primary intraocular malignancy of adults.

Block 2

Answers

2-1. The answer is a. (*Murray RK, pp 249–263. Scriver, pp 1971–2006.*) Lack of the enzyme homogentisate oxidase causes the accumulation of homogentisic acid, a metabolite in the pathway of degradation of phenylalanine and tyrosine. Homogentisate, like tyrosine, contains a phenol group. It is excreted in the urine, where it oxidizes and is polymerized to a dark substance upon standing. Under normal conditions, phenylalanine is degraded to tyrosine, which is broken down through a series of steps to fumarate and acetoacetate. The dark pigment melanin is another end product of this pathway. Deficiency of homogentisate oxidase is called alkaptonuria (black urine—203500), a mild disease discovered by Sir Archibald Garrod, the pioneer of biochemical genetics. Garrod's geneticist colleague, William Bateson, recognized that alkaptonuria, like nearly all enzyme deficiencies, exhibits autosomal recessive inheritance.

2-2. The answer is a. (*Kumar, pp 545–547. Behrman, p 1726.*) Hemangiomas are benign tumors of blood vessels that histologically reveal the presence of red blood cells (erythrocytes) within the lumen of the proliferating vessels. Hemangiomas may be subclassified as capillary or cavernous. The juvenile (strawberry) hemangioma is a fast-growing lesion that appears in the first few months of life, but most completely regresses by the age of 5 years. Unless near the eye, definitive therapy is usually not indicated, as the possible techniques, such as surgery, cryotherapy, laser therapy, and injection of sclerosing drugs, all cause more scarring than is produced by spontaneous resolution.

2-3. The answer is e. (*Levinson, pp 15–16, 100–102. Ryan, p 31.*) Oxygen, when it is metabolized, gives rise to hydrogen peroxide (H_2O_2) and superoxide-anion (O_2). Both of these by products are extremely toxic to cells. Peroxide is produced by many bacteria, particularly facultative anaerobes that use flavoprotein intermediates. H_2O_2 is degraded by peroxidases, as illustrated in equation 2. Superoxide is detoxified by a critical enzyme known as *superoxide dismutase*. Such metabolism also results in H_2O_2 production (equation 1). *Peroxidase* and *catalase* are often used interchangeably to describe H_2O_2 reactions. However, in equation 2 when the H_2A reactant is another H_2O_2 molecule, the enzyme is known as *catalase*. If H_2A is another intermediate, then the enzyme is known as *peroxidase*.

2-4. The answer is d. *(Ganong, pp 5–6.)* The osmolality of a substance is the number of osmoles per kg of solvent. One osmole (Osm) equals the gram molecular weight of a substance divided by the number of free moving particles that each molecule liberates in solution. Osmotically active substances in the body are dissolved in water, and the density of water is 1. Thus, osmolar concentrations can be expressed as osmoles (or milliosmoles) per liter of water. If the osmolality is zero, there are no free moving particles, and thus, the molecule is as diffusible as water through the membrane.

2-5. The answer is a. *(Kumar, pp 215–218. Damjanov, pp 400–401.)* Type IV hypersensitivity reactions do not involve antibody formation, but instead are mediated by T cells (cell-mediated hypersensitivity). There are two subtypes of type IV hypersensitivity reactions, one of which involves CD4 cells [delayed-type hypersensitivity (DTH)] and the other of which involves CD8 cells (cell-mediated cytotoxicity). The classic example of a DTH reaction is the tuberculin skin test (Mantoux reaction), in which a local area of erythema and induration peaks at about 48 h following intracutaneous injection of tuberculin. Other examples of DTH reactions include granulomatous inflammation, poison ivy reactions and contact dermatitis (often the result of sensitivity to nickel, which can be found in some watchbands).

The formation of granulomas (with epithelioid cells) is another example of a type IV hypersensitivity reaction. The pathomechanisms involved in the formation of granulomas is as follows. Upon first exposure to the antigen in DTH reactions, macrophages ingest the antigen and process it in association with class II antigens (HLA-D) to helper T cells (CD4), which differentiate into CD4 T_H1 cells based on the actions of interleukin-12 secreted by macrophages and dendritic cells. Upon reexposure to the antigen, these CD4 T_H1 cells are activated and secrete biologically active factors (the lymphokines). Specifically, T_H1 cells secrete gamma-interferon, interleukin 2, and TNF-alpha. Gamma-interferon is the main cytokine that is responsible for DTH reactions. It activates macrophages (epithelioid cells) and forms granulomas (caseating or noncaseating). Interleukin 2 activates other CD4 cells, while TNF-alpha causes endothelial cells to increase production of prostacyclin and ELAM-1.

Note that type I hypersensitivity reactions involve IgE antibodies, secreted from plasma cells, that attach to the surface of mast cells and basophils. Initially an allergen binds to antigen-presenting cells, which then stimulate T_H2 cells to secrete IL-4, IL-5, and IL-6. IL-5 stimulates the production of eosinophils, while IL-4 stimulates B cells to transform into plasma cells and produce IgE. The activation of mast cells and basophils causes them to secrete many substances, such as histamine. Finally, leukotrienes C4, D4, and E4 increase vascular permeability and cause vasoconstriction and bronchospasm.

2-6. The answer is e. *(Brooks, pp 466–469. Levinson, pp 283–291. Murray PR—2005, pp 678–685. Ryan, p 549.)* In a small number of patients with acute hepatitis B infection, HBsAg can never be detected. In others, HBsAg becomes negative before the onset of the disease or before the end of the clinical illness. In such patients with acute hepatitis, hepatitis B virus infection may be established only by the presence of anti–hepatitis B core IgM (anti–HBc IgM), a rising titer of anti–HBc, or the subsequent appearance of anti–HBsAg.

HBsAg positive, anti–HBs and anti–HBc negative would identify an early acute HBV infection. HBsAg and anti–HBc positive could indicate an acute or chronic HBV infection. IgM anti–HBc could differentiate between these conditions. HBsAg negative and anti–HBs positive tests indicate immunity due to natural infection or vaccination. Hepatitis symptoms and negative HBsAg, anti–HBs and anti–HBc test would indicate another infectious agent, toxic injury to the liver or possible disease of the biliary tract.

2-7. The answer is e. *(Moore and Dalley, pp 21–22, 729–730.)* The clavicle is the most frequently broken bone in body. Greenstick fractures of the clavicle are extremely common in children as a result of falling on outstretched arms. Colles' fracture is also common from falling on outstretched arms, but there are no physical findings to support a Colles' fracture [(**answer a**); fracture of the distal radius, occasionally including the ulna] in this boy, [nor scaphoid fracture (**answer b**)]. The sternoclavicular joint (**answer d**) is extremely stable and is rarely dislocated. Fracture of the surgical head of the humerus (**answer c**) is *not* indicated by the physical findings.

2-8. The answer is d. *(Murray RK, pp 49–59. Scriver, pp 4571–4636.)* Isozymes are multiple forms of a given enzyme that occur within a given species. Since isozymes are composed of different proteins, analysis by electrophoretic separation can be done. Lactate dehydrogenase is a tetramer composed of any combination of two different polypeptides, H and M. Thus the possible combinations are H4, H3M1, H2M2, H1M3, and M4. Although each combination is found in most tissues, M4 predominates in the liver and skeletal muscle, where as H4 is the predominant form in the heart. White and red blood cells as well as brain cells contain primarily intermediate forms. The M4 forms of the isozyme seem to have a higher affinity for pyruvate compared with the H4 form. Following a myocardial infarction, the H4 (LDH1) type of lactate dehydrogenase rises and reaches a peak approximately 36 hours later. Elevated LDH1 levels may signal myocardial disease even when the total lactate dehydrogenase level is normal.

2-9. The answer is a. *(Ganong, p 17. Kasper et al., pp 2340, 2510–2512.)* Connexin is a membrane-spanning protein that is used to create gap junction channels. The gap junction channel creates a cytoplasmic passage between two cells. Each cell membrane contains half of the channel. The channel, called a connexon, is constructed from six connexin molecules that form a cylinder with a pore at its center. Charcot-Marie-Tooth (CMT) disease comprises a heterogeneous group of inherited peripheral neuropathies. Approximately 1 in 2500 persons has some form of CMT, making it one of the most frequently occurring inherited neurological syndromes. Transmission is most frequently autosomal dominant but it may also be autosomal recessive or X-linked, like the mutation affecting the connexin 32 (Cx32), located in the folds of the Schwann cell cytoplasm around the nodes of Ranvier. This localization suggests a role for gap junctions composed of Cx32 in ion and nutrient transfer around and across the myelin sheath of peripheral nerves.

2-10. The answer is g. *(Afifi, pp 47–58, 422–424, 426–430, 476–477. Siegel and Sapru, pp 8–13, 287–289, 312–315.)* This figure is a midsagittal section of the brain. A major portion of the anterior commissure (E) contains fibers mediating olfactory signals that arise from the olfactory bulb and decussate to the contralateral olfactory bulb. The septum pellucidum (G) forms the medial wall of the lateral ventricle, which in fact separates the lateral ventricle on one side from that on the opposite side. The cingulate gyrus (H) is a prominent structure on the medial aspect of the cerebral cortex and constitutes a component of the limbic lobe. As part of the limbic system, its functions relate in part to the regulation of emotional behavior. Accordingly, tumors of this region have resulted in marked changes in emotionality. The primary visual cortex lies on both banks of the calcarine fissure. Cells located on the upper bank of this fissure (B) receive inputs from the lateral geniculate nucleus that relate to the lower visual field. Therefore, a lesion of this region would result in a lower visual field deficit.

The major output pathway of the hippocampal formation is the fornix system of fibers (A), which arises from cells in its subicular cortex and adjoining regions of the hippocampus. These fibers are then distributed to the anterior thalamic nucleus, mammillary bodies, and septal area. Accordingly, the most effective way of activating the output pathways of the hippocampal formation would be to stimulate these fibers of the fornix. The basilar portion of the pons (D) lies in the ventral half of this region of the brainstem. It receives inputs from each of the lobes of the cerebral cortex, which it then relays to the cerebellar cortex. As noted in the answer to Question 2, this circuit mediates functions associated with the regulation of voluntary movements of the limbs. Disruption of any part of this circuit, whether at the level of the internal capsule or basilar pons, would affect inputs from the cerebral cortex to the hemispheres of the cerebellar cortex, thus eliminating key inputs necessary for the expression of smooth, coordinated movements. With respect to the neurons located on the lower bank of the calcarine fissure (C), they receive inputs from the lateral geniculate nucleus that relate to the upper retinal (or temporal) visual fields. Therefore, a lesion of this region would produce an upper quadrantanopia (i.e., loss of one-quarter of the visual field). The corpus callosum (F) constitutes the major channel by which the cerebral cortex on one side can communicate with the cortex of the opposite side. In order to stop the spread of seizures from one hemisphere to the other (when the seizures are severe), cutting of the corpus callosum is carried out.

2-11. The answer is c. (*Brunton, pp 487–488, 753. Craig, pp 393–395. Katzung, pp 256, 475–478.*) There is a clinically important relationship between serum sodium concentrations and the concentration-dependent effects of lithium. In essence, Li^+ and Na^+ compete with one another, such that in the presence of hyponatremia the effects of the lithium may be increased to the point of causing toxicity. (Conversely, hypernatremia can counteract lithium's therapeutic effects.) Of the drugs listed, hydrochlorothiazide (and other thiazides and such thiazide-like agents as metolazone) poses the greatest risk of causing hyponatremia. (And you should consider the ultimate renal effects of ACE inhibition to lower serum Na^+ levels further when used with a diuretic. ACE inhibitors used without a diuretic are not at all as likely to cause hyponatremia.)

There are no clinically significant pharmacodynamic or pharmacokinetic interactions between nitroglycerin or HMG CoA reductase inhibitors and the SSRIs (fluoxetine, sertraline, others) or lithium.

2-12. The answer is a. *(Brooks, pp 477–479. Levinson, pp 285–289. Murray PR—2005, pp 679, 684. Ryan, pp 547–549.)* The e antigen is related to the hepatitis B virus and is associated with viral replication (Dane particle). Possession of the e antigen suggests active disease and thus an increased risk of transmission of hepatitis to others. HBsAg and e antigen are components of hepatitis B only and are not shared by other hepatitis viruses.

2-13. The answer is c. *(Kumar, p 1158. McPhee, pp 544–546.)* The visual pathway extends from the retina through the optic nerve, then the optic chiasm, through the optic tract, through the lateral geniculate body, and then through the optic radiations of the temporal and parietal lobes to end in the occipital lobes. Lesions in any of these areas produce characteristic visual field defects. For example, bitemporal hemianopsia (loss of vision in the periphery, also called "tunnel vision") is classically produced by lesions that involve the optic chiasm. The pituitary gland, which normally weighs about 0.5 g, lies in a bone depression (the sella turcica) and is covered by dura (diaphragma sellae). Anterior to the diaphragma sellae is the optic chiasm. Pituitary tumors may easily compress the optic chiasm and result in bilateral loss of peripheral vision.

Involvement of the optic nerve produces blindness in one eye (mononuclear anopsia), while involvement of the optic tract on one side results in homonymous hemianopsia (loss of the same side of the visual field in both eyes). A lesion involving the temporal lobe optic radiations produces a homonymous superior field defect, while a lesion involving the parietal lobe optic radiations produces a homonymous inferior field defect.

2-14. The answer is c. *(Ganong, pp 569–570, 582–583.)* The magnitude of the cardiac output is regulated to maintain an adequate blood pressure and to deliver an adequate supply of oxygen to the tissues. In anemia, a greater cardiac output is required to supply oxygen to the tissues because the oxygen-carrying capacity of the blood is reduced. The reduced blood viscosity increases the velocity and thus the turbulence of the blood flow, which makes systolic murmurs common in anemic patients. In aortic regurgitation, the stroke volume will be increased, but a portion of the blood ejected by the heart will return to the heart during diastole. Thus, the output delivered to the tissues does not increase despite the fact that the blood ejected by the heart has increased. In hypertension, third-degree heart block, and cardiac tamponade (decreased filling of the heart due to accumulation of fluid within the pericardium), cardiac output will be normal or reduced.

2-15. The answer is b. *(Brooks, pp 542–547. Levinson, pp 259–264. Murray PR—2005, pp 611–615. Ryan, p 501.)* The symptoms described are consistent with influenza virus infection. The titers of antibody on November 6 and 30 show low levels of antibody against swine influenza, but indicate at least a measurable amount. The 160 titer on December 20 reflects a definitive diagnostic rise in antibody against swine influenza (>1:4 rise between acute and convalescent sera).

The previous titers (10 or 1:10) most likely represent cross-reacting antibodies from a non-swine influenza virus hemagglutinin or neuraminidase enzymes, which could account for cross-reacting antibodies.

2-16. The answer is a. *(Murray RK, pp 136–144. Scriver, pp 1489–1520.)* Hereditary fructose intolerance (229600) is caused by deficiency of aldolase B that converts fructose-1-phosphate to dihydroxyacetone phosphate and glyceraldehydes. Fructose can be converted to fructose-1-phosphate (by fructokinase, the block in essential fructosuria, 229800) but accumulates with its phosphate and is diverted to fructose-1,6-bisphosphate. These compounds allosterically inhibit glycogen phosphorylase and cause hypoglycemia in the presence of abundant glycogen stores. The abnormal sequestration of phosphate interferes with ATP generation from AMP, depleting cellular energy sources with severe effects on liver or kidney. Affected individuals become nauseated when eating fructose and exhibit a natural aversion to fruits. If diagnosis is postponed and fructose is not minimized in the diet, they can undergo progressive liver and kidney failure with malnutrition and death. Countries like Belgium that use fructose in hyperalimentation solutions may observe patients with milder fructose intolerance who decompensate in the face of high serum concentrations.

2-17. The answer is a. *(Murray RK, pp 122–129, 173–179. Scriver, pp 2297–2326.)* Fatty acids are bound to coenzyme A as thiol esters for synthesis or degradation, each proceeding in two-carbon steps. The serially repeated steps in fatty acid oxidation involve (1) removal of two hydrogens to form a double bond between the carbons adjacent to the acid group (acyl-CoA dehydrogenase), (2) addition of water to the double bond so that a hydroxyl is on the second carbon (enoyl-CoA hydratase), oxidation of the hydroxyl group to a ketone (3-hydroxyacylCoA dehydrogenase), and removal of acetyl CoA (thiolase) to leave a fatty acyl CoA that is two carbons shorter. At least three groups of these sequentially acting enzymes are present in the mitochondrion, specific for very long or long chain, medium chain, or short chain fatty acids. Children with very long or long chain oxidation enzyme deficiencies, e.g. very long chain fatty acyl CoA dehydrogenase deficiency (VLCAD, 201475) accumulate fat in their heart and liver and have energy deficits in heart and muscle due to inadequate fat oxidation. Severely affected children often die of cardiac failure in the newborn period, and their enzyme deficiency combined with the maternal heterozygote state may cause HELLP syndrome in the last trimester of pregnancy, a variant of toxemia or preeclampsia that can be fatal. Premature delivery may be necessary for maternal health, and therapy with low-fat diets, frequent feeding (to minimize need for fat oxidation), and carnitine (to maximize transport of fatty acyl CoAs into mitochondria) may be attempted with the affected child.

2-18. The answer is e. *(Kandel, pp 879–880.)* The carotid sinus reflex involves several neuronal elements. The afferent side of the reflex begins with stretch receptors in the walls of the carotid sinus. These receptors signal pressure as a result of stretch of the low-capacitance vessel. This causes an afferent volley of action potentials to pass along the glossopharyngeal nerve into the medulla, where the fibers synapse with neurons in the solitary nucleus. These neurons, in turn, synapse upon neurons in the dorsal motor nucleus (and nucleus ambiguus) of the vagus nerve whose axons innervate the heart. Activation of this reflex results in a decrease in heart rate and force of contraction. As a consequence of the decrease in cardiac output, there is an ensuing decrease in blood pressure as well.

2-19. The answer is c. *(Casals, pp 1476–1483.)* If the brother has a child with cystic fibrosis, then he must be a carrier of the cystic fibrosis gene, meaning there is a 50% chance that the husband is a CF carrier. Congenital absence of the ejaculatory ducts is increased in carriers of CF. If the ejaculatory ducts are absent, then there should be *no* sperm from the vas deferens (normally 0.5 mL of the semen volume) and *no* products of the seminal vesicles (normally 2.0 mL of the semen volume). The seminal vesicle is responsible for fructose normally present in the ejaculate. Prostatic secretions are normally slightly acidic. The normal physical of the husband rules out hypospadias **(answer b),** bilateral cryptorchidism **(answer a),** and hydrocele **(answer d).** The congenital absence of the prostate gland is extremely rare **(answer e).**

2-20. The answer is e. *(Goldman, pp 1284–1285. Kumar, p 521.)* Increased serum lipids (hyperlipidemia) may be a primary genetic defect or may be secondary to another disorder, such as diabetes mellitus, alcoholism, the nephrotic syndrome, or hypothyroidism. Secondary hypertriglyceridemia in patients with diabetes mellitus usually occurs secondary to increased blood levels of VLDL. The reason for this is that with decreased levels of insulin with diabetes mellitus there is increased mobilization of free fatty acids from adipose tissue (increased lipolysis). This increases delivery of free fatty acids to the liver, which increases production and secretion of VLDL by the liver. This is a type IV hyperlipidemia pattern. Ethanol can also produce a type IV pattern due to increased VLDL. This is because ethanol also increases lipolysis of adipose tissue, which increases delivery of free fatty acids to the liver. Ethanol also increases the esterification of fatty acid to triglycerides in the liver and inhibits the release of lipoproteins from the liver.

2-21. The answer is c. *(Sadler, pp 172, 176–179. Moore and Persaud, Developing pp 168, 214.)* The child in the vignette is suffering from DiGeorge anomaly, which results in the absence of the thymus and parathyroid glands, which arise from the third and fourth pairs of branchial pouches. The absence of the thymus results in a deficiency in T lymphocyte–dependent areas of the immune system. These areas include the deep cortex of the lymph nodes, periarterial lymphatic sheath (PALS) of the spleen, and interfollicular areas of the Peyer's patches. Parathyroid hormone (PTH) stimulates the development of osteoclasts and the formation of ruffled borders in osteoclasts. The absence of PTH results in: i) a drastic reduction in numbers and activity of osteoclasts, ii) reduced Ca^{2+} levels in the blood, iii) denser bone, iv) spastic contractions of muscle called tetany, and v) excessive excitability of the nervous system. The parafollicular (C) cells arise from the ultimobranchial body that migrates into the thyroid gland and should form normally.

2-22. The answer is d. *(Ganong, pp 65–67. Kasper et al., p 1359.)* Titin is a large protein that connects the Z lines to the M lines, thereby providing a scaffold for the sarcomere. Titin contains two types of folded domains that provide muscle with its elasticity. The resistance to stretch increases throughout a contraction, which protects the structure of the sarcomere and prevents excess stretch.

2-23. The answer is d. *(Brooks, pp 273–275. Levinson, pp 140–141. Murray PR—2005, pp 347–351. Ryan, pp 379–380.)* Until recently, both erythromycin and ciprofloxacin were the drugs of choice for *C. jejuni* enterocolitis. Recently, resistance to the quinolones (ciprofloxacin) has been observed. Ampicillin is ineffective against this gram-negative, curved rod. While Pepto-Bismol may be adequate for a related ulcer-causing bacterium,

Helicobacter, it is not used for *C. jejuni.* While the pathogenesis of *C. jejuni* suggests an enterotoxin, an antitoxin is not available.

2-24. The answer is b. *(Lewis, pp 135–154. Scriver, pp 193–202.)* Many common disorders tend to run in families but are not single-gene or chromosomal disorders. These disorders exhibit multifactorial determination, a theoretical mechanism envisioned as the interaction of multiple genes (polygenic inheritance) and environmental factors. For quantitative traits like height, it is easy to visualize how the alleles at multiple loci plus environmental factors (e.g., nutrition) might make additive contributions toward a given stature. For qualitative traits such as cleft lip/palate and other congenital anomalies, a threshold is envisioned that divides normal from abnormal phenotypes. Individuals with more clefting alleles, in combination with an unfavorable intrauterine environment, can cross the threshold and manifest the anomaly. Environmental factors in multfactorial determination are thus prenatal as well as postnatal. For adult diseases like coronary artery disease, strokes, or hypertension, the quantitative trait can be viewed as degree of artery occlusion or blood pressure and the threshold as events like myocardial or cerebral infarction. The likelihood of inheriting hypertension-promoting alleles is increased if there are several affected relatives as in the family under discussion, translating the usual 3–5% risk for a multifactorial disorder in a first-degree relative to the 5–10% risk estimated in answer b. Recurrence risks for multifactorial disorders are modified by family history because the multiple predisposing alleles cannot be determined by testing. Current research is attempting to find single nucleotide polymorphisms (SNPs) that travel with these multiple predisposing alleles, allowing more definitive susceptibility testing and risk prediction for the occurrence and transmission of multifactorial traits.

2-25. The answer is e. *(Kumar, pp 603, 607–609. Rubin, pp 575–576.)* Inflammation of the myocardium (myocarditis) has numerous causes, but most of the well-documented cases of myocarditis are of viral origin. The most common viral causes are coxsackieviruses A and B, echovirus, and influenza virus. Patients usually develop symptoms a few weeks after a viral infection. Most patients recover from the acute myocarditis, but a few may die from congestive heart failure or arrhythmias. Sections of the heart show patchy or diffuse interstitial infiltrates composed of T lymphocytes and macrophages. There may be focal or patchy acute myocardial necrosis. Bacterial infections of the myocardium produce multiple foci of inflammation composed mainly of neutrophils. Giant cell myocarditis, which was previously called Fiedler's myocarditis, is characterized by granulomatous inflammation with giant cells and is usually rapidly fatal. In hypersensitivity myocarditis, which is caused by hypersensitivity reactions to several drugs, the inflammatory infiltrate includes many eosinophils, and the infiltrate is both interstitial and perivascular. Beriberi, one of the metabolic diseases of the heart, is a cause of high-output failure and is characterized by decreased peripheral vascular resistance and increased cardiac output. Patients have dilated hearts, but the microscopic changes are nonspecific. Hyperthyroid disease and Paget's disease are other causes of high-output failure.

2-26. The answer is a. (*Damjanov, pp 714–716. Kumar, pp 447–449.*) Protein-energy malnutrition (PEM) in underdeveloped countries leads to a spectrum of symptoms from kwashiorkor at one end to marasmus at the other. Marasmus, caused by a lack of caloric intake (i.e., starvation), leads to generalized wasting, stunted growth, atrophy of muscles, and loss of subcutaneous fat. There is no edema or hepatic enlargement. These children are alert, not apathetic, and are ravenous. In contrast, children with kwashiorkor, which is characterized by a lack of protein despite adequate caloric intake, have peripheral edema, a "moon" face, and an enlarged, fatty liver. The peripheral edema is caused by decreased albumin and sodium retention, while the fatty liver is caused by decreased synthesis of the lipoproteins necessary for the normal mobilization of lipids from liver cells. Additionally, these children have "flaky paint" areas of skin and abnormal pigmented streaks in their hair ("flag sign"). In children with marasmus, the skin is inelastic due to loss of subcutaneous fat. In either severe kwashiorkor or marasmus, thymic atrophy may result in the reduction in number and function of circulating T cells. B cell function (i.e., immunoglobulin production) is also depressed, so that these children are highly vulnerable to infections.

2-27. The answer is b. (*Ganong, pp 651–652, 688-689. Kasper et al., p 1511. Levitzky, pp 41–42, 58–59, 263. Stead et al, pp 255–256, 263–265.*) During a forced vital capacity (FVC), the patient is asked to breathe in as much air as possible (up to the total lung capacity), and then exhale all of the gas in her lung as fast as possible, which, in this case is 3.5 L. The $FEV_{1.0}$ is the volume of gas expelled from the lung during the first second, which, in this case, is 2 L. The ratio of the $FEV_{1.0}$ to the FVC in this patient is 2 L/3.5 L, which equals 0.57. Normally, $FEV_{1.0}$/FVC should be ≥ 0.8. The decreased $FEV_{1.0}$/FVC is indicative of an obstructive impairment. Obstructive lung diseases, such as asthma, are characterized by a greater-than-normal total lung capacity (TLC), residual volume (RV), and functional residual capacity (FRC). The inspiratory and expiratory reserves (inspiratory capacity and expiratory volume) are decreased, as is the vital capacity and the maximum voluntary ventilation.

2-28. The answer is a. (*Kumar, pp 91, 94, 1327. Alberts, pp 1299–1300.*) Satellite cells in skeletal muscle proliferate and reconstitute the damaged part of the myofibers. They are supportive cells for maintenance of muscle and a source of new myofibers after injury or after increased load. There is no dedifferentiation of myocytes into myoblasts **(answer b)**, or fusion of damaged myofibers to form new myotubes **(answer c)**. Hypertrophy, not hyperplasia **(answer d)**, occurs in existing myofibers in response to increased load. Proliferation of fibroblasts may occur in the damaged area but leads to fibrosis, not repair of skeletal muscle. Fibroblasts do *not* differentiate into myocytes **(answer e)**. The multinucleate organization of skeletal muscle is derived developmentally by fusion and not by amitosis (failure of cytokinesis after DNA synthesis). Mitotic activity is terminated after fusion occurs. In the development of skeletal muscle, myoblasts of mesodermal origin undergo cell proliferation. Myocyte cell division ceases soon after birth. Myoblasts, which are mononucleate cells, fuse with each other end to end to form myotubes. This process requires cell recognition between myoblasts, alignment, and subsequent fusion.

2-29. The answer is d. (*Lewis, pp 135–154. Scriver, pp 2863–2914. Murray RK, pp 219–230.*) This man has familial hypercholesterolemia (143890), an autosomal dominant phenotype defined by studying men who experienced heart attacks at young ages. Mutations in the LDL receptor lead to decreased cellular cholesterol uptake and increased serum cholesterol. Since LDL has a high cholesterol content, the LDL fraction is elevated compared to the HDL fraction on lipoprotein electrophoresis. In normal individuals, the LDL is taken up by its specific receptor and imported via caveolae to the cell interior. Cholesterol then produces feedback inhibition on the rate-limiting enzyme of cholesterol synthesis (hydroxymethylglutaryl CoA reductase) and also leads to a decrease in the number of LDL receptors. In rare cases, two individuals with familial hypercholesterolemia marry and produce a child with homozygous familial hypercholesterolemia. These children develop severe atherosclerosis and xanthomas (fatty tumors) at an early age.

2-30. The answer is c. (*Kumar, pp 34, 37–41, 423, 905.*) Hyalin is a nonspecific term that is used to describe any material, inside or outside the cell, that stains a red homogenous color with the routine H&E stain. There are many different substances that have the appearance of hyalin. Alcoholic hyaline inclusions (Mallory bodies) are irregular eosinophilic hyaline inclusions that are found within the cytoplasm of hepatocytes. Mallory bodies are composed of prekeratin intermediate filaments. They are a nonspecific finding and can be found in patients with several diseases other than alcoholic hepatitis, such as Wilson's disease, and in patients who have undergone bypass operations for morbid obesity. Immunoglobulins may form intracytoplasmic or extracellular oval hyaline bodies called Russell bodies. Excess plasma proteins may form hyaline droplets in proximal renal tubular epithelial cells or hyaline membranes in the alveoli of the lungs (hyaline membrane disease). The hyalin found in the walls of arterioles of kidneys in patients with benign nephrosclerosis is composed of basement membranes and precipitated plasma proteins. Lipofuscin is an intracytoplasmic aging pigment that has a yellow-brown, finely granular appearance with H&E stains. Its appearance does not resemble that of hyaline material.

2-31. The answer is b. *(Young, p 133. Junqueira, p 158. Kierszenbaum, pp 28–29. Kasper, pp 1042–1044. Moore and Dalley, pp 85–87.)* Kinesin is a motor protein that uses energy from ATP hydrolysis to move vesicles (– → +) from the cell body in the dorsal root ganglion (shown in the photomicrograph) in an anterograde direction toward the axon terminal **(answer d).** The patient in question has shingles caused by the herpes virus known as the varicella-zoster virus (VZV). Shingles begins as erythematous maculopapular eruptions and rapidly evolves to vesicles; it often presents with fever. The patient had chickenpox as a child. Chickenpox is also caused by VZV. The virus is stored in the dorsal root ganglion, primarily in the satellite cells surrounding the perikarya (cell bodies). Kinesin walks along the microtubule toward the plus end of the microtubule. The dyneins **(answers a and c)** are minus-end directed microtubule motors that move organelles, including vesicles, in a retrograde direction toward the cell body (in this case toward the cell bodies of the dorsal root ganglia). The dyneins involved in axonal transport are the cytoplasmic dyneins as compared to the axonemal dyneins seen in cilia and flagella. Myosin II **(answer e)** is an actin-based motor protein that generates the force of muscle contraction. The Tzanck test is a method of testing for the virus; it can detect the presence of the herpesvirus in the cells scraped from a lesion. It cannot detect the difference between herpes simplex virus (HSV) and VZV. PCR of the DNA is required for absolute detection.

The patient's shingles involve dermatomal segment T4, which surrounds the nipple. The nipples are normally found in the middle of T4, although T5 may also innervate this region. A dermatome is the area of skin supplied by nerves originating from a single spinal nerve root.

2-32. The answer is e. *(Kasper et al., p 1361.)* Phospholamban is a protein contained within the sarcoplasmic reticulum (SR) that inhibits the activity of the SR calcium pump. Inactivation of phospholamban results in an increase in calcium sequestration by the SR. Increasing the concentration of calcium within the SR increases the force of the ventricular contraction.

2-33. The answer is b. *(Brooks, pp 352–354. Levinson, pp 93, 177, 484s. Murray—2005, pp 459–461. Ryan, pp 477–478.)* Coxiella burnetii is a rickettsial organism that causes upper respiratory infections in humans. These can range from subclinical infection to influenza-like disease and pneumonia. Transmission to humans occurs from inhalation of dust contaminated with rickettsiae from placenta, dried feces, urine, or milk, or from aerosols in slaughterhouses. *C. burnetii* can also be found in ticks, which can transmit the agent to sheep, goats, and cattle. No skin rash occurs in these infections. Treatment includes tetracycline and chloramphenicol.

2-34. The answer is c. *(Damjanov, pp 1536–1541. Kumar, pp 735–737. Rubin, pp 637–639.)* The segmented or beaded, often dumbbell-shaped bodies are ferruginous bodies that are probably asbestos fibers coated with iron and protein. The term ferruginous body is applied to other inhaled fibers that become iron-coated; however, in a patient with interstitial lung fibrosis or pleural plaques, ferruginous bodies are probably asbestos bodies. The type of asbestos mainly used in America is chrysotile, mined in Canada, and it is much less likely to cause mesothelioma or lung cancer than is crocidolite (blue asbestos), which has limited use and is mined in South Africa. Cigarette smoking potentiates the relatively mild carcinogenic effect of asbestos. In contrast, laminated spherical (Schaumann's) bodies are found in granulomas of sarcoid and chronic berylliosis, while *Candida* species histologically may show elongated chains of yeast without hyphae (pseudohyphae), and silica particles are very small and are birefringent.

2-35. The answer is a. *(Adams, pp 799, 1383. Afifi, pp 125–127, 141–143. Siegel and Sapru, pp 501–504.)* Emma had a stroke resulting from occlusion of medial branches of the left vertebral artery, presumably secondary to atherosclerosis (i.e., cholesterol deposits within the artery, which eventually occlude it). The resulting syndrome is called the medial medullary syndrome, because the affected structures are located in the medial portion of the medulla. These structures include the pyramids, the medial lemniscus, the medial longitudinal fasciculus, and the nucleus of the hypoglossal nerve and its outflow tract. Emma's symptoms resulted from damage to the aforementioned structures and may have been caused by the same process (atherosclerosis) that resulted in her heart disease. The weakness of her right side was caused by damage to the medullary pyramid (at the level of the hypoglossal nerve) on the left side. Her face was spared because fibers supplying the face exited above the level of infarct. However, a lesion in the corticospinal tract of the cervical spinal cord above C5 could cause arm and leg weakness and spare the face, because facial fibers exit at the pontine-medulla border. A lesion in the inferior portion of the precentral gyrus of the left frontal lobe would cause right-sided weakness, but would include the face, because this area is represented more inferiorly than are the extremities. Her unsteady gait was a result of the weakness of her right side, but may also have been the result of the loss of position and vibration sense on that side from damage to the medial lemniscus (as demonstrated by the inability to identify the position of her toe with her eyes closed, and the inability to feel the vibrations of a tuning fork). Without position sense, walking becomes unsteady because it is necessary to feel the position of one's feet on the floor during normal gait. Damage to both the medial lemniscus and pyramids at this level causes problems on the contralateral side because this lesion is located rostral to the level where both of these fiber bundles cross to the opposite side of the brain. Damage to the descending component of the MLF could only affect head and neck reflexes, but not gait. Gait is also unaffected by pain inputs. Deviation of the tongue occurs because fibers from the hypoglossal nucleus innervate the genioglossus muscle on the ipsilateral side of the tongue. This muscle normally protrudes the tongue toward the contralateral side. Therefore, if one side is weak, the tongue will deviate toward the side ipsilateral to the lesion when protruded.

2-36. The answer is a. (*Young, pp 47–57. Junqueira, pp 226–235.*)
   Neutrophil. The neutrophil (**A**) contains neutrophilic granules. Neutrophils are involved in the acute phase of inflammation and are responsible for the phagocytosis of invading bacteria. Neutrophils contain lysozyme and alkaline phosphatase within their granules. They die soon after phagocytosing bacteria and are added to the pus, which consists of dead neutrophils, serum, and tissue fluids.

Basophil. The basophil (**B**) is about the same size as the neutrophil (**A**) and contains granules of variable size that may obscure the nucleus. The nucleus of the basophil is irregularly lobed with condensed chromatin. Basophils are involved in the attraction of eosinophils to the site of infection. This occurs in parasitic and nonparasitic infections and involves chemoattraction by histamine and eosinophil-chemoattractant factor of anaphylaxis (ECF-A). Basophils are similar in structure and function to the connective tissue mast cell. Basophils are also phagocytic granulocytes, but are involved in inflammation through the release of histamine and heparin. Immunoglobulin E (IgE) produced by plasma cells becomes bound to the cell surface of mast cells and basophils on first exposure. At the time of secondary exposure, the antigen binds to the IgE and stimulates the degranulation of mast cell and basophil granules releasing histamine and heparin. Basophils and mast cells are involved in anaphylactic and immediate **hypersensitivity reactions.**

Eosinophil. The eosinophil (**C**) is bilobed with more regular granules than the basophil (**B**). Eosinophils have less phagocytic ability than neutrophils and may kill parasites by either phagocytosis or exocytotic release of granules. Eosinophils contain major basic protein, histaminase, acid phosphatase, and other lysosomal enzymes. Eosinophils are essential for the destruction of parasites such as trichinae and schistosomes.

Monocyte. The monocyte (**D**) contains an eccentric nucleus, which is often kidney-shaped. The chromatin generally has a ropelike appearance and, therefore, is less condensed than the chromatin of a lymphocyte (**F**). The monocyte has some phagocytic activity in the blood, but its major role is as a source of macrophages throughout the body including Langerhans cells (skin), microglia (brain), and Kupffer cells (liver).

Megakaryocyte. The megakaryocyte (**E**) is a large cell with a multilobular appearance and is the source of platelets. Megakaryocytes fragment to form the platelets, which are key elements of the blood.

Lymphocyte. The lymphocyte (**F**) is considered an agranular cell with an ovoid nucleus and scanty cytoplasm. The shape and the arrangement of chromatin vary, depending on the classification of the lymphocyte: small, medium, or large. Small and medium are involved in chronic inflammation, whereas, large lymphocytes are the source of T and B cells. Lymphocytes are either T or B cells based on their education in the thymus or bone marrow. Plasma cells differentiate from B lymphocytes that undergo mitosis and form a plasma cell and a memory cell after exposure to appropriate antigen. An antigen-presenting cell and a specific subtype of T lymphocyte called a helper T cell are required for B cell differentiation into antibody-producing plasma cells.

2-37. The answer is a. *(Brooks, pp 637–639. Murray PR—2005, pp 712–714.)* Valley fever is caused by *C. immitis.* It is grown on Sabouraud's agar, and the infection is endemic in the semiarid regions of the southwestern United States, as well as Central and South America. Hyphae form chains of arthroconidia (arthrospores) which often develop in alternate cells of a hypha. Individual arthroconidia are released from chains, become airborne and are resistant to harsh environmental conditions. Following inhalation, arthroconidia become spherical, enlarge forming spherules that contain endospores. Such spherules have a thick, refractive cell wall and are diagnostic of *C. immitis.* Blastospores represent conidial formation through a budding process, as seen in yeast or chains of *Cladosporium.* Chlamydospores are large, thick-walled spherical conidia produced from terminal hyphal cells (*C. albicans*). Sporangiospores are sexual structures characteristic of zygomycetes (mitotic spores produced within an enclosed sporangium, of ten supported by one sporangiophore (*Rhizopus, Mucor*).

2-38. The answer is c. *(Brunton, pp 161–163, 171t–172t, 257–259. Craig, pp 105–106, 349–351. Katzung, pp 81–90.)* Amphetamines (dextroamphetamine, methamphetamine, amphetamine, and several related drugs) can be classified as indirect-acting sympathomimetics (adrenomimetics). They are taken into the adrenergic nerve ending by the amine pump, displace NE from its storage vesicles (via processes that are not dependent on an action potential) and cause the stored neurotransmitter to be released into the synaptic space. At that point, all the expected effects of NE on its receptors and effectors occur. These drugs have no direct effects, whether as an agonist or antagonist, on the adrenergic receptors. Their actions are wholly dependent on intraneuronal NE stores.

2-39. The answer is c. *(Murray RK, pp 481–497. Scriver, pp 3897–3964.)* Prolonged vitamin C deficiency (scurvy) usually occurs with severe malnutrition (famine, prisoners of war, alcoholism, extreme food fadism). Exclusive feeding of cow's milk, as may occur in areas of famine with poor supplies of maternal milk, can result in infantile scurvy with the symptoms described in the question. X-rays of the limbs are helpful in diagnosing scurvy, with a white line at the metaphysis and occasional subperiosteal hemorrhage. These radiologic features may be seen in copper deficiency associated with hyperalimentation, emphasizing the role of ascorbic acid (vitamin C) as a coenzyme for proline/lysine hydroxylases that modify collagen and also require copper.

The causes of hemorrhagic disease of the newborn are desribed in the previous answer, and vitamin K deficiency is almost never seen after the newborn period because of wide dietary availability. Deficiencies of the fat-soluble vitamins A, E, and D can occur with intestinal malabsorption, but avid fetal uptake during pregnancy usually prevents infantile symptoms. Vitamin D deficiency (rickets) can also cause a series of rib lumps (rosary) and is more likely with darker skin pigmentation but has other symptoms. Hypervitaminosis A can cause liver toxicity but not bleeding, and deficiency of vitamin E can be associated with anemia in prematures but is unknown in older children and adults.

2-40. The answer is c. (*Kandel, pp 523–543. Siegel and Sapru, pp 274–278.*) Cells in the lateral geniculate nucleus respond very much like ganglion cells in the retina because of the point-to-point projection pathway from the retina to the lateral geniculate. Accordingly, lateral geniculate cells have small concentric receptive fields that are either on-center or off-center in which the cells respond best to small spots of light that are in the center of the receptive field. On the other hand, cells in the visual cortex display a much greater complexity in their responses to images in the visual field. Instead of responding to small spots of light, they respond to lines and borders in the different areas of the visual field. In particular, the simple cell responds as a function of the retinal position in which the line-stimulus is located, as well as its orientation (e.g., whether it is in a vertical or horizontal position). As a result, when a bar of light is positioned in the appropriate part of the visual field with the appropriate orientation, the cells in area 17 will respond maximally. When either of these parameters is altered, the firing pattern of the cell will be reduced or totally inhibited. Complex cells lack clear excitatory and inhibitory zones (i.e., these neurons respond to bars of light in a given orientation but they are not position specific). Hypercomplex cells are stimulated by bars of light of specific lengths or by specific shapes.

2-41. The answer is d. (*Murray RK, pp 190–196. Scriver, pp 4029–4240.*) Leukotrienes C_4, D_4, and E_4 together compose the slow-reacting substance of anaphylaxis (SRS-A), which is thought to be the cause of asphyxiation in individuals not treated rapidly enough following an anaphylactic shock. SRS-A is up to 1000 times more effective than histamines in causing bronchial muscle constriction. Anti-inflammatory steroids are usually given intravenously to end chronic bronchoconstriction and hypotension following a shock. The steroids block phospholipase A_2 action, preventing the synthesis of leukotrienes from arachidonic acid. Acute treatment involves epinephrine injected subcutaneously initially and then intravenously. Antihistamines such as diphenhydramine are administered intravenously or intramuscularly.

2-42. The answer is d. *(Kumar, p 109. Lobov, pp 11205–11210).* Angiostatin and endostatin are cleavage products of plasminogen and type XVIII collagen respectively and function as anti-angiogenic peptides. Vascular endothelial growth factor (VEGF, **answer a**) stimulates the recruitment and growth of endothelial cells through the VEGF-R located on endothelial cell precursors as well as endothelial cells. Platelet-derived growth factor (PDGF) recruits smooth muscle cells **(answer b)** and transforming growth factor-beta (TGF-β) stimulates and stabilizes extracellular matrix production. Recruitment and proliferation of periendothelial cells **(answer e)**, smooth muscle cells, pericytes, and fibroblasts are required for development and maturation of new blood vessels. The angiopoietins (Ang) 1 and 2 bind their receptor, Tie2, a receptor tyrosine kinase which regulates endothelial cell proliterative status. Ang 1 binds Tie2 leading to periendothelial cell recruitment and therefore vascular maturation.

Ang 2 is found in organs of the female reproductive tract and blocks Ang 1 effects when VEGF is absent. The result is regression of the blood vessel. Ang 2 in the presence of VEGF leads to loosening of the surrounding cells permitting multiplication of endothelial cells and angiogenesis.

2-43. The answer is f. *(Lewis, pp 1–20, 75–94. Scriver, pp 3–45.)* It is important that the pedigree be an accurate reflection of the family history and that information not be recorded unless specifically mentioned. Pedigree B in Fig. 41 omits the double line needed to indicate consanguinity, and pedigree C assumes that the father's affected cousin is the offspring of his uncle rather than being unspecified. Pedigree F correctly illustrates the birth order (third) of the affected female (indicated by arrow) and the consanguinity (double line) represented by the first-cousin marriage. Cystic fibrosis is an autosomal recessive disease that causes progressive lung disease and intestinal malabsorption due to deficiencies of multiple pancreatic enzymes (219700). Autosomal recessive diseases are much more common with consanguinity or inbreeding because the related couple has a greater chance to inherit the same rare allele.

2-44. The answer is e. *(Ganong, pp 709–712. Widmaier et al., pp 536.)* The renal threshold for glucose is the plasma concentration at which glucose first appears in the urine. The graph shows that glucose is excreted at a plasma concentration of 300 mg/dL. (This is higher than the typical value of 200 mg/dL.)

Glucose appears in the urine at a filtered load less than the T_{max} for glucose because of the differences in the reabsorptive capacity of the nephrons. Some nephrons can only reabsorb a small amount of glucose. When their reabsorptive capacity is exceeded, glucose is excreted. Other nephrons can absorb much more glucose. The T_{max} represents the average reabsorptive capacity of all the renal nephrons. The T_{max} for glucose is the maximum rate of glucose reabsorption from the kidney. Typically, the T_{max} is 375 mg/min. However, the T_{max} in this patient is 500 mg/min. The higher-than-normal reabsorptive capacity accounts for the lower-than-expected urinary concentration. The T_{max} is calculated by subtracting the amount of glucose excreted from the filtered load at any plasma concentration at which the amount of glucose excreted increases linearly as plasma glucose concentration increases. For example, when the plasma glucose concentration is 600 mg/dL, the filtered load of glucose is 600 mg/min, the amount of glucose excreted is 100 mg/min, and the amount of glucose reabsorbed (the T_{max}) is 500 mg/min.

2-45. The answer is a. *(Brooks, pp 720, 739–740. Levinson, pp 61–62, 66. Murray PR—2005, p 843. Ryan, pp 854–855.)* Many sputum specimens are cultured unnecessarily. Sputum is often contaminated with saliva or is almost totally made up of saliva. These specimens rarely reveal the cause of the patient's respiratory problem and may provide laboratory information that is harmful. The sputum in the question appears to be a good specimen because there are few epithelial cells. The pleomorphic, gram-negative rods are suggestive of *Haemophilus,* but culture of the secretions is necessary. Normal flora from a healthy oral cavity consists of gram-positive cocci and rods, with few or no PMNs.

2-46. The answer is c. *(Murray RK, pp 318–319. Lewis, pp 178–184. Scriver, pp 3–45.)* Special DNA structures at the end of chromosomes, called telomeres, consist of repetitive DNAs including a particular 6-base pair repeat (5'-TTAGGG-3') at each chromosome terminus. A special DNA polymerase called telomerase replicates these terminal repeats using a complementary RNA primer that makes it analogous to the viral enzyme reverse transcriptase. The number of 6-base pair repeats is normally in the thousands, but has been noted to shorten in tumor tissues and in normal tissues as a function of aging. The adjacent repetitive DNAs in telomeres, like those comprising centromeres, can be generally distributed or unique to the particular chromosome. Multicolor, fluorescent DNA probes to these unique telomeric DNAs allow labelling of the various chromosome ends and can detect rearrangements by Flourescent *In Situ* Hybridization (FISH) showing a shift of signal from telomere to chromosome interior. Such rearrangements may not change the length or banding pattern of the chromosome arm and will not be obvious on routine karyotypes. Telomere array analysis is thus useful on children with mental disability and malformations who are suspected to have a chromosome aberration but prove to have a normal routine karyotype.

2-47–2-50. The answers are 47-a, 48-d, 49-b, 50-c. (*Levinson, pp 67–81. Ryan, pp 195–198, 201–202, 204, 643–644.*) The antibiotics in these questions have significantly different modes of action. Recent evidence suggests that while penicillin inhibits the final cross-linking of the cell wall, it also binds to penicillin-binding proteins and inhibits certain key enzymes involved in cell-wall synthesis. The mechanism is complex. Amdinocillin, although classified as a penicillin, selectively binds to PBP-2. Binding to PBP-2 results in aberrant cell-wall elongation and spherical forms, seen when *E. coli,* for example, is exposed to mecillinam.

Because amphotericin binds to sterols (such as ergosterol, a compound of fungal membrane) in the cell membrane, its range of activity is predictable; that is, it is effective against microorganisms that contain sterol in the cell membrane (such as molds, yeasts, and certain amebas). These polyene antibiotics cause reorientation of sterols in the membrane, and membrane structure is altered to the extent that permeability is affected. If sterol synthesis is blocked in fungi, then amphotericin is not effective. This occurs when fungi are exposed to miconazole, another antifungal antibiotic.

Chloramphenicol can be either bacteriocidal or bacteriostatic, depending on the organism. It is bacteriostatic against organisms such as *S. typhi,* but bacteriocidal against encapsulated organisms that cause meningitis such as *H. influenzae, S. pneumoniae,* and *N. meningitidis.* Bacterial ribosomes are spherical particles. Protein synthesis takes place on the ribosome by a complex process involving various ribosomal subunits, tRNA, and mRNA. Chloramphenicol, in contrast to the aminoglycosides and tetracycline, attaches to the 50S ribosome subunit. The enzyme peptidyl transferase, found in the 50S subunit, is inhibited. Removal of the inhibition—in this case, chloramphenicol—results in full activity of the enzyme.

Trimethoprim (TMP), a diaminopyrimidine, is a folic acid antagonist. Although TMP is commonly used in combination with sulfa drugs, its mode of action is distinct. TMP is structurally similar to the pteridine portion of dihydrofolate and prevents the conversion of folic acid to tetrahydrofolic acid by inhibition of dihydrofolate reductase. Fortunately, this enzyme in humans is relatively insensitive to TMP.

Block 3

Answers

3-1. The answer is C. *(Nolte, pp 263–287. Siegel and Sapru, pp 13–15, 223–250, 280–285, 330–339, 447–453.)* This figure is a ventral view of the brainstem. Fibers that arise from the dorsal motor nucleus and nucleus ambiguus (in part) exit the brain on the lateral side of the medulla as part of the vagus nerve (K) and innervate the myenteric plexus and smooth muscles of the stomach, which normally function to produce gastric secretions. Cutting some of these fibers would result in a reduction in gastric secretions. The tumor affected the motor component of the trigeminal nerve. (H) The motor root lies medial to the sensory root and innervates the muscles of mastication. The mammillary bodies (A), which lie on the ventral surface of the brain at the caudal aspect of the hypothalamus, receive many of their inputs from the hippocampal formation and project to the anteroventral thalamic nucleus as the mammillothalamic tract, which in turn send their axons to the cingulate gyrus and then back to the hippocampal formation, forming what is referred to as the Papez circuit. This circuit has been associated with memory functions and the regulation of emotional behavior. The facial nerve (C) exits the brain at the level of the ventrolateral aspect of the caudal pons, and its special visceral efferent component innervates the muscles of facial expression. Damage to this nerve causes loss of facial expression on the side of the face ipsilateral to the affected nerve.

The cerebral peduncle (G) is situated in the ventrolateral aspect of the midbrain and contains fibers of cortical origin that project to all levels of the neuraxis of the brainstem and spinal cord. A lesion in this region would affect UMNs that control motor functions associated with both the body and the head region, producing diminution in strength of the muscles of the ipsilateral head and paralysis of the contralateral leg and arm. Note that the selection of choice E, the pyramids, would not have been correct, since the fibers present at this level can only terminate within the medulla or spinal cord, and therefore could not account for the loss of muscle strength associated with the head. First-order somatosensory fibers from the region of the face (I) enter the brain laterally at the level of the middle of the pons as the sensory root of the trigeminal nerve. Damage to this nerve would cause loss of sensation associated with the face. The oculomotor nerve (B) exits the brain at the level of the ventromedial aspect of the midbrain, and some fibers of the general somatic efferent component of this nerve innervate the medial rectus. Damage to this component results in a loss of ability for medial gaze, and the eye will additionally be directed downward because of the unopposed action of cranial nerve IV. Another component of the oculomotor nerve, the general visceral efferent, constitutes the preganglionic parasympathetic neuron in a disynaptic pathway whose postganglionic division innervates the pupillary constrictor muscles. Accordingly, damage to the preganglionic division results in loss of pupillary constriction, which normally occurs in the presence of light as well as in accommodation, and the eye will dilate because of the unopposed action of the sympathetic fibers. The abducens nerve (J) exits the brain at a ventromedial position at the level of the medulla-pontine border, and its fibers innervate the lateral rectus muscle. Damage to this nerve results in a lateral gaze paralysis.

The optic chiasm (F) contains fibers that cross over to reach the lateral geniculate nucleus on the side contralateral to the retina from which they originated. Such fibers are associated with the temporal (i.e., lateral) visual fields. Therefore, damage to the optic chiasm will cause blindness in the lateral half of each of the visual fields. Such a deficit is referred to as *bitemporal hemianopsia*. First-order neurons from the labyrinth organs (D) (i.e., semicircular canals, saccule, and utricle) convey information concerning the position of the head in space along the vestibular component of the eighth nerve into the central nervous system (CNS). This nerve enters the brain laterally at the level of the upper medulla. Damage to this nerve could result in symptoms such as ringing in the ear, nystagmus, loss of balance, and dizziness. The hypoglossal nerve (L) exits the brain at the level of the middle of the medulla between the pyramid and the olive. These fibers innervate muscles that move the tongue toward the opposite side. For this reason, a lesion of the hypoglossal nucleus or its nerve will result in a deviation of the tongue to the side of the lesion because of the unopposed action of the contralateral hypoglossal nerve, which remains intact.

3-2. The answer is a. (*Kandel, pp 910–918. Simon, pp 47, 258. Siegel and Sapru, pp 460–463.*) The seizure described in this patient has progressed from a complex partial seizure to a generalized seizure. As indicated previously, this type of seizure involves all of the limbs. The patient falls to the ground and typically loses consciousness. As stated in the answer to Question 444, the other choices involve seizures that are characterized differently than what was described in the progression of this case.

3-3. The answer is a. (*Brunton, pp 204, 211, 214, 538–540. Craig, pp 128, 130, 371. Katzung, pp 105, 1010–1011.*) Patients with Alzheimer's disease present with progressive impairment of memory and cognitive functions such as a lack of attention, disturbed language function, and an inability to complete common tasks. Although the exact defect in the central nervous system (CNS) has not been elucidated, evidence suggests that a reduction in cholinergic nerve function or receptor activation plays an important role in the etiology. At the very least, increasing central cholinergic receptor activation seems to reduce symptom severity.

Tacrine has been found to be somewhat effective in patients with mild-to-moderate symptoms of this disease for improvement of cognitive functions. The drug is primarily a reversible cholinesterase inhibitor that increases the concentration of functional ACh in the brain. However, the pharmacology of tacrine is complex; the drug also acts as a muscarinic receptor modulator in that it has partial agonistic activity, as well as weak antagonistic activity on muscarinic receptors in the CNS. In addition, tacrine appears to enhance the release of ACh from cholinergic nerves, and it may alter the concentrations of other neurotransmitters such as dopamine and NE.

Of all the reversible cholinesterase inhibitors, only tacrine and physostigmine cross the blood-brain barrier in sufficient amounts to make these compounds useful for disorders involving the CNS. Physostigmine has been tried as a therapy for Alzheimer's disease; however, it is more commonly used to antagonize the effects of toxic concentrations of drugs with antimuscarinic properties, including atropine, antihistamines, phenothiazines, and tricyclic antidepressants. Neostigmine, pyridostigmine, and ambenonium are used mainly in the treatment of myasthenia gravis; edrophonium is useful for the diagnosis of this disease because of its fast onset and short duration.

3-4. The answer is c. (*Brooks, pp 562–566. Levinson, pp 262–264, 269–270. Murray PR—2005, pp 598–603. Ryan, pp 519–520.*) Measles (rubeola) caused by a paramyxovirus is an acute, highly infectious disease characterized by a maculopapular rash. German measles (rubella—a togavirus) is an acute, febrile illness characterized by a rash as well as suboccipital lymphadenopathy. Incubation time for measles is 9 full days after exposure. Onset is abrupt and symptoms mostly catarrhal. Koplik's spots, pale, bluish-white spots in red areolas, can frequently be observed on the mucous membranes of the mouth and are pathognomonic for measles.

3-5. The answer is e. (*Ganong, pp 333–334. Stead et al., pp 69–70.*) The islets of Langerhans, which constitute 1 to 2% of the pancreatic weight, secrete insulin, glucagon, somatostatin, and pancreatic polypeptide. Each is secreted from a distinct cell type, A, B, D, and F, respectively. The islets are scattered throughout the pancreas, but are more plentiful in the tail than in the body or head.

3-6. The answer is a. (*Young, pp 95, 164, 168. Junqueira, pp 79–80, 370–372.*) The cyst in the vignette is an epidermoid or sebaceous cyst and the gland shown in the photomicrograph is a sebaceous gland, located in the dermis and associated with a hair follicle. Secretion from sebaceous glands is classified as holocrine (i.e., shedding of the disintegrated cell along with sebum into the hair follicle). Blockage of sebaceous gland ducts, presumably from injury, infection or irritation, results in cyst formation. Sebaceous cysts are prone to infection and can have foul-smelling drainage with inflammation and pain. The lesion usually consists of an enlarged sebaceous gland with numerous lobules grouped around a centrally located sebaceous duct, which has become obstructed causing the cyst. The photomicrograph represents a microscopic section obtained from thin skin. The presence of sebaceous glands/hair follicles identifies the section as thin skin. Sebaceous glands and hair follicles are not found in thick skin. Another difference between thick and thin skin is the virtual absence of the stratum lucidum in thin skin. There are two types of sweat glands: merocrine and apocrine. The merocrine glands release their secretion through exocytosis with conservation of membrane (**answer b**). In anal, areolar, and axillary regions, sweat glands are apocrine (**answer c**); the apical part of the cell is released with the secretion. Endocrine secretion occurs into the blood (**answer d**); autocrine secretion is self-stimulation (**answer e**). For example, activated T cells stimulate their own proliferation by secreting IL-2 and synthesizing IL-2 receptors that bind the IL-2.

3-7. The answer is b. (*Murray RK, pp 5–13. Scriver, pp 3–45. Lewis, pp 185–204.*) Proteins can be effective buffers of body and intracellular fluids. Buffering capacity is dependent on the presence of amino acids having ionizable side chains with pKas near physiologic pH. In the example given, only histidine has an ionizable imidazolium group that has a pK close to neutrality (pK = 6.0). Valine and leucine are amino acids with uncharged, branched side chains. Lysine has a very basic amino group (pK = 10.5) on its aliphatic side chain that is positively charged at physiologic pH, and aspartic acid has a side chain carboxyl (pK = 3.8) that is negative at pH 7.

3-8. The answer is c. (*Brunton, pp 263–270. Craig, pp 111–113. Katzung, pp 144–146, 148.*) Tamsulosin is a selective α_1-adrenergic blocker, and presumably its affinity is greater for α receptors on smooth muscles in the prostate (hence, its use for BPH, due to relaxation of smooth muscles there) than for those in the peripheral vasculature. Nonetheless, its pharmacologic profile is most similar to that of prazosin, which can be considered the prototypic α_1-selective adrenergic blocker that is mainly used to treat hypertension because it competitively blocks vasoconstriction caused by α agonists such as epinephrine and norepinephrine. (Remember: drugs with a generic name that ends in "-osin" or "-zosin" are selective α_1-adrenergic blockers: for example, tamsulosin, prazosin, terazosin, doxazosin.)

So, of the answers listed above, orthostatic hypotension is the most likely side effect. Among the many classes of adrenergic drugs, bradycardia would most likely be caused by a β blocker (or lesser prescribed drugs such as reserpine, a catecholamine depletor), or a muscarinic agonist or cholinesterase inhibitor, and certainly not by a drug that has no direct cardiac effects and is more likely to elicit reflex cardiac stimulation secondary to reduced blood pressure. There are no known interactions between α blockers and atorvastatin or related drugs. Photophobia is an unlikely problem: it is usually caused by drugs that cause mydriasis (e.g., α-adrenergic agonists or antimuscarinics), and if anything tamsulosin is likely to prevent the mydriasis that is a common cause of photophobia. Exacerbations of emphysema, whether due to bronchoconstriction or other causes, is unlikely too. From an autonomic perspective, epinephrine is the main bronchodilator substance (via β_2 activation), ACh is the main autonomic bronchoconstrictor (via muscarinic activation). Tamsulosin affects neither.

3-9. The answer is b. (*Young, p 261. Junqueira, pp 290–295, 298–300.*) The patient in the scenario is suffering from celiac disease, an allergic response to gliadin. The result is villous atrophy and crypt and Brunner gland (the structures labeled with the asterisks in the photomicrograph) hyperplasia. The presence of the mucus and bicarbonate (HCO_3^-) secreting Brunner's glands in the submucosal layer of the small intestine is an identifying feature of the duodenum. The Brunner's gland secretions function to neutralize the acidic pH of the stomach and establish the appropriate pH for function of the enzymes in the pancreatic juice. Parietal cells are unique to the stomach and synthesize acid (**answer a**) and intrinsic factor (required for vitamin B_{12} absorption from the small intestine). Chief cells in the fundic glands produce pepsinogen (**answer c**) that is activated by acid to form pepsin. Paneth cells in the base of the crypts make lysozyme (**answer d**) and modulate the flora of the small intestine. Enterokinase (**answer e**) is made by the duodenal mucosa and is instrumental in the conversion of pancreatic zymogens to their active form (e.g., trypsinogen to trypsin).

3-10. The answer is d. *(Simon et al., pp 163–164.)* In this case, there is a loss of superficial abdominal reflexes, which require that spinal segments T8–T12 be intact. The test for these reflexes is to stroke a quadrant of the abdominal wall with an object such as a wooden stick. The normal response is for the muscle of the quadrant stimulated to contract and for movement of the umbilicus in the direction of the stimulus.

3-11. The answer is b. *(Ganong, pp 391–393, 710. Stead et al., pp 246–249.)* Between 85 and 90% of the filtered phosphate is reabsorbed in the proximal tubule by a sodium-dependent secondary active transport system. The transporter is electrically neutral, requiring two Na^+ molecules for every HPO_4^{2-} molecule that it transports. The transporter is inhibited by parathyroid hormone (PTH). The decreased reabsorption of phosphate results in an increased clearance from the plasma. PTH is released from the parathyroid gland in response to lowered plasma Ca^{2+} concentrations. In addition to inhibiting the reabsorption of phosphate from the proximal tubule, PTH increases the reabsorption of Ca^{2+} from the loop of Henle.

3-12. The answer is c. *(Afifi, pp 91–103. Siegel and Sapru, p 156.)* The patient received a diagnosis of *Brown-Séquard syndrome*, or hemisection of the spinal cord. The lesion is not at the cervical level because motor functions of the upper limbs were considered normal. The examiner can pinpoint the location of the lesion by using the "sensory level," or level at which the loss of pain and temperature begin, by remembering that the lesion affects fibers that have entered the spinal cord one or two levels below it, and then cross to the contralateral side. Therefore, a loss of sensory function at the T10 level indicates a lesion at the T8 or T9 level, a level at which motor deficits may be helpful in diagnosis. In lesions of the thoracic spinal cord, muscles innervated by thoracic nerves are difficult to test. The examiner still expects weakness in the lower extremities, and this helps to make the diagnosis. If the lesion involved the lumbar level, there would be a flaccid paralysis of the lower limb. The disorder could not have been the result of a peripheral nerve injury, because such a possibility could not account for the preservation of pain and temperature in the right leg but with a loss of conscious proprioception associated with that limb. Brown-Séquard syndrome may occur as a result of different types of tumors, infections of the spinal cord, or as a result of a knife or bullet wound.

3-13. The answer is a. *(Kasper, pp 2109–2111. Greenspan, pp 81, 91–92, 257–258. Kierszenbaum, p 504. Kumar, pp 1169–1171.)* The patient is suffering from Hashimoto's thyroiditis in which there is extensive infiltration of the thyroid gland. Autoantibodies develop to thyroglobulin and thyroid peroxidase, an iodine transporter and/or the TSH receptor. In cases where there are autoantibodies to TSH receptor, the TSH receptor activity is blocked, resulting in hypothyroidism compared to the hyperthyroidism, which occurs in Graves' disease (see question 227). The antibodies are to a different site on the receptor, resulting in the different overall effect. $CD8^+$ T cells are also directed against that site. T3 and T4 levels may be elevated early in the disease **(answer b)** process due to disruption of the follicles and release of hormones; however, the overall effect is hypothyroidism. Destruction of thyroid hormone receptors **(answer c)** would lead to hyperthyroidism. Calcitonin is secreted by the C cells in the thyroid and is not affected by the thyroiditis **(answer d)**. Glucocorticoid levels are not elevated **(answer e)**.

3-14. The answer is d. *(Brunton, pp 578–579. Craig, p 327. Katzung, pp 512, 1070t.)* Dextromethorphan is, indeed, chemically related to codeine, but it lacks many effects you probably associate with codeine or other opioids, except one: it has excellent antitussive activity. This cough-suppressant effect presumably occurs via some ill-defined central mechanism, but does not involve agonist actions on opioid receptors. Dextromethorphan does not have analgesic effects (a); alter gut motility (b); or have effects on the bladder musculature that might relieve nocturia. Very high doses of dextromethorphan can cause CNS depression, but regardless of the dose it is not used as a sedative or other agent for controlling symptoms of ADD/ADHD. Finally, unlike codeine and most other opioids, dextromethorphan lacks addictive properties or potential.

3-15. The answer is e. *(Scriver, pp 1521–1551. Murray RK, pp 145–152.)* Under circumstances of intense muscular contraction, the rate of formation of NADH by glycolysis exceeds the capacity of mitochondria to reoxidize it. Consequently, pyruvate produced by glycolysis is reduced to lactate, thereby regenerating NAD^+. Since erythrocytes have no mitochondria, accumulation of lactate occurs normally. Lactate goes to the liver via the blood, is formed into glucose by gluconeogenesis, and then reenters the bloodstream to be reutilized by erythrocytes or muscle. This recycling of lactate to glucose is called the Cori cycle. A somewhat similar phenomenon using alanine generated by muscles during starvation is called the glucose-alanine cycle. All of the other substances listed—oxaloacetate, glycerol, and pyruvate—can be made into glucose by the liver. In muscle, glycogenolysis is synchronized with contraction by epinephrine (through cyclic AMP) and calcium activation of phosphorylase. In those with muscle-specific phosphorylase defects (glycogen storage diseases V and VII), glucose is not mobilized as efficiently from glycogen, causing decreased contractile efficiency (cramping, fatigue), decreased yield of lactate from glycolysis, and maintenance of serum glucose by compensating liver metabolism.

3-16. The answer is c. (*Brunton, pp 503–506, 523. Craig, p 381. Katzung, p 387.*) Vigabatrin (γ-vinyl GABA) is useful in partial seizures. It is an irreversible inhibitor of GABA aminotransferase, an enzyme responsible for the termination of GABA action. This results in accumulation of GABA at synaptic sites, thereby enhancing its effect.

3-17. The answer is e. (*Ganong, pp 706–708. Kasper et al., pp 246–249, 1701, 2312, 2336.*) Clearance is a measure of how much plasma is totally cleared of a substance. It is calculated using the formula

$$\text{Clearance} = U_{\text{uric acid}} \times V/P_{\text{uric acid}} = 36 \text{ mg/dL} \times 1 \text{ mL/min} / 0.6 \text{ mg/dL}$$

$$= 60 \text{ mL/min}$$

The boy's hypouricemia is an inherited defect in the ability to reabsorb uric acid by the anion/urate exchangers on proximal tubule cells rather than an increased secretion of uric acid. Patients with hypouricemia sometimes develop exercise-induced acute renal failure. Although the mechanism is not known, some investigators suggest that uric acid has an important antioxidant role in the kidney and that the oxygen radicals produced during prolonged exercise are responsible for the acute renal failure in patients with low uric acid levels.

3-18. The answer is c. (*Kumar, pp 238–239.*) The combination of trouble swallowing, hypertension, and sclerosis of the skin should raise the possibility of progressive systemic sclerosis (scleroderma), a multisystem disease that involves the cardiovascular, gastrointestinal, cutaneous, musculoskeletal, pulmonary, and renal systems through progressive interstitial fibrosis. Small arterioles in the aforementioned systems show obliteration caused by intimal hyperplasia accompanied by progressive interstitial fibrosis. In the skin, the changes begin in the fingers and hands and consist of sclerotic atrophy, which is characterized by increased dermal collagen, epidermal atrophy, and loss of skin adnexal structures. Two antinuclear antibodies are unique to systemic sclerosis. One is Scl-70, which is found in diffuse progressive systemic sclerosis, and the other is an anticentromere antibody found in the CREST syndrome, a variant of progressive systemic sclerosis. The CREST syndrome is characterized by calcinosis, Raynaud's syndrome (episodic ischemia of digits), esophageal dysmotility, sclerodactyly, and telangiectasia. Pulmonary hypertension and primary biliary cirrhosis are common in the CREST syndrome, but the kidneys are usually spared. In contrast to the histologic findings with systemic sclerosis, a conjunctival biopsy that reveals noncaseating granulomas is suggestive of sarcoidosis; a peripheral nerve biopsy that reveals rare acid-fast bacteria is diagnostic of leprosy; and a temporal artery biopsy that reveals fragmentation of the internal elastic lamina is characteristic of temporal arteritis.

3-19. The answer is a. *(Brooks, pp 642–644. Levinson, pp 333–337. Murray PR—2005, pp 765–769. Ryan, pp 672–683.)* The key diagnostic finding is the morphology of the yeast isolated from the granulomatous, supurative lesions of the lung. *Blastomyces dermatitidis*, which causes blastomycosis, grows in the yeast form in infected tissues. The bud of growing yeast is attached to the parent cell by a broad base. Although the fungi that cause all other diseases listed in the question grow in yeast form in infected tissues, most buds are attached to the parent cell by a narrow base.

3-20. The answer is d. *(Afifi, pp 59–89. Nolte, p 227. Siegel and Sapru, pp 155–157.)* The fact that the disorder affected the neuronal cell bodies of the ventral horn indicates that the patient will present with an LMN paralysis. The affected neurons from L1–L4 innervate the muscles of the lower limb; therefore, the LMN paralysis would affect the leg normally innervated by these neurons.

3-21. The answer is e. *(Junqueira, pp 385–386, 392–393. Kumar, pp 996–1004.)* Tubulointerstitial nephritis uveitis (TINU) is an autoimmune disease in which autoantibodies are targeted against the renal tubular cells. The transmission electron micrograph illustrates a proximal convoluted tubule cell, the primary site for reduction of the tubular fluid volume by reabsorption from the glomerular filtrate. The elaborate microvilli at the apical surface and the extensive endocytic vacuoles are "designed" for protein reabsorption and are the distinguishing features of proximal convoluted tubule cells. Numerous mitochondria, within basal folds, provide energy for transport. In the distal tubule, there are very few microvilli.

The afferent arterioles contain the juxtaglomerular cells, modified arterial smooth muscle cells that produce renin (**answer d**), a major factor in blood pressure regulation. The thin loop of Henle is responsible for the production of the countercurrent multiplier (**answer b**), which allows the kidneys to produce a hyperosmotic medulla. The multiplier moves Na^+ and Cl^- out of the ascending limb (which is impermeable to water) and into the medullary interstitial fluid. Subsequently, the descending limb, which is permeable to water, takes up the Na^+ and Cl^- from the interstitium. The vasa rectae adjust their osmolarity to that of the medulla.

The distal convoluted tubule (DCT) has the highest concentration of Na^+, K^+-ATPase. The DCT pumps Na^+ against a concentration gradient and is relatively impermeable to water, leading to the production of a hypotonic tubular fluid. The distal tubules empty into the connecting and collecting ducts, which are permeable to water under the regulation of ADH (**answer a**). ADH stimulation increases collecting duct permeability to water, allowing the production of hyperosmotic urine. Without ADH, the urine leaving the kidney would be hypo-osmotic. The collecting duct principal cells are the ADH responsive cells and contain fewer mitochondria and basal infoldings than occur in the cells of the distal convoluted tubule. Aldosterone (**answer c**) also acts on the principal cells and secondarily on the thick ascending limb of Henle to increase reabsorption of Nacl.

3-22. The answer is c. (*Murray RK, pp 80–101. Scriver, pp 2261–2296.*) Under conditions of plentiful oxygen (aerobic metabolism), pyruvate formed from glycolysis in the cytosol is metabolized to acetylCoA. Acetyl CoA enters the mitochondria and the citric acid cycle in the conversion of oxaloacetate to citrate, generating NADH and $FADH_2$ reducing equivalents that generate ATP through oxidation in the mitochondrial respiratory chain. In respiratory chain disorders, the disrupted electron transport chain does not function as well, causing more pyruvate to be converted to lactate in muscle with muscle weakness and cramping. Lactate from exercising muscle is normally converted to glucose by the liver, but excess lactate produced in severe respiratory chain disorders accumulates in serum to lower the pH (acidosis). Mitochondria are called the powerhouses of the cell since they contain the citric acid cycle and the respiratory chain that generates abundant ATP through oxidative phosphorylation.

3-23. The answer is b. (*Ross and Pawlina, p 787. Young, pp 341, 351–355. Junqueira, pp 444–451. Kierszenbaum, p 578.*) The secretory phase of the menstrual cycle depends on progesterone secretion and follows the proliferative (follicular) phase. The menstrual phase occurs after the secretory phase. During the follicular phase (approximately days 4 to 16), estrogen produced by the ovaries drives cell proliferation in the base of endometrial glands and the uterine stroma. The proliferative phase culminates with ovulation. The secretory phase (approximately days 16 to 25) is characterized by high progesterone levels from the corpus luteum, a tortuous appearance of the uterine glands, and apocrine secretion by the gland cells. During this phase, maximum endometrial thickness occurs. The menstrual phase (approximately days 26 to 30) is characterized by decreased glandular secretion and eventual glandular degeneration because of decreased production of both progesterone and estrogen by the theca lutein cells. Contraction of coiled arteries and arterioles leads to ischemia and necrosis of the stratum functionale. The events of the menstrual cycle are shown in the figure below.

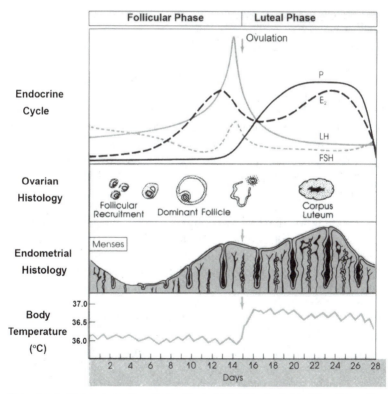

(Reproduced, with permission, from Kasper DL, et al (eds.). Harrison's Principles of Internal Medicine, 16th ed. New York, NY: McGraw-Hill, 2005: 2201.)

3-24. The answer is D. *(Siegel and Sapru, pp 225, 233–235.)* The cranial nerve in question is the glossopharyngeal nerve (cranial nerve IX). As noted in answer to the previous question, the special visceral efferent component supplies the muscles of the pharynx and the general visceral efferent component supplies the parotid gland. Therefore, damage to this nerve would affect swallowing and gag reflex as well as one's ability to salivate. This nerve exits the brain at the level of the upper medulla in a lateral position just caudal to cranial nerve VIII.

3-25. The answer is d. *(Brunton, pp 860–862. Craig, pp 155, 228–229. Katzung, pp 172–174.)* Hydralazine predominately dilates arterioles, with negligible effects on venous capacitance. It typically lowers blood pressure "so well" that it can trigger the following two unwanted cardiovascular responses that need to be dealt with:

1. Reflex cardiac stimulation (involving the baroreceptor reflex) is common, and it is typically managed with a β-adrenergic blocker (unless it is contraindicated). An alternative approach would be to use either verapamil or diltiazem (but not a dihydropyridine-type calcium channel blocker such as nifedipine, which would not suppress—and, in fact might aggravate—the reflex cardiac stimulation).

2. The renin-angiotensin-aldosterone system is activated. One consequence of this unwanted compensatory response would be increased renal sodium retention that would expand circulating fluid volume and counteract hydralazine's blood pressure–lowering effects. This is typically managed with a diuretic. A thiazide often is sufficient to combat the renal sodium retention, but a more efficacious diuretic (loop diuretic) may be necessary.

Captopril (or another ACE inhibitor, or an angiotensin receptor blocker such as losartan) might be a suitable add-on (it would cause synergistic antihypertensive effects and prevent aldosterone-mediated renal effects). However, combining it with nifedipine (dihydropyridine) is irrational. As noted above, given the "pure" vasodilator actions of nifedipine and no cardiac-depressing activity whatsoever (as we get with verapamil or diltiazem), the net effect on heart rate would be either no suppression of the tachycardia or a worsening of it.

Digoxin, alone or with virtually any other drug, is not rational. There is no indication that there is need for inotropic support in this patient.

Spironolactone, alone or with digoxin, would be of little benefit. One could argue that by virtue of the spironolactone's ability to induce diuresis by blocking aldosterone's renal tubular effects, it would counteract hydralazine's ability to lead to renal sodium retention. That may be true, but spironolactone (with or without digoxin) will do nothing desirable to the unwanted tachycardia.

Nitroglycerin would add to hydralazine's antihypertensive effects, but it would probably aggravate the reflex cardiac stimulation and also increase the unwanted renal response (via a hemodynamic mechanism).

Both triamterene and amiloride are potassium-sparing diuretics. The combination of two diuretics in this class is generally irrational (it can lead to hyperkalemia). Either might beneficially combat a propensity for renal sodium retention in response to hydralazine. But, as with any diuretic alone, either or both would do little if anything to control the cardiac response.

Vitamin K was included as a foil. If you are associating hydralazine with some vitamin-related problem, you should be thinking of vitamin B_6 (pyridoxine): hydralazine can interfere with B_6 metabolism, causing such symptoms as peripheral neuritis, and so prophylactic B_6 supplementation is often used along with long-term hydralazine therapy.

3-26. The answer is d. (*Adams, p 1383.*) Dysarthria is slurred speech, occurring from lesions affecting innervation of the tongue, lips, and palate. We are given evidence that his tongue was weak in that it pointed to the right. The interruption of fibers traveling to the hypoglossal nerve from the left side eventually innervates the right genioglossus muscle, which pulls the tongue to the left. Dysarthria is a motor phenomenon, unlike aphasia, which is a disruption of language. Language is primarily generated in the cerebral cortex; therefore, because the lesion spares the cortex, there were no signs of aphasia.

3-27 The answer is e. (*Brooks, pp 645–647. Levinson, pp 338–341. Murray PR—2005, pp 781–786. Ryan, pp 660–664.*) C. albicans is the most important species of *Candida* and causes thrush, vaginitis, skin and nail infections, and other infections. It is part of the normal flora of skin, mouth, GI tract, and vagina. It appears in tissues as an oval budding yeast or elongated pseudohyphae. It grows well on laboratory media and is identified by germ-tube formation. A vaccine is not available, and serologic and skin tests have little value.

3-28. The answer is e. (*Brunton, pp 272–275, 864. Craig, pp 230–231. Katzung, p 175.*) Nitroprusside is likely to elicit baroreceptor reflex-mediated rises of heart rate and contractility. It may be significant and dangerous for any patient, more so for patients with ischemic heart disease, and potentially deadly for patients with aneurysms, such as our patient. For aortic aneurysm patients, the problem is not the rise of heart rate, but rather of left ventricular contractility (left ventricular dP/dt). The bounding aortic pressure pulse with each systole favors rupture of the aneurysm, and use of a β blocker such as propranolol is an effective and common way to minimize the risk (and, of course, reflex cardiac stimulation overall). Atropine (a) is an illogical choice. It will increase heart rate (and, indirectly, contractility) further by removing parasympathetic tone on the SA node. Diazoxide (b) is a rapidly acting antihypertensive/vasodilator, given as an IV bolus in situations where safe nitroprusside use (and the invasive monitoring it normally requires) is not practical. Diazoxide, like nitroprusside, triggers reflex cardiac stimulation as blood pressure falls. The drug also has some direct cardiac-stimulating effects (not involving antimuscarinic or adrenergic-agonist effects). Diazoxide also tends to cause hyperglycemia (an oral dosage form of the drug is sometimes prescribed to manage blood glucose levels in patients prone to developing hypoglycemia.) Furosemide (c) is a loop diuretic that is an important adjunct in such conditions as hypertensive crisis due to volume overload, heart failure, and acute pulmonary edema. However, the volume depletion and hypotension it would cause would exacerbate the clinical situation we have described. The prompt diuresis and fall of blood pressure may also trigger unwanted baroreceptor-mediated cardiac stimulation. Phentolamine (d), an α-adrenergic blocker, would be irrational. It is a powerful vasodilator (indeed, it is often used for vasoconstrictor drug-induced hypertensive emergencies) that would add to—unfavorably—nitroprusside's prompt antihypertensive effect and the reflex cardiac stimulation that is so dangerous for our patient.

3-29. The answer is d. (*Adams, pp 802–805. Afifi, pp 163–168, 180–182. Siegel and Sapru, p 190.*) This is an example of the locked-in syndrome, or pseudocoma, caused by an infarction of the basilar pons. Because the tracts mediating movement of the limbs and face run through this region, the patient is unable to move the face, as well as both arms and legs. Consciousness and eye movements are preserved. The pontine basilar pons is supplied mainly by the basilar artery. Complete occlusion of this artery causes deficits on both sides, since this artery supplies both sides of the pons. Sensory loss, including loss of proprioception (feeling the movement of a limb), also occurs as a result of damage to the medial lemniscus bilaterally. This tract contains fibers from the dorsal columns and also runs through the pontine tegmentum. Patients with the locked-in syndrome are often mistaken for comatose patients due to their inability to move or speak. If the lesion spares the reticular formation, an area mediating consciousness in the pons, the patient will remain alert.

3-30. The answer is b. *(Waxman, pp 169–170.)* The middle cerebral artery supplies a large portion of cerebral cortex, including portions of the frontal, parietal, and temporal lobes. These regions include the Broca's and Wernicke's areas and the precentral motor and postcentral sensory regions. Decreased blood flow in these regions explains the observed motor and sensory deficits. The anterior choroidal artery **(answer a)** is a branch of the internal carotid artery and is primarily distributed to the basal ganglia, hippocampus, and choroid plexus of the lateral ventricle. The posterior communicating artery **(answer c)** connects the internal carotid and vertebral arterial systems. The ophthalmic artery **(answer d)** is a direct branch of the internal carotid artery that enters the orbit along with the optic nerve. Although the anterior cerebral artery **(answer e)** has a wide distribution and anastomoses with branches of both the middle and posterior cerebral arteries, it primarily supplies medial and superior portions of the cortex.

3-31. The answer is e. *(Ganong, pp 313, 509, 544–545. Stead et al., p 374.)* Vitamin K is a fat-soluble vitamin produced by intestinal bacteria that is essential for maintaining normal clotting of blood. The vitamin is essential for hepatic synthesis of prothrombin and factors VII, IX, and X. Common causes of vitamin K deficiency include cholestasis, and factors that limit fat absorption.

3-32. The answer is c. *(Brooks, pp 514–519. Levinson, pp 294–296. Murray PR—2005, p 703. Ryan, p 591.)* Saint Louis encephalitis virus has structural and biologic characteristics in common with other Flaviviruses. It is the most important arboviral disease in North America. Saint Louis encephalitis virus was first isolated from mosquitoes in California. Patients who contract the disease usually present with one of three clinical manifestations: febrile headache, aseptic meningitis, or clinical encephalitis.

3-33. The answer is a. *(Parslow, pp 221–223. Levinson, pp 65, 117–118, 227, 437–438, 439.)* ELISA (enzyme-linked immunosorbent assay) methods can be used to detect either antigens or antibodies. If antigen is to be detected, then specific antibody is initially bound to the plate (see A in the diagram presented with the question). If antibody is to be detected, then antigen is bound to the solid phase. The bound antigen and antibody then "captures" the analyte to be detected. One of the major causes for high background in

ELISA tests is the failure to wash off unbound antigen or antibody (see B in the diagram presented with the question). ELISA is routinely used to screen patient sera for different antibodies (including anti–HIV-1 antibodies). In this case, the well is initially coated with HIV-1 antigen, and the patient sera is tested for anti–HIV-1 antibodies.

3-34. The answer is e. (*Kandel, pp 919–927. Siegel and Sapru, pp 468–470.*) The pyramidal cell is a cell in the cortex that uses glutamate, an excitatory neurotransmitter, whereas most other types of cortical neurons use GABA, an inhibitory neurotransmitter. The spike, one identifying feature of an epileptic seizure seen on an EEG recorded on the scalp, is initiated by a depolarization shift, which is thought to be generated by EPSPs.

3-35. The answer is a. (*Moore and Dalley, pp 973, 1137.*) This condition is most likely due to an aneurysm of the left posterior cerebral artery compressing cranial nerve III. The woman's symptoms, ptosis of the upper eyelid, an eye that is rotated down (because superior oblique muscle, innervated by CN IV is still functioning) and out (because the lateral rectus muscle, innervated by CN VI is still functioning) with a dilated pupil (because sympathetics, which innervate the dilator pupili muscles are still V_3 functioning) are all consistent with loss of function of cranial nerve III. An aneurysm in either the posterior cerebral or superior cerebellar artery often can compress cranial nerve III as it exits the midbrain. An aneursym of the right anterior cerebral artery (**answer b**) would be very unlikely to cause a problem for the left third cranial nerve. A tumor within the left optic canal (**answer c**) would effect the left optic nerve which passes through it. Cranial nerve III passes into the orbit through the superior orbital fissure along with CN IV, V_1, and VI. Neither glaucoma (**answer d**) nor parotid gland tumor (**answer e**) would present with those symptoms.

3-36. The answer is d. (*Brunton, pp 726–727. Craig, pp 455, 466–467. Katzung, pp 329–330.*) The precise mechanism of action by which nedocromil or the related drug cromolyn works is not known, but the most likely explanation is "stabilization" of immunologically sensitized mast cells. This may involve calcium channel blockade: calcium entry into mast cells is a critical step in their immunologically mediated activation. There is no direct or indirect interaction with antigens (c) or mast cell antibodies, but the drug does suppress the release of preformed mast cell mediators. Nedocromil and cromolyn have no histamine receptor-blocking activity (a), nor vasoconstrictor or other decongestant effects (b). They do not inhibit synthesis of histamine, leukotrienes, or other vasodepressor, bronchoconstrictor, or inflammatory mediators in mast cells or elsewhere.

3-37. The answer is a. (*Murray RK, pp 122–129, 173–179. Scriver, pp 2297–2326.*) Fatty acid oxidation is a major source of energy after glycogen is depleted during fasting. Fatty acids are first coupled with coenzyme A, transferred for mitochondrial import as acylcarnitines, and degraded in steps that remove two carbons. The fatty acyl CoA dehydrogenases, enoyl hydratases, hydroxyacyl CoA dehydrogenases, and thiolases that carry out each oxidation step are present in three groups with specifities for very long/long, medium, and short chain fatty acyl esters. As would be expected, deficiencies of long-chain oxidizing enzymes have more severe consequences than those for short chains since they impair many more cycles of two-carbon removal. Long chain deficiencies may be lethal in the newborn period, while medium or short chain deficiencies may be undetected until a child goes without food for a prolonged time and must resort to extensive fatty acid oxidation for energy. Medium chain coenzyme A dehydrogenase (MCAD) deficiency (201450) can be fatal if not recognized, and sometimes presents as Sudden Unexplained Death Syndrome (SUDS—usually at older ages than Sudden Infant Death Syndrome—SIDS—that is mostly from respiratory problems). The deficit of acetyl CoA from fatty acid oxidation impacts gluconeogenesis with hypoglycemia, and the energy deficit leads to heart, liver, and muscle disease that may be lethal. Unlike most causes of hypoglycemia, the impaired fatty acid oxidation does not produce ketones (nonketotic hypoglycemia). Carnitine is tied up as medium chain acylcarnitines and is secondarily deficient in fatty acid oxidation disorders. Rare primary carnitine deficiencies (as in answer option e) impair oxidation of all fatty acids because they cannot be imported into mitochondria.

3-38. The answer is b. (*Murray RK, pp 237–241. Scriver, pp 2961–3062.*) The porphyrias are a group of inborn errors that affect synthesis of porphyrins, the precursors of heme in hemoglobin. Defective synthesis of heme would not elevate heme breakdown products of the heme catabolic pathway, including bilirubin to conjugated bilirubin diglucuronide (in liver), bilirubin diglucuronide to urobilinogen and stercobilin (by bacteria in stool), and reabsorption of urobilinogen to be excreted in urine as urobilin. Delta-aminolevulinic acid (ALA) is synthesized from succinyl CoA and glycine followed by condensation of two ALA molecules to form porphobilinogen (PBG) with a 5-member pyrrole ring. Four molecules of PBG are converted to the four-ring uroporphyrin by hydroxymethylbilane synthase, the primary defect in acute intermittent porphyria (176000). Deficiencies in other enzymes of the pathway from ALA to heme cause symptoms varying from anemia to photosensitivity to the well-known but rarely encountered presentation with abdominal pain and neuropsychiatric symptoms.

3-39. The answer is c. *(Moore and Dalley, p 1019.)* He suffers from sinusitis, which has eroded through the wall on the frontal sinus, and since the frontalis muscle is *not* attached to bone, allows pus to leak into the upper eyelid. Inflammation of the mucous membrane that lines the sinuses may sometimes lead to a build up of pus that can block the normal drainage pathways. If pressure builds, erosion of the bony wall of the sinus can occur. In this instance, the anterior wall of the frontal sinus was compromised and pus escaped into the forehead and into the upper eyelid, since the frontalis muscle, a normal barrier, attaches only into skin of the forehead. In order to allow movement, the skin of the eyelid is only attached to underlying structures by loose areolar connective tissue, through which infections easily spread. Intravenous antibiotics were initiated. The swelling spontaneously reduced after the first week of treatment and no visible defects were noted 1 month later. Trigeminal neuralgia or tic douloureux **(answers a and b)** is characterized by sudden sharp pains over the distribution of one or more branches of the trigeminal nerve. Although pain is perceived within the ophthalmic division, the teenager would *not* suffer from sudden sharp twinges of pain, rather a dull constant pain from swollen tissue. Bell's palsy **(answer d)** is generally caused by a herpes simplex virus infection of the facial nerve within the facial canal that causes unilateral facial paralysis, which would limit one's ability to close the upper eyelid, *not* raise it. A sty **(answer e)** is an inflammation of the sebaceous gland, associated with each eyelash or cilia. A chalazion is an inflammation of a Meibomian or tarsal gland, which lies on the inner surface of the eyelid. This could cause a bulge in the upper eyelid but does *not* fit with the other clinical findings.

3-40. The answer is a. *(Brooks, pp 214, 315. Levinson, pp 179–180, 484s. Murray PR—2005, p 398. Ryan, p 479.)* While the essential information (i.e., the evidence that the child in question was scratched by a cat) is missing, the clinical presentation points to a number of diseases, including cat-scratch disease (CSD). Until recently, the etiologic agent of CSD was unknown. Evidence indicated that it was a pleomorphic, rod-shaped bacterium that had been named *Afipia.* It was best demonstrated in the affected lymph node by a silver impregnation stain. However, it now appears that *Afipia* causes relatively few cases of CSD and that the free-living rickettsia primarily responsible is *Rochalimaea henselae,* which has recently been renamed *B. henselae.*

3-41. The answer is d. (*Kumar, pp 686–690. Rubin, pp 1140–1147.*) The diagnosis of Hodgkin's disease (HD) depends on the clinical findings added to the total histologic picture, which includes the presence of binucleated giant cells with prominent acidophilic "owl-eye" nucleoli known as Reed-Sternberg (RS) cells. These malignant cells characteristically stain with both the CD15 and CD30 immunoperoxidase stains. Note that cells similar in appearance to RS cells may also be seen in infectious mononucleosis, mycosis fungoides, and other conditions. Thus, while RS cells are necessary for histologic confirmation of the diagnosis of Hodgkin's disease, they must be present in the appropriate histologic setting of the different types of HD, which includes lymphocyte predominance, nodular sclerosis, mixed cellularity, and lymphocyte depletion. The most common type of HD is the nodular sclerosis variant. This type is characterized morphologically by the presence of the lacunar variant of RS cells and by bands of fibrous tissue that divide the lymph node into nodules. Unlike the other subtypes of Hodgkin's disease, it is more common in females. Young adults are classically affected and the disease typically involves the cervical, supraclavicular, or mediastinal lymph nodes. Involvement of extranodal lymphoid tissue is unusual. Variant RS cells with a multilobed, puffy nucleus ("popcorn" cells) are seen in the lymphocyte-predominant subtype.

3-42 The answer is e. (*Brooks, p 148. Levinson, pp 32–38. Murray PR—2005, p 193.*) Organisms may be transmitted in a number of ways, such as by air, food, hands, sexual contact, and infected needles. However, for each disease or disease category, there is usually a portal of entry not always unique to the organism. The skin is a tough integument and, infact, is resistant to most infectious organisms except those that may break down human skin. Breaches of the skin as by wounds, burns, and the like predispose patients to a variety of infections such as tetanus caused by wound contamination with spores of *C. tetani,* or direct infection by *Staphylococcus, Streptococcus,* or gram-negative rods (such as *Serratia* or *Pseudomonas*). The respiratory tract is a common portal of entry to such airborne organisms as *M. tuberculosis.* This is why respiratory precautions must be taken when patients are harboring viable *M. tuberculosis.* The gastrointestinal tract is usually infected from ingestion of contaminated food or water (*Shigella, Salmonella, Campylobacter*) or by an alteration of the normal microbial flora such as with *C. difficile* disease. The genital tract may become infected either by sexual contact or by alteration of the genital environment, as often occurs with yeast infections. Several bacteria such as *N. gonorrhoeae*, *Chlamydia*, and *T. pallidum* are transmitted by direct sexual contact with infected partners.

3-43. The answer is b. *(Afifi, pp 154–156. Nolte, pp 340–342. Siegel and Sapru, pp 184–186.)* The principal ascending pathway of the auditory system listed in this question (that was affected by the stroke) is the lateral lemniscus. It transmits information from the cochlear nuclei to the inferior colliculus. The trapezoid body is a commissure that contains some of the fibers of the lateral lemniscus that cross from the cochlear nuclei of one side of the brainstem en route to the inferior colliculus of the other side. The trapezoid body is present at the level of the caudal pons. The brachium of the superior colliculus, trigeminal lemniscus, and medial lemniscus do not transmit auditory sensory information.

3-44. The answer is d. *(Moore and Dalley, pp 120–124.)* The lobe indicated by the asterisk is the left upper (or superior) lobe. The general orientation when viewing CTs is that the observer is looking up from the patient's feet. Therefore, the patient's left is on your right, thus it can't be a part of the right lung **(answers a, b, c)**. In addition, on the left, the inferior (lower) lobe **(answer e)** begins relatively high in the thoracic cavity and is posterior to the upper lobe.

3-45. The answer is e. *(Ganong, pp 474–475. Kasper et al., p 231.)* The colon is the major site for the generation and absorption of short-chain fatty acids. They are products of bacterial metabolism of undigested complex carbohydrates derived from fruits and vegetables. In addition to exhibiting trophic effects on the colonic mucosa, they are believed to promote sodium absorption from the colon. The mechanism of action remains controversial.

3-46. The answer is c. *(Ganong, pp 477–478.)* Iron is transported in the blood bound to the β globulin, transferrin. Excess iron is stored in all cells, but especially in hepatocytes where it combines with apoferritin. The stored form is called ferritin. The rate of iron absorption is extremely slow, with a maximum of only a few milligrams per day. Iron is absorbed primarily in the ferrous form. Therefore, ferrous iron compounds, rather than ferric compounds, are effective in treating iron deficiency.

3-47. The answer is b. *(Ganong, pp 487–495. Stead et al., pp 121–123.)* Somatostatin, located within the gastric antral mucosa, is the principal paracrine secretion involved in the inhibitory feedback of gastric acid secretion by parietal cells. Somatostatin has a short half-life of several minutes, which limits its clinical use, but the analog octreotide (Sandostatin) should be administered subcutaneously to inhibit the secretion of gastrin and gastric acid and visceral blood flow in patients with bleeding esophageal varices secondary to portal hypertension, after stabilizing with IV fluids, as acute variceal bleeds have a 50% mortality. Acid secretion is stimulated by acetylcholine (via M_3 muscarinic receptors), histamine (via H_2 receptors) and gastrin (directly via gastrin receptors and principally via stimulation of histamine secretion by enterochromaffin-like [ECL] cells). Gastrin secretion is stimulated by the amino acids and peptides produced by pepsin's action in protein digestion.

3-48. The answer is b. *(Ganong, p 490. Kasper et al., pp 1741–1742. Stead et al., pp 106–107.)* Important inhibitory neurotransmitters in the gastrointestinal tract include vasoactive intestinal peptide and nitric oxide. Relaxation of gastrointestinal smooth muscle occurs following activation of nonadrenergic, noncholinergic (NANC) enteric nerve fibers. Acetylcholine, substance P, and dopamine are excitatory neurotransmitters. Somatostatin is a paracrine secretory product with multiple effects on gastrointestinal function.

3-49. The answer is d. *(Ganong, pp 475–477. Stead et al., pp 139–140.)* Most water and electrolyte absorption occurs in the jejunum, with the duodenum serving primarily as the site of osmotic equilibration of chyme. Water absorption is passive and occurs as the direct result of active sodium absorption. The small intestine and colon absorb approximately 9 to 12 L of fluid per 24-hour period, most of which comes from gastrointestinal secretions. In contrast to the small intestine, the colon has a limited capacity to absorb water (approximately 3 to 6 L per day); most water absorption in the colon occurs in the proximal colon.

3-50. The answer is c. *(Ganong, pp 500–503, 782–783. Kasper et al., pp 238–243, 1764–1765, 1831–1833. Stead et al., pp 124–127.)* Infectious hepatitis is a systemic infection predominantly affecting the liver. When jaundice appears, serum bilirubin rises, and, in most instances, total bilirubin is equally divided between the conjugated (direct) and unconjugated (indirect) fractions. The bilirubin in serum represents a balance between input from production of bilirubin and hepatic/biliary removal of the pigment. Hyperbilirubinemia may result from (1) overproduction of bilirubin; (2) impaired uptake, conjugation, or removal of bilirubin; or (3) regurgitation of unconjugated or conjugated bilirubin from damaged hepatocytes or bile ducts. Alkaline phosphatase, which is excreted in bile, increases in patients with jaundice due to bile duct obstruction, but generally not when the jaundice is due to hepatocellular disease. Bile acids are synthesized in the liver by a series of enzymatic steps that also involve cholesterol catabolism. Liver disease decreases bile acid synthesis.

Block 4

Answers

4-1. The answer is e. (*Kumar, pp 606–607. Rubin, pp 581–583.*) Restrictive (constrictive) cardiomyopathy is associated in the United States with amyloidosis and endocardial fibroelastosis. The latter disorder is so named because of the infiltration and deposition of material in the endomyocardium and the layering of collagen and elastin over the endocardium. This deposition affects the ability of the ventricles to accommodate blood volume during diastole. Grossly this abnormality has a "cream cheese" appearance. Endocardial fibroelastosis occurs mainly in infants during the first 2 years of life; there may be associated aortic coarctation, ventricular septal defects, mitral valve defects, and other abnormalities. In contrast, endomyocardial fibrosis (not fibroelastosis) is a form of restrictive cardiomyopathy that is found mainly in young adults and children in Southeast Asia and Africa. It differs from endocardial fibroelastosis in the United States in that elastic fibers are not present.

4-2. The answer is a. (*Lewis, pp 241–266. Scriver, pp 3–45.*) Aneuploidy involves extra or missing chromosomes that do not arise as increments of the haploid chromosome number n and thus would fit the 90,XX cell line since tetraploidy without aneuploidy would imply a 92,XXXX or 92,XXYY karyotype. Polyploidy involves multiples of n, such as triploidy (3n = 69,XXX) or tetraploidy (4n = 92,XXXX). Diploidy (46,XX) and haploidy (23,X) are normal karyotypes in gametes and somatic cells, respectively. A 92,XXXX/90,XX karyotype represents mosaicism with a tetraploid cell line and an aneuploid line with tetraploidy minus two X chromosomes, which was observed in a patient with features of Turner syndrome. The mental disability, unusual in Turner syndrome, may reflect the usual trend towards greater severity when sex chromosome aneuploidy involves more extra chromosomes (e.g., 47,XXY Klinefelter to 48,XXXY and 49,XXXXY Klinefelter variants).

4-3. The answer is d. (*Ganong, pp 542–544. Kasper et al., p 666. Stead et al., p 160.*) The citrate ion has three anionic carboxylate groups that avidly chelate calcium and reduce the concentration of free calcium in blood. Because free calcium (Ca^{2+}) is required for multiple steps in both coagulation pathways, citrate is a useful anticoagulant in vitro. The citrate ion is rapidly metabolized; thus, blood anticoagulated with citrate can be infused into the body without untoward effects. Oxalate, another calcium-chelating anticoagulant, is toxic to cells.

4-4. The answer is b. *(Brooks, pp 305–306. Levinson, pp 145–146, 478s. Murray PR—2005, pp 422–425. Ryan, pp 324–325.)* B. fragilis is a constituent of normal intestinal flora and readily causes wound infections often mixed with aerobic isolates. These anaerobic, gram-negative rods are uniformly resistant to aminoglycosides and usually to penicillin as well. Reliable laboratory identification may require multiple analytical techniques. Generally, wound exudates smell bad owing to production of organic acids by such anaerobes as B. fragilis. Black exudates or a black pigment (heme) in the isolated colony is usually a characteristic of *Bacteroides* (*Porphyromonas*) *melaninogenicus*, not B. fragilis. Potent neurotoxins are synthesized by the gram-positive anaerobes such as C. tetani and C. botulinum.

4-5. The answer is d. *(Brooks, pp 349–356. Levinson, pp 176–178. Murray PR—2005, pp 449–456. Ryan, pp 475–476.)* The disease described is epidemic typhus or louse-borne typhus. It is caused by R. prowazekii and is spread by the human body louse, *Pediculus humanus*. Lice obviously occur most readily in unsanitary conditions brought on by war or natural disasters, where normal healthy living conditions are unavailable. Rickettsial diseases respond to tetracycline treatment and vector control. The organisms replicate in endothelial cells, resulting in vasculitis. Recrudescent disease (recurrence in later years) has been demonstrated in people exposed to epidemic typhus during World War II. This form of disease is generally milder, and convalescence is shorter.

4-6. The answer is c. *(Adams, pp 43–48, 1312–1318. Siegel and Sapru, pp 70, 74.)* This patient does not have a UMN lesion (spinal cord or above) because of the absent reflexes and ascending paralysis bilaterally involving all of the extremities. Lesions in the brain almost always give unilateral findings, and spinal cord lesions provide clues which identify the distinct level of spinal cord involvement. The damage cannot be in the muscle, because the patient has sensory involvement as well. This case is an example of Guillain-Barré syndrome, or an inflammatory disease of the peripheral nerve resulting from demyelination. Inflammatory cells are found within the nerves, as well as segmental demyelination and some degree of Wallerian degeneration. This damage can cause an ascending paralysis and sensory loss, affecting the arms, face, and legs. The CSF often has a high protein level, making a spinal tap a useful test for the diagnosis of Guillain-Barré syndrome. Nerve conduction studies are also helpful in making the diagnosis. Most neurologists believe Guillain-Barré syndrome to be an immunological reaction directed against the peripheral nerve, and some patients have a history of having had some type of infection prior to developing Guillain-Barré syndrome. However, a clear-cut cause is rarely found. Despite a known cause, most patients recover from Guillain-Barré syndrome, although the speed of recovery varies. Treatment is currently available (administration of gamma globulin), and, if instituted early in the course of the disease, decrease in the length of the illness is possible.

4-7. The answer is d. (*Murray, pp 14–20. Scriver, pp 1971–2006. Lewis, pp 185–204.*) Leucine and isoleucine have nonpolar methyl groups as side chains. As for any amino acid, titration curves obtained by noting the change in pH over the range of 1–14 would show a pK of about 2 for the primary carboxyl group and about 9.5 for the primary amino group; there would be no additional pK for an ionizable side chain. Recall that the pK is the point of maximal buffering capacity when the amounts of charged and uncharged species are equal (see answer to question 104). Aspartic and glutamic acids (second carboxyl group), histidine (imino group), and glutamine (second amino group) all have ionizable side chains that would give an additional pK on the titration curve. The likely diagnosis here is maple syrup urine disease, which involves elevated isoleucine, leucine, and valine together with their ketoacid derivatives. The ketoacid derivatives cause the acidosis, and the fever suggests that the metabolic imbalance was worsened by an infection.

4-8. The answer is c. (*Afifi, pp 125–133. Martin, pp 42–44. Siegel and Sapru, pp 233–235.*) The axons of the nucleus ambiguus of cranial nerve X innervate the soft palate and pharynx. As noted in Question 204, damage to these neurons would frequently cause dysphagia, hoarseness, and paralysis of the soft palate.

4-9. The answer is b. (*Moore and Dalley, pp 270–271.*) Meckel's (ileal) diverticuli are the most common congenital abnormality of the digestive system. They are a remnant of the herniation and rotation of the midgut and at times the diverticulum remains attached to the umbilicus by a connective tissue stalk, as is mostly likely the case here. The diverticulum generally extends 2 inches from the ileum; about 2 ft from the ileocecal valve and usually manifests itself by bleeding prior to the first 2 years of life. There may be two types of ectopic tissue present in the diverticulum: either acid secreting epithelium (stomach; detected with radioactive technetium injected into the venous blood stream which then accumulates within the diverticulum) or pancreatic epithelium. (The rule of "2" helps remind you of the characteristics of Meckel's diverticulum.) The appendix (**answer a**) is a diverticulum off the cecum, *not* the ileum. Diverticuli (**answer c**) can cause blood in the stool but would be extremely rare in a toddler. Internal hemorrhoids (**answer d**) would generally be detected in a rectal exam, especially in a toddler and is *not* associated with "currant jelly" stools. The blood would more likely be black if a duodenal ulcer (**answer e**) were present, which would also be very rare in a toddler.

4-10. The answer is b. (*Kumar, pp 588–591. McPhee, pp 281–283.*) Aortic stenosis (AS) is usually the result of a bicuspid aortic valve (AV), degenerative calcification of a bicuspid valve, or rheumatic heart disease. Patients with aortic stenosis may present with angina (chest pain), syncopal episodes with exertion, and heart failure. Angina results from the mismatch between increased oxygen demand of the hypertrophied left ventricle (LV) and decreased blood flow, while syncope results from the inability to increase stroke volume as necessary with a stenotic AV. AS is the most common valvular disease that is associated with angina and syncope. The characteristic heart murmur of AS is a crescendo-decrescendo midsystolic ejection murmur that has a paradoxically split S_2. In order to pump the blood into the aorta across a stenotic AV, the pressure in the LV must be much greater than the resultant pressure in the aorta. In order to produce this increased pressure, the LV undergoes concentric hypertrophy, which increases contractility. This concentric hypertrophy also makes the wall of the LV stiffer (decreased compliance). This stiff LV is unable to dilate until the time the LV starts to fail.

4-11. The answer is b. (*Ganong, pp 505–506. Kasper et al., pp 2220–2226.*) Removal of the terminal ileum can lead to diarrhea and steatorrhea. The terminal ileum contains specialized cells responsible for the absorption of primary and secondary bile salts by active transport. Bile salts are necessary for adequate digestion and absorption of fat. In the absence of the terminal ileum there will be an increase in the amounts of bile acids and fatty acids delivered to the colon. Fats and bile salts in the colon increase the water content of the feces by promoting the influx (secretion) of water into the lumen of the colon. Amino acids are absorbed in the jejunum. Iron is primarily absorbed in the duodenum. Gastrointestinal neuroendocrine tumors are derived from the diffuse neuroendocrine system of the GI tract, which is composed of amine- and acid-producing cells with different hormonal profiles, depending on the site of origin. The tumors they produce are generally divided into carcinoid tumors (ectodermal stem cells) and pancreatic endocrine tumors. One third of all primary gut tumors are carcinoid. Carcinoid tumors are frequently classified according to their anatomic area of origin (foregut, midgut, hindgut). Small intestinal (midgut) carcinoid tumors arise from the argentaffin cells of the crypts of Lieberkühn in the terminal ileum, and have a high serotonin content. Small intestinal carcinoids are the most common cause of the carcinoid syndrome (classic triad: cutaneous flushing, diarrhea, bronchospasm, right heart valvular lesions), which is manifest when they metastasize, but only occurs in 5 to 10% of carcinoid tumors.

4-12. The answer is d. (*Brooks, pp 155, 225. Levinson, pp 44, 104. Murray PR—2005, pp 228–233. Ryan, pp 263–264.*) Certain strains of staphylococci elaborate an enterotoxin that is frequently responsible for food poisoning. Typically, the toxin is produced when staphylococci grow on foods rich in carbohydrates and is present in the food when it is consumed. The resulting gastroenteritis is dependent only on the ingestion of toxin and not on bacterial multiplication in the gastrointestinal tract. Characteristic symptoms are nausea, vomiting, abdominal cramps, and explosive diarrhea. The illness rarely lasts more than 24 hours.

4-13. The answer is a. (*Brunton, pp 164, 269–270, 855, 857; Craig, p 231; Katzung, pp 146–147.*) The figure approximates what is likely to happen following administration of a β blocker to a patient with a pheochromocytoma.

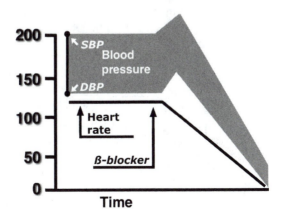

To answer this question correctly you must integrate your basic knowledge of both autonomic pharmacology and cardiovascular physiology. With a pheochromocytoma we have what might be described as "massive" amounts of catecholamines—mainly epinephrine—being released from the tumor into the bloodstream. Germane to our problem, then, is excessive stimulation of cardiac rate, contractility, impulse conduction, and automaticity (β_1); intense vasoconstriction (α); and vasodilation in some vascular beds (β_2).

Nonetheless, while the patient we've described is not at all healthy, he is still alive before we give the β blocker. But what happens after we give the β blocker is critical. The β blocker does nothing to block the α-mediated vasoconstriction, so in terms of only vascular effects BP will remain very high. If you wish to opine that blocking β_2-mediated vasodilation will raise BP a bit, that's fine; we've shown that in the figure. (Remember: Usually effective doses of a β blocker will either lower BP [most common response], or not affect it at all, in patients with essential hypertension. If pressure rises in response to a β blocker, *suspect pheochromocytoma*.)

Nonetheless, there will not be a sudden and significant rise or normalization of BP and/or cardiac function (b, c, d). Likewise, heart rate will not rise significantly (e); it can't: the β_1 receptors necessary for that to occur are blocked.

Next you must recall that the inotropic state of the heart (i.e., of the left ventricle, LV) is critical. This is critical because LV peak systolic pressure must exceed aortic pressure in order to establish the LV-aortic pressure gradient to expel blood into the aorta, and propel blood throughout the circulation. If aortic diastolic pressure exceeds LV peak systolic pressure, blood will not flow out of the heart. But until we give the β blocker, the heart can maintain (for a while) its function thanks to catecholamine-mediated stimulation.

But when we give just a β blocker to the pheochromocytoma patient we have done little if anything to lower the already high aortic pressure, and simultaneously have inhibited cardiac contractility, rate, and other key parameters. The function of the heart as a pump is suppressed. It now faces a very high aortic pressure, and ultimately it fails. Cardiac output falls, the patient develops cardiogenic shock, and is then likely to die.

This is why, when treating hypertension associated with a pheochromocytoma, we give an α blocker first. Blood pressure will fall. We then deal with the excessive cardiac stimulation (which may be intensified, *via* the baroreceptor reflex, in response to a sudden and significant BP fall) by giving a suitable β blocker immediately thereafter.

4-14. The answer is e. *(Brunton, pp 269–271. Craig, pp 94, 111–113, 231–232. Katzung, pp 144t, 145, 147–148, 172.)* This is an apt description of an α-adrenergic blocker, and not at all descriptive of the actions or effects of any other drug listed. Prazosin can be considered the prototype of the α-adrenergic blockers, at least those that selectively block α_1 receptors (in comparison with phentolamine and several other drugs, which block both α_1 and α_2 receptors). It's not likely your patient was taking prazosin itself (or a related drug like doxazosin or terazosin). That is because those drugs not only exert significant inhibitory effects on smooth muscle of the prostate capsule and urethra, but also on the peripheral vasculature. They could be (and sometimes are) used for benign prostatic hypertrophy. If the patient is also hypertensive, one drug may help both conditions. If blood pressure is normal, or controlled well with other antihypertensives, then prazosin or doxazosin may lower pressure too much (unless we change dosages or drugs). More likely your patient is taking tamsulosin. It's clearly in the same class as prazosin, but seems to have more selectivity for smooth muscles in the urinary tract, and fewer or milder peripheral vascular actions that would tend to lower blood pressure and trigger the other responses we noted.

4-15. The answer is d. *(Murray RK, pp 270–285. Scriver, pp 2961–3104.)* Once bile is excreted into the gut, bilirubin diglucuronide is hydrolyzed and reduced by bacteria to form urobilinogen, which is colorless. Much of the urobilinogen of the stools is further oxidized by intestinal bacteria to stercobilin, which gives stools their characteristic brown color. Some urobilinogen is reabsorbed by the gut into the portal blood, transported to the kidney, and converted and excreted as urobilin, which gives urine its characteristic yellow color. The woman has usual risk factors for cholecystitis (inflammation of the gall bladder) remembered as fair, fat, and forty. The inflammation can block excretion of conjugated bilirubin into the intestine, reducing oxidation to stercobilin and producing white (acholic) stools.

4-16. The answer is c. *(Kumar, pp 754–756. Mandell, pp 2746–2755.)* In the approximate center of the photomicrograph is the classic refractile, double-walled spherule of the deep fungus *Coccidioides immitis*, which is several times the diameter of the largest inflammatory cell nearby. Coccidioidomycosis is endemic in California, Arizona, New Mexico, and parts of Nevada, Utah, and Texas, where it resides in the arid soils and is contracted by direct inhalation of airborne dust. If inhaled, it produces a primary pulmonary infection that is usually benign and self-limiting in immunologically competent persons, often with several days of fever and upper respiratory flulike symptoms. However, certain ethnic groups, such as some African Americans, Asians, and Filipinos, are at risk of developing a potentially lethal disseminated form of the disease that can involve the central nervous system. If the large, double-walled spherule containing numerous endospores can be demonstrated outside the lungs (e.g., in a skin biopsy), this is evidence of dissemination. Antibodies of high titers are detectable by means of complement fixation studies in patients undergoing spontaneous recovery. Amphotericin B is usually reserved for treating high-risk and disseminated infection. The cultured mycelia of the organism on Sabouraud's agar present a hazard for laboratory workers.

4-17. The answer is a. (*Kumar, pp 1240–1241.*) Actinic (solar) keratoses, found on sun-damaged skin, microscopically show hyperkeratosis, parakeratosis, atypia of the epidermal keratinocytes, and degeneration of the elastic fibers in the dermis (referred to as solar elastosis). Clinically, actinic keratoses appear as irregular erythematous brown papules. When the atypia of the intraepidermal keratinocytes is extreme (full thickness), the lesion is referred to as Bowen's disease (carcinoma in situ). Obviously in this lesion there is no invasion into the underlying dermis, which, if present, would be diagnostic of a squamous cell carcinoma. Keratoacanthoma, a benign tumor, may resemble squamous cell carcinoma both clinically and histologically, but penetration of the dermis never extends deeper than adjacent hair follicles. The lesion is cup-shaped with central keratin; biopsy or excision excludes squamous carcinoma.

4-18. The answer is e. (*Gilroy, pp 201–215, 357–362. Siegel and Sapru, p 156. Simon, pp 170–171, 179.*) In ALS, there is damage initially to ventral horn cells of the spinal cord, producing LMN signs. As the disease progresses, there is involvement of UMNs located in the lateral columns of the spinal cord (i.e., corticospinal dysfunction), thereby producing UMN signs such as an increase in tendon reflexes and the presence of an extensor plantar response. Sensory neurons are not involved in this disorder.

4-19. The answer is d. (*Brooks, pp 223–230. Levinson, pp 104–105, 469s. Murray PR—2005, pp 221–236. Ryan, p 268.*) S. aureus is a well-known pathogen that is very opportunistic and commonly causes abscess lesions. It routinely may resist phagocytosis by WBCs due to protein A. Osteomyelitis and arthritis, either hematogenous or traumatic, are commonly caused by S. aureus, especially in children. Salmonella are gramnegative. S. saprophyticus is a common skin flora and is usually not pathogenic. *S. pneumoniae* is seldom or never involved in osteomyelitis infections, as is true for *L. monocytogenes.*

4-20. The answer is c. (*Kumar, pp 240–245. Flake, pp 1806–1810, 1996.*) Patients with severe combined immunodeficiency disease (SCID) have defects of lymphoid stem cells involving both T and B cells. These patients have severe abnormalities of immunologic function with lymphopenia. They are at risk for infection with all types of infectious agents, including bacteria, mycobacteria, fungi, viruses, and parasites. Patients have a skin rash at birth, possibly due to a graft-versus-host reaction from maternal lymphocytes. Patients are particularly prone to chronic diarrhea, due to rotavirus and bacteria, and to oral candidiasis. The most common form of SCIDs is X-linked and related to a mutation in the common gamma chain subunit of cytokine receptors. In particular, the cytokine receptor that is mainly responsible for this defect is the receptor for interleukin-7. The remaining cases of SCIDs have an autosomal recessive inheritance (Swiss type of SCIDs) and lack the enzyme adenosine deaminase (ADA) in their red cells and leukocytes. This leads to accumulation of adenosine triphosphate and deoxyadenosine triphosphate, both of which are toxic to lymphocytes.

The Wiskott-Aldrich syndrome (WAS) is also an X-linked recessive disorder, but it is characterized by the combination of recurrent pyogenic infections, eczema, and thrombocytopenia. WAS is associated with a mutation in a gene on the X chromosome that codes for the Wiskott-Aldrich syndrome protein (WASP). The immune abnormalities associated with WAS are characterized by progressive loss of T-cell function and decreased IgM. The other immunoglobulin levels are normal or increased. There are decreased numbers of lymphocytes in the peripheral blood and paracortical (T cell) areas of lymph nodes. Both cellular and humoral immunity are affected, and, because patients fail to produce antibodies to polysaccharides, they are vulnerable to infections with encapsulated organisms.

In patients with chronic granulomatous disease (CGD), another X-linked recessive disorder, the neutrophils and macrophages have deficient H_2O_2 production due to abnormalities involving the enzyme NADPH oxidase. These individuals have frequent infections that are caused by catalase-positive organisms, such as *S. aureus*, because the catalase produced by these organisms destroys the little hydrogen peroxide that is produced.

Finally, hyper-IgM immunodeficiency is paradoxically a T-cell disorder as a defect in CD40L prevents T lymphocytes from inducing isotype switching in B lymphocytes. Therefore, there is decreased levels of IgG, IgE, and IgA but increased levels of IgM. The most common form of this disease is X-linked (XLM).

4-21. The answer is b. (*Murray RK, pp 580–597. Scriver, pp 3127–3162.*) Ferrous iron (Fe^{2+}) is the form absorbed in the intestine by ferritin, transported in plasma by transferrin, and stored in the liver in combination with ferritin or as hemosiderin. There is no known excretory pathway for iron, either in the ferric or ferrous form. For this reason, excessive iron uptake over a period of many years may cause hemochromatosis (235200), the likely diagnosis for this man. This is a condition of extensive hemosiderin deposition in the liver, myocardium, pancreas, and adrenals. The resulting symptoms include liver cirrhosis, congestive heart failure, diabetes mellitus, and changes in skin pigmentation.

4-22. The answer is d. (*Brunton, pp 223, 227–228. Craig, p 342. Katzung, p 433.*) While this may seem like a trick question, the point is that even with markedly deficient cholinesterase activity, the succinylcholine eventually will be metabolized and its effects will disappear. All that needs to be done is to maintain adequate mechanical ventilatory support.

Succinylcholine exerts its effects by activating nicotinic receptors on skeletal muscle (powerfully but normally briefly, owing to prompt metabolism) and depolarizing the myocytes. Atropine will not work. It blocks only muscarinic receptors. Bethanechol is a muscarinic agonist. Although it may have some nicotinic activating actions at extraordinarily high doses, that effect would add to, not resolve, the effects of the succinylcholine.

Some texts note that under some conditions succinylcholine can cause what is termed Phase II block: a type of neuromuscular blockade that is curare-like (i.e., nondepolarizing). Because nondepolarizing blockade can be (and is, clinically) reversed with acetylcholinesterase inhibitors (mainly neostigmine; physostigmine would work but is not used because of its CNS effects), the implication is that we could administer a cholinesterase inhibitor here and reverse the paralysis. However, this so-called Phase II block is a manifestation of excessive (toxic) doses of succinylcholine and is not likely to apply here. Regardless, the approach is to give nothing and to ventilate the patient as long as needed, as noted.

4-23. The answer is e. (*Ganong, pp 30–34. Kasper et al., pp 2339, 2536–2537.*) Electrically excitable gates are those that respond to a change in membrane potential. The most notable electrically excitable gates are those on the sodium and potassium channels that produce the nerve action potential. The potassium channel gate is opened by depolarization. Ventricular muscle SR releases its calcium in response to an increase in intracellular calcium. The gates opened by ACh are chemically excitable gates.

In rods, sodium channels are closed when cGMP is hydrolyzed. Electrically excitable gates do not regulate the active transport of glucose.

4-24. The answer is b. *(Sadler, pp 169–172. Moore and Persaud, Developing, pp 354–355, 372–373. See diagram provided after the answer for question 14.)* The presence of a murmur could be indicative of any of the conditions. The presence of a continuous machine-like murmur is indicative of a patent ductus arteriosus (PDA). Usually, as in this case, the premature baby with PDA does not acutely become cyanotic and ill, although brief desaturations can occur that become more persistent. The ventilator requirements are increased due to increasing pCO_2 (as the lungs become "wet," the pCO_2 increases). The diastolic blood pressure usually drops and there is a widened pulse pressure (usually greater than 20). The PDA was always there, it is just that her pulmonary vascular resistance relaxed enough to allow more left-to-right shunting and more blood flow to the lungs (less to the body). An atrial septal defect (ASD), such as a persistent foramen ovale, could be eliminated from the diagnosis because the murmur would be heard as an abnormal splitting of the second sound during expiration **(answer a).** A patent foramen ovale is a common echo finding in premature babies and is usually not followed up unless it appears remarkable to the pediatric cardiologist or there is a persistent murmur. A patent foramen ovale might result in only minimal or intermittent cyanosis during crying or straining to pass stool. A murmur caused by a ventricular septal defect (VSD, **answer c**), occurs between the first and second heart sounds (S_1 and S_2) and is described as holosystolic (pansystolic) because the amplitude is high throughout systole. Pulmonary stenosis would be heard as a harsh systolic ejection murmur **(answer d).** Coarctation of the aorta **(answer e)** would result in a systolic murmur. PDA refers to the maintenance of the ductus arteriosus, a normal fetal structure. In the fetus, the ductus arteriosus allows blood to bypass the pulmonary circulation, since the lungs are not involved in CO_2/O_2 exchange until after birth. The placenta subserves the function of gas exchange during fetal development. The ductus arteriosus shunts flow from the left pulmonary artery to the aorta. High oxygen levels after birth and the absence of prostaglandins from the placenta cause the ductus arteriosus to close in most cases within 24 hours. A PDA most often corrects itself within several months of birth, but may require infusion of indomethacin (a prostaglandin inhibitor) as a treatment, insertion of surgical plugs during catheterization, or actual surgical ligation.

4-25. The answer is a. *(Kumar, pp 149, 181–183. Rubin, pp 263–264.)* Fragile X syndrome is one of four diseases that are characterized by long repeating sequences of three nucleotides. The other diseases are Huntington's disease, myotonic dystrophy, and spinal and bulbar muscular atrophy. The fragile X syndrome, which is more common in males than females, is one of the most common causes of familial mental retardation. Additional clinical features of this disorder include developmental delay, a long face with a large mandible, large everted ears, and large testicles (macroorchidism). Examination of the DNA from patients with fragile X syndrome reveals multiple tandem repeats of the nucleotide sequence CGG on the X chromosome. Normally these repeats average up to 50 in number, but in patients with fragile X syndrome there are more than 230 repeats. This number of repeats is called a full mutation. Normal transmitting males (NTMs) and carrier females have between 50 and 230 CGG repeats. This number of repeats is called a premutation. During oogenesis, but not spermatogenesis, premutations can be converted to mutations by amplification of the triplet repeats. This explains the much higher incidence of mental retardation in grandsons rather than brothers of NTMs (Sherman's paradox), as the premutation is amplified in females but not in males. Since the premutation is not amplified in males, no daughters of NTMs are affected. An additional finding associated with these repeat units is anticipation, which refers to the fact that the disease is worse in subsequent generations.

4-26. The answer is d. (*Parslow, p 703. Levinson, pp 390, 413–418.*) Maternal transfer of antibody (secretory IgA in the colostrum of breast milk), however, is passive but still confers specific immunity. It is termed *passive acquired* immunity. Natural immunity is nonspecific. The natural immune functions described are not specific for a certain antigen. For example, certain proteins such as C-reactive protein (CRP) are acute-phase reactants. While elevated CRP is seen in infection, it is not disease-specific.

4-27. The answer is e. (*Murray RK, pp 556–579. Scriver, pp 5493–5524.*) The major problem in myasthenia gravis is a marked reduction of acetylcholine receptors on the motor endplate where cranial nerves form a neuromuscular junction with muscles. In these patients, autoantibodies against the acetylcholine receptors effectively reduce receptor numbers. Normally, acetylcholine molecules released by the nerve terminal bind to receptors on the muscle endplate, resulting in a stimulation of contraction by depolarizing the muscle membrane. The condition is improved with drugs that inhibit acetylcholinesterase.

4-28. The answer is b. (*Kumar, pp 674–676. Rubin, pp 1135–1137.*) Some of the non-Hodgkin's lymphomas are associated with involvement of the peripheral blood (leukemic phase). More than half of the patients with small lymphocytic lymphoma (SLL) have involvement of the bone marrow with spillage of neoplastic cells into the peripheral blood, where they appear as mature lymphocytes, many of which are smudged. The clinical picture is then similar to that of chronic lymphocytic leukemia (CLL). Follicular NHLs also commonly involve the bone marrow, but spillage into the peripheral blood is much less common than in SLL. Still, when the malignant small cleaved lymphocytes, which are also called centrocytes, are found within the peripheral blood, they have a characteristic cleaved appearance that is described as "buttock cells." Lymphoblastic lymphoma is another type of lymphoma that frequently involves the bone marrow and peripheral blood. The clinical picture then is similar to that of T-cell acute lymphoblastic leukemia (ALL). In contrast, multiple myeloma and Hodgkin's disease do not have malignant cells in the peripheral blood.

4-29. The answer is d. (*Lewis, pp 241–266. Scriver, pp 3–45.*) The hallmarks of children with chromosomal anomalies are mental disability (developmental delay in children) with multiple congenital anomalies. The described individual has learning problems that are not yet described as mental disability, and many such children are mistakenly assumed to have poor motivation rather than cognitive problems that could be defined by IQ testing. Parents also may resist the classification as mental disability, particularly when the harsher term retardation is used. The hand changes can be classified as minor anomalies rather than major birth defects that cause cosmetic or surgical problems, but minor anomalies are significant in that several indicate abnormal development and an increased possibility of a birth defect pattern or syndrome. The physician was astute to suspect a chromosomal anomaly with subtle cognitive and physical changes, and this boy would be typical of 47,XYY individuals with tall stature, variable anomalies, and aggressive or antisocial behaviors. Other indications for peripheral blood chromosome studies include couples with three or more pregnancy losses, relatives of individuals with chromosome rearrangements, and children with ambiguous external genitalia. Fetal chromosomes will be considered with triple/quad screen and/or ultrasound abnormalities, while bone marrow/solid tumor chromosomes are now examined in most cancers as a guide to tumor type, chemotherapy, and prognosis.

4-30. The answer is d. (*Brooks, pp 196–203. Levinson, pp 103–114, 145–146, 180–182. Murray PR—2005, pp 83–88. Ryan, p 143.*) An understanding of normal, or indigenous, microflora is essential in order to appreciate the abnormal. Usually, anatomic sites contiguous to mucous membranes are not sterile and have characteristic normal flora.

The skin flora differs as a function of location. Skin adjacent to mucous membranes may share some of the normal flora of the gastrointestinal system. Overall, the predominant bacteria on the skin surface are *S. epidermidis* and *Propionibacterium,* an anaerobic diphtheroid.

The mouth is part of the gastrointestinal tract, but its indigenous flora shows some distinct differences. While anaerobes are present in large numbers, particularly in the gingival crevice, the eruption of teeth at 6–9 months of age leads to colonization by organisms such as *S. mutans* and *Streptococcus sanguis,* both α-hemolytic streptococci. An edentulous person loses β-hemolytic streptococci as normal flora.

The gastrointestinal tract is sterile at birth and soon develops characteristic flora as a function of diet. In the adult, anaerobes such as *B. fragilis* and *Bifidobacterium* may outnumber coliforms and enterococci by a ratio of 1000:1. The colon contains 10^{11}–10^{12} bacteria per gram of feces.

Soon after birth, the vagina becomes colonized by lactobacilli. As the female matures, lactobacilli may still be predominant, but anaerobic cocci, diphtheroids, and anaerobic, gram-negative rods also are found as part of the indigenous flora. Changes in the chemical or microbiologic ecology of the vagina can have marked effects on normal flora and may promote infection such as vaginitis or vaginosis.

4-31. The answer is a. (*Brunton, pp 436t, 447–448, 453, 616, 731. Craig, p 388. Katzung, pp 484i, 487t, 489t, 493t.*) Bupropion is marketed, under different trade names, for two main purposes: anxiety relief, and suppression of the cravings for nicotine. Since too many physicians prescribe by brand-name products, and ignore the active generic drug, such problems as the one we described in our scenario, due to accidental duplication and overdoses of a drug, are more common than you'd like to believe. One of the main consequences of bupropion overdose is seizures. Chlordiazepoxide (b) is a benzodiazepine that is not indicated for depression or as a stop-smoking aid. If anything, the drug will suppress, rather than cause, seizures. Fluoxetine (c) and imipramine (d) are antidepressants, but they are not normally prescribed as smoking-cessation aids, nor are they marketed in products approved for that use. Lithium (e) is a mood-stabilizing drug used in bipolar illness. It is not at all likely to have been approved for managing depression or for smoking cessation.

4-32. The answer is b. (*Ganong, pp 65–68, 77. Kasper et al., pp 2532–2537.*) Dystrophin is a large protein that forms a rod, which connects the thin filaments of actin to the transmembrane protein β-dystroglyan in the sarcolemma. β-Dystroglyan is connected to laminin in the extracellular matrix by α-dystroglyan. The dystroglycans are also associated with a complex of four transmembrane glycoproteins, called sarcoglycans. The dystrophin-glycoprotein complex adds strength to the muscle by providing a scaffolding for the fibrils and connecting them to the extracellular environment. Muscular dystrophy is the term used for some 50 diseases that cause progressive skeletal muscle weakness. Duchenne's and Becker's muscular dystrophy are two types resulting from mutations in the dystrophin gene.

4-33. The answer is b. *(Afifi, 117–135. Nolte, pp 254–276. Siegel and Sapru, pp 227–235, 302–306, 316–320, 361.)* Different groups of neurons of the solitary complex (B) respond to taste stimuli and to inputs that signal sudden changes in blood pressure. The medial vestibular nucleus (C) receives direct vestibular inputs from the otolith organ and semicircular canals. Axons of medial vestibular neurons descend to the spinal cord in the MLF and serve to regulate reflexes associated with the head. The inferior vestibular nucleus (D) also receives vestibular inputs, but does not project its axons to the spinal cord. The inferior olivary nucleus (H) receives inputs from the red nucleus and spinal cord, and it projects its axons through the inferior cerebellar peduncle (where it constitutes its largest component) to the contralateral cerebellar cortex, where they synapse with the dendrites of Purkinje cells.

The nucleus ambiguus (G) is a special visceral efferent nucleus that is situated in a position ventrolateral to that of the hypoglossal nucleus. Its axons innervate the muscles of the larynx and pharynx and, therefore, are essential for the occurrence of such responses as the gag reflex. The pyramids (I), located on the ventromedial aspect of the brainstem, contain fibers that arise from the sensorimotor cortex. These neurons serve as essential UMNs that mediate voluntary control of motor functions. The hypoglossal nucleus (A), a general somatic efferent nucleus, is located in the dorsomedial aspect of the medulla. Its axons innervate the muscles of the tongue and cause extrusion of the tongue toward the opposite side, but when this structure is damaged, the tongue protrudes to the side of the lesion when extended. Fibers contained in the inferior cerebellar peduncle (E) comprise the largest single-most input into the cerebellum (approximately 40% of afferents) and these fibers arise from cells located in both the spinal cord and the brainstem.

4-34. The answer is e. *(Parslow, pp 636, 638–642.)* HIV infection affects mainly the immune system and the brain. The main immunologic feature of HIV infection is progressive depletion of the CD4 subset of T lymphocytes

(T helper cells), causing a reversal in the normal CD4:CD8 ratio, leading to immunodeficiency. Currently, ELISA is the basic screening test to detect anti-HIV antibodies. Repeated reactive ELISA tests should be confirmed using either Western blot or immunofluorescence. The Western blot detects specific antibodies against the various HIV proteins (antigens).

4-35. The answer is e. (*Kumar, pp 816–820. Rubin, pp 688–694.*) Benign peptic ulcers are associated with the effects of acid and may occur anywhere in the gastrointestinal tract exposed to acid-peptic activity. Over 98% of cases occur in the stomach or duodenum, with duodenal cases outnumbering gastric cases 4 to 1. Peptic ulcers tend to be solitary lesions, but ulcers associated with Zollinger-Ellison syndrome are typically multiple and frequently involve distal duodenum and jejunum. Duodenal ulceration appears to be related to hypersecretion of acid. Gastric ulceration typically occurs in a setting of normo- or hypochlorhydria with abnormality of mucosal defense mechanisms, back-diffusion of acid, and possibly local ischemia. *H. pylori* is present in up to 100% of patients with duodenal ulcers and about 75% of patients with gastric ulcers.

Note that gastric ulcers can be either benign peptic ulcers or malignant ulcers associated with gastric cancers. Certain gross and microscopic characteristics help to differentiate benign peptic ulcers from malignant ulcers. Benign peptic ulcers tend to be round and regular with punched-out straight walls. The margins are only slightly elevated and rugae radiate outward from the ulcer. Raised peripheral margins are quite characteristic of malignant lesions, which are also irregular in appearance. Most benign peptic ulcers are located in the first portion of the duodenum or the stomach. The anterior wall of the duodenum is a more common location than the posterior wall, while benign gastric ulcers are most commonly located on the lesser curvature. The location of the ulcer, however, does not differentiate a benign ulcer from a malignant ulcer. Most benign ulcers are less than 2 cm in diameter, but they can be large. Most malignant ulcers are large, but they too can be less than 2 cm in diameter. Therefore, size can not be used to tell a benign ulcer from a malignant ulcer. Also both benign and malignant ulcers can erode through the wall of the stomach and perforate into the peritoneal cavity.

Histologically the surface of a benign ulcer shows acute inflammation and necrotic fibrinoid debris, while the base has active granulation tissue overlying a fibrous scar. Grossly, the floor of the ulcer is smooth. The gastric epithelium adjacent to the benign ulcer is reactive and is characterized by numerous mitoses and epithelial cells with prominent nucleoli. Malignant ulcers obviously have malignant cells infiltrating at the margins of the ulcer. Additionally, *H. pylori* may be seen with either type of ulcer, and its presence is not diagnostic for the type of ulcer. It is also found in 20% of the general population.

4-36. The answer is a. *(Alberts, pp 872–874, 1015. Kumar, pp 42, 95, 110, 1198, 1204. Rubin, pp 86–88, 103.)* Platelet-derived growth factor (PDGF) stimulates chemotaxis of monocytes and macrophages as well as fibroblasts to the site of a wound. PDGF also induces proliferation of vascular smooth muscle cells **(answer b)** to facilitate blood vessel repair and fibroblasts **(answer c)** to synthesize type I collagen. PDGF stimulates the formation of granulation tissue **(answer d)** consisting of new connective tissue and small blood vessels that form in the wound site. Type II collagen **(answer e)** is synthesized by chondrocytes in hyaline and elastic cartilage. Wound healing is a complex process initiated by damage to capillaries in the dermis. The clot forms through the interaction of integrins on the surface of blood platelets with fibrinogen and fibronectin. Fibrin is the primary protein that constructs the three-dimensional structure of the clot. A scar is formed as a very dense region of type I collagen fibers. Macrophages remove debris at the wound site and are also involved in the remodeling of the scar. All wound healing processes are slower in diabetics, and the presence of advanced-glycation end products (AGE) and their interaction with the receptor for AGE (RAGE) as well as the endogenous ligand for RAGE (ENRAGE) appear to contribute to inhibited healing in diabetes. AGE are produced by the nonenzymatic glycation and oxidation of proteins/lipids and alter those molecules and therefore the function and structure of tissues and organs such as the kidney (diabetic nephropathy), peripheral nerves (neuropathy), and the retina (diabetic retinopathy).

4-37. The answer is c. *(Kumar, pp 799–800, 812.)* Several congenital abnormalities of the gastrointestinal tract present with specific symptoms. Infants with congenital hypertrophic pyloric stenosis present in the second or third week of life with symptoms of regurgitation and persistent severe vomiting. Physical examination reveals a firm mass in the region of the pylorus. Surgical splitting of the muscle in the stenotic region is curative. Diaphragmatic hernias, if large enough, may allow abdominal contents—including portions of the stomach, intestines, or liver—to herniate into the thoracic cavity and cause respiratory compromise. Congenital aganglionic megacolon (Hirschsprung's disease) is caused by failure of the neural crest cells to migrate all the way to the anus, resulting in a portion of distal colon that lacks ganglion cells and both Meissner's submucosal and Auerbach's myenteric plexuses. This results in a functional obstruction and dilation proximal to the affected portion of colon. Symptoms of Hirschsprung's disease include failure to pass meconium soon after birth followed by constipation and possible abdominal distention.

4-38. The answer is b. *(Brooks, pp 597–601, 433. Levinson, pp 296, 209, 306, 244–255. Murray PR—2005, pp 523–532, 541. Ryan, pp 559–561.)* Primary HSV-1 infections are usually asymptomatic. Symptomatic disease occurs most frequently in small children (1–5 years old). Buccal and gingival mucosa are most often involved, and lesions, if untreated, may last 2–3 weeks. Acyclovir treatment is effective therapy and should be started immediately. The classic location of latent HSV-1 infection is the trigeminal ganglia. Reactivation results in sporadic vesicular lesions and may also be treated with acyclovir. B cell activation would be unusual, and there appears to be no greater risk for cancer development than that seen in the general population.

4-39. The answer is c. *(Young, pp 184–187.)* The child in the vignette is suffering from Turner's syndrome, gonadal dysgenesis in which the XO karyotype results in multiple medical problems. The short stature has recently been attributed to the short stature homeobox gene SHOX which can affect various stages of endochondral development. The light micrograph illustrates a developing long bone. The zone shown is the region of chondrocyte hypertrophy, and the cells synthesize alkaline phosphatase, which calcifies the cartilage matrix. This secretion results in the eventual death of these cells that depend on diffusion to obtain oxygen and nutrients from the matrix. During development of the long bones of the body, specific zones are established, as a cartilage model of a long bone is converted to mature bone. The zones from the epiphysis toward the center of the shaft (diaphysis) are as follows: resting zone, proliferative zone, hypertrophy zone, and zone of calcified cartilage that is used as the scaffolding for the deposition of bone. The periosteal bud represents the ingrowth of blood vessels (angiogenesis) bringing, bone marrow precursors and osteoprogenitor cells into the diaphysis. Angiogenesis is required for bone formation. Bone is formed by the action of osteoblasts forming type I collagen, noncollagenous proteins (e.g., osteocalcin, osteopontin, and osteonectin), and alkaline phosphatase, which plays an essential role in mineralization of the osteoid. Cyclins are synthesized by cells passing through the cell cycle, cells in the proliferative zone **(answer a)**; acid phosphatase **(answer b)** is synthesized by osteoclasts; and type I collagen and osteocalcin **(answers d and e)** are synthesized by osteoblasts.

4-40. The answer is a. *(Lewis, pp 377–396. Scriver, pp 2297–2326. Murray RK, pp 180–189.)* Catastrophic metabolic disease often begins after the first few feedings, when the baby is exposed to nutrients that cannot be metabolized and are toxic. Often there are misguided attempts to encourage feeding, which further poison the child. Inborn errors of carbohydrate, amino acid, or organic/fatty acid metabolism can present in the newborn period. They are characterized by a similar pattern of symptoms that include spitting up, vomiting, exaggeration of the usual physiologic jaundice, lethargy progressing to coma, hypoglycemia, acidosis, hyperammonemia, and, in the case of maple syrup urine disease or isovaleric acidemia, unusual odors. Disorders of fatty acid oxidation worsen during fasting to cause carnitine depletion, failure of fatty acid oxidation, and excretion of dicarboxylic acid intermediates. Deficiencies in medium-chain fatty acid oxidation are milder, and may present after a period of illness with calorie deprivation in children aged 2–6 years. Urea cycle disorders worsen during fasting (catabolic breakdown) or protein feeding, producing excess ammonia, rapid breathing, and respiratory alkalosis. Galactosemia worsens on exposure to lactose-containing formula, producing hypoglycemia, liver failure, and excretion of urinary sugars (reducing substances). Tyrosinemia and maple syrup urine disease are amino acid disorders that worsen after protein feeding and produce elevated levels of tyrosine or branch-chain amino acids (leucine, isoleucine, valine). Tyrosinemia is associated with severe liver failure and maple syrup urine disease with severe acidosis due to conversion of excess amino acids to ketoacids.

4-41. The answer is d. *(Moore and Dalley, pp 321–324.)* The diffuse central abdominal pain in the patient presented is probably referred pain from the loop of small bowel incarcerated within the herniated peritoneal sac that then undergoes ischemic necrosis. Compression of the bowel results in compromise of the blood supply and subsequent ischemic necrosis [thus not **(answer e)**]. The visceral afferent fibers from the distal small bowel travel along the blood vessels to reach the superior mesenteric plexus and lesser splanchnic nerves, which they follow to the T10–T11 levels of the spinal cord. The pain, therefore, is referred to (appears as if originating from) the T10–T11 dermatomes, which supply the umbilical region. Because the gut develops as a midline structure, visceral pain tends to be centrally located regardless of the adult location of any particular region of the gut. As a result of dilation **(answer c)** of the inguinal canal by the hernial sac, however, the patient also experiences localized somatic pain mediated by the iliohypogastric, ilioinguinal **(answer b)**, and genitofemoral nerves **(answer a)**, but this was *not* what the question asked.

4-42. The answer is h. *(Nolte, pp 52–60, 62–69. Siegel and Sapru, pp 6–8, 331–335, 475–491.)* This figure is a lateral view of the cerebral cortex. Cells in the "arm" area of the primary motor cortex (H) project their axons to the cervical level of the spinal cord and are activated at the time when a response of this limb occurs. The leg region of the left primary somatosensory cortex (A) lies immediately caudal to the central sulcus, is almost devoid of pyramidal cells, is referred to as a *granulous cortex*, and receives inputs from the right leg. Damage to this region would result in loss of vibration sensibility (as well as tactile sensation and two-point discrimination) from the right leg. Damage to the cells situated in the region of the dorsal border of the superior temporal gyrus and the adjoining area of the inferior parietal lobule (Wernicke's area; C) causes impairment in the appreciation of the meanings of written or spoken words.

The primary, secondary, and tertiary auditory receiving areas in the cortex are located mainly in the superior temporal gyrus (D). It is the final receiving area for inputs from the medial geniculate nucleus, which represents an important relay in the transmission of auditory signals to the cortex. Damage to this region of the cortex would result in some hearing loss. An additional area of the cortex governing speech (F) is called the *motor speech area*, or *Broca's area*. It is situated in the inferior aspect of the frontal lobe immediately rostral and slightly ventral to the precentral gyrus. Lesions of this region produce impairment of the ability to express words in a meaningful way or to use words correctly. The orbital frontal cortex (E) lies in a position inferior and rostral to Broca's motor speech area. This region governs higher-order intellectual functions and some aspects of emotional behavior. Damage to this region often results in personality changes and emotionality. The caudal aspect of the middle frontal gyrus (G) contains cells that, when activated, produce conjugate deviation of the eyes. This action is believed to be accomplished, in part, by virtue of descending projections to the superior colliculus, pretectal region, and horizontal gaze center of the pons. A lesion of this region would result in loss of capacity to produce voluntary horizontal movement of the eyes in one direction. Lesions of the posterior parietal lobe (B) of the nondominant hemisphere will produce a disorder of body image, referred to as sensory neglect. The patient will frequently fail to recognize or neglect to shave or wash those body parts. The patient may even fail to recognize the presence of a hemiparesis involving that part of the body as well. The precentral gyrus (H) constitutes the primary motor cortex. Lesions of this region produce a UMN paralysis involving a contralateral limb.

4-43. The answer is c. (*Damjanov, pp 2630–2634. Kumar, pp 1305–1309.*) Pannus is the name given to describe the classic destructive joint lesion found in individuals with rheumatoid arthritis. This lesion is characterized by proliferation of the synovium (hyperplasia) along with numerous chronic inflammatory cells. The thickened synovial membrane may develop villous projections, which can destroy the joint cartilage. Nodular collections of lymphocytes resembling follicles are characteristically seen along with numerous plasma cells. Palisades of proliferating cells may surround areas of necrosis. This latter histologic appearance can be seen in subcutaneous nodules (rheumatoid nodules), but rheumatoid arthritis most frequently affects the small joints of the hands and feet. Larger joints are involved later. In contrast to a pannus, gummas are seen with syphilis, while tophi are found with gout. Finally, eburnation describes the "polished" appearance of the bone affected by degenerative joint disease, while spondylosis refers to a degenerative process of the vertebrae that can compress the spinal cord and its nerve roots.

4-44. The answer is b. (*Lewis, pp 361–391. Murray RK, pp 396–414. Scriver, pp 233–238.*) Succinylcholine is metabolized by a plasma enzyme formerly called pseudocholinesterase [now called butyrylcholinesterase (BChE) to designate its favored substrate]. Approximately 1 in 100 individuals are homozygous for a variant of BChE that has 60% activity, whereas 1 in 150,000 individuals are homozygous for a variant with 33% activity. The latter group exhibits prolonged recovery from succinylcholine-induced anesthesia, a phenotype known as succinylcholine apnea (177400). As with most enzyme defects, succinylcholine apnea exhibits autosomal recessive inheritance. The parents will be heterozygous for a BChE variant but have not undergone anesthesia to display the phenotype.

4-45. The answer is b. (*Lewis, pp 241–266. Scriver, pp 3–45.*) The recurrence risk for simple extra or missing chromosomes (whole chromosome aneuploidies) is about 1% in addition to the maternal age-related risk. It is not known why the risk for aneuploidy increases slightly after an affected child is born, but parental karyotypes are almost always normal. Parental chromosome studies are thus not indicated in this case, especially with the low degree of mosaicism that might have arisen after conception. The empiric risk of 1% is comparable to that of women over 35 (ironically called advanced maternal age!) for fetal chromosome aberrations, so prenatal diagnosis should be discussed as an option for the parents. The school should not be given a copy of the karyotype unless the parents request it and sign a release of medical records. Some parents prefer to keep diagnoses of genetic disease or attention deficit-hyperactivity disorders confidential so their child will not be labeled as different by school personnel. Trisomy 8 mosaicism can have a very mild phenotype, so special education should not be recommended unless cognitive testing demonstrates a lower IQ (below 75 is often required for special education).

4-46. The answer is b. (*Craig, p 327. Brunton, pp 122, 578–579. Katzung, p 512.*) Dextromethorphan is a centrally acting antitussive drug that is about as efficacious a cough-suppressant as codeine. However, unlike codeine (c) and hydrocodone (d; another useful antitussive in some cases), dextromethorphan is not an opioid and lacks analgesic effects or the potential for ventilatory suppression or abuse. Diphenhydramine (c) and promethazine (e) also have antitussive action. However, they, too, can cause generalized CNS and ventilatory depression. They also exert significant antimuscarinic effects. Although that may be good in terms of inhibiting ACh-mediated bronchoconstriction, it may also cause thickening of airway mucus, favoring mechanical plugging of the airways with viscous mucus deposits that cannot be removed normally by mucociliary transport or coughing. Note warnings for all pediatric patients, specifically because of the risk of serious (and sometimes fatal) respiratory depression. This warning was not specifically targeted at pediatric patients with asthma. Nonetheless, asthma patients (and younger ones especially) are particularly vulnerable to drugs that suppress ventilatory drive, and so the warning should elicit extra vigilance.

4-47. The answer is c. (*Brunton, pp 361–362, 407. Craig, pp 295–296, 355–360. Katzung, pp 319–322.*) The term asthma derives from a Greek word that means, literally, "to pant." In severe asthma attacks such as the one we describe here the hyperpnea precedes the likely development of ventilatory depression and, ultimately, ventilatory arrest. It is a sometimes successful and sometimes futile physiologic response elicited to increase ventilatory oxygen uptake and eliminate excess CO_2, although it may be insufficient to raise arterial O_2 saturation adequately and more than sufficient to induce metabolic alkalosis from excess CO_2 loss. Nonetheless, it is a "protective" response, and breathing too quickly, even inefficiently, is better than not breathing at all. This leads to the admonition: Never give a drug that can depress ventilation or the normal ventilatory drive to an asthma patient unless he or she has a protected airway and ventilation can be controlled and supported mechanically. IV midazolam (or the IV administration of virtually any other benzodiazepine, opioid, or barbiturate) will allay anxiety, but will also tend to suppress ventilatory drive and hasten the onset of ventilatory arrest. In the scenario described here, diazepam is the wrong drug to give. Albuterol (a) or a similar β_2 agonist bronchodilator, whether given by inhalation or parenterally, would not be expected to worsen the boy's ventilatory status. They should not be the only drugs relied on, but they would be appropriate adjunctive treatments, as would be all the rest for the stated purposes. As an important aside, you may recall that atropine (b) and other drugs with antimuscarinic activity have bronchodilator activity, but also tend to make airway mucus secretions more viscous, leading to airway mucus plugging. In the context of this scenario, with the administration of other drugs that we listed, and the availability of airway suctioning devices as needed, the mucus-thickening effects of an antimuscarinic should not be a problem with which we cannot easily deal by way of airway suctioning and the administration of mucus-thinning (mucolytic) drugs. Glucocorticoids (d) and nebulized saline would be valuable, if not essential, adjuncts to this boy's therapy.

4-48. The answer is c. (*Brunton, pp 721–722, 1598–1599, 1603–1604. Craig, pp 464–465. Katzung, pp 328–329, 332.*) It usually takes a couple of weeks of inhaled corticosteroid use "as directed" to suppress airway inflammation, and the resulting bronchoconstriction, well enough that the patient can sense clinical improvement (fewer or milder asthma symptoms). Unless the patient is forewarned about this slow onset, and urged to remain compliant, they are likely to believe the drug is ineffective and therefore not worth taking. Clearly, inhaled corticosteroids do not cause the obvious "rush"—the prompt, dramatic, and unmistakable symptom relief that typically occurs with adrenergic bronchodilators. Nonetheless, given adequate time, the inhaled steroids usually prove to be the key to effective long-term control of asthma. Inhaled corticosteroids act locally; little enters the systemic circulation; such side effects as fluid retention, weight gain (e), and hyperglycemia, that are typical with systemic steroids (e.g., prednisone), rarely occur or become problematic. Inhaled steroids do not cause cardiac stimulation (a), diarrhea (b), or drowsiness (d).

4-49. The answer is e. (*Brunton, pp 728–730. Craig, p 463. Katzung, pp 325–327.*) Theophylline, a methylxanthine, is a caffeine–like drug that is becoming outmoded as therapy for asthma in most adolescents and adults. It should probably not be prescribed by any physician other than a pulmonologist who is familiar with the limitations and problems with this class of drugs. A low margin of safety, extreme dependence on adequate liver function (for metabolism), susceptibility to numerous clinically significant drug interactions, and a lack of airway anti inflammatory activity, are among the reasons why without proper dosage adjustments and monitoring it is all too easy, and common, for blood levels to fall into subtherapeutic ranges or, as we see here, into toxic ranges. The earliest signs and symptoms of excess involve CNS stimulation (jitteriness, tremors, difficulty sleeping, anxiety). As blood levels rise the CNS is increasingly stimulated. Seizures may occur, and when they do the inability to breathe during the seizures is the main cause of death. Thus, answer b is incorrect. Theophylline tends to cause tachycardia, increases of cardiac contractility and, potentially, tachyarrhythmias. Bradycardia (a) is not at all likely. Theophylline is not hepatotoxic (c); it does not cause paradoxical bronchospasm (d), even when serum levels are very high or truly toxic.

4-50. The answer is b. (*Brunton, p 722. Craig, p 467. Katzung, pp 127, 325, 332.*) When pulmonary function deteriorates so much that respiratory acidosis ensues (because sufficient amounts of CO_2 aren't being eliminated by ventilation) and severe hypoxia develops (because of inadequate oxygen transfer), acute tolerance (in essence, desensitization) develops to the bronchodilator effects of drugs with β_2- agonist activity—all of them. If this point is forgotten, repeated administration of a β_2 agonist will lead to increasing degrees of cardiac stimulation (rate, contractility, automaticity, conduction) because under these conditions they lose their selectivity for β_2 receptors and also begin activating β_1 receptors very effectively. (They become isoproterenol-like in their profiles.)

Even epinephrine won't work as an efficacious bronchodilator under these conditions, and repeated injections of it will do little more than cause further cardiac stimulation plus vasoconstriction via α activation. Through mechanisms that are not quite clear, administering suitable doses of a parenteral steroid under these conditions of acidosis and hypoxia "restores" a substantial degree of airway responsiveness to β agonists. Giving a steroid (plus oxygen, which helps correct the underlying blood gas and pH changes) is essential.

Giving diphenhydramine, even though it blocks the bronchoconstrictor effects of both ACh and histamine, will not do much good for the acute and life-threatening signs and symptoms. Giving cromolyn will prove largely worthless and certainly not life-saving.

Block 5

Answers

5-1. The answer is d. (*Brunton, pp 12–29. Craig, pp 52–53. Katzung, pp 44–50.*) The dose to give equals the product of the target blood concentration and the drug's clearance.

$$D = C_{desired} \times Cl$$

To simplify things, let's get the units of volume the same for both clearance and concentration. The clearance of 0.08 L/min = 80 mL/min. Therefore

$$D = 8 \text{ mcg/mL} \times 80 \text{ mL/min} = 640 \text{ mcg/min}$$

The stated dosing interval is 4 h, so

$$640 \text{ mcg/min} \times 60 \text{ min/h} \times 4 \text{ h} = 153,500 \text{ mcg}$$

which (rounded) is closest to 150 mg.

5-2. The answer is a. (*Ganong, pp 87–88. Kasper et al., pp 842–844.*) Botulinum toxin inhibits the release of acetylcholine from α-motoneurons by blocking one of the proteins responsible for the fusion of the synaptic channel with the presynaptic membrane. Botulinum toxin also inhibits the release of acetylcholine from the neurons of the autonomic nervous system. Botulinum and tetanus toxin are released from the same class of bacteria (*Clostridium*). Tetanus toxin produces an increase in skeletal muscle contraction by blocking the release of inhibitory neurotransmitter from spinal interneurons.

5-3. The answer is b. (*Moore and Dalley, p 400.*) Cystocele. Bulges in the anterior wall of the vagina are most likely due to the bladder falling posteriorly into the anterior vaginal wall. A bulge on the posterior wall of the vagina would most likely be a rectocele **(answer b)**. Cervical cancer **(answer c)** generally would *not* present as described. A didelphic uterus **(answer d)** is a duplication of the uterus as result of failure of the right and left paramesonephric ducts to fuse in the midline. An indirect inguinal hernia (**answer e**) would generally present as a mass within the labia major.

5-4. The answer is c. *(Simon, pp 173–183.)* The most likely cause of the condition in this patient is a cervical disk prolapse. This disorder would produce pain in the neck and arm, which increases with movement of the head. It would also cause loss of some sensation in the thumb and other fingers, as well as weakness in both finger extension and of the biceps reflex. Syringomyelia would produce bilateral segmental loss of pain and temperature. A knife wound completely severing the nerve would result in a functional loss similar to that experienced with an LMN paralysis. Polio results in loss of LMNs, thus also producing an LMN (flaccid) paralysis. One of the effects of AIDS is that it produces damage to the lateral and dorsal columns, resulting in the appearance of a UMN disorder.

5-5. The answer is b. *(Brooks, pp 645–647. Levinson, pp 331–341. Murray PR—2005, pp 716, 781–784. Ryan, pp 660–664.)* Candida species are normal flora of the skin, mucous membranes, and gastrointestinal tract. The risk of endogenous infection is ever present. Candidiasis is the most common systemic mycosis. Oral thrush develops in most patients with AIDS. Other risk factors include antibiotic use and cellular immunodeficiency. *Mucor* and *Rhizopus* are primarily dermatophytes, while *Aspergillus* is usually derived from an environmental source. While *Aspergillus* is a significant opportunist, the numbers of cases are much lower than those observed to be caused by *Candida*. *Cryptococcus* is usually acquired by inhalation.

5-6. The answer is c. *(Kumar, pp 1187–1188. Rubin, pp 1180–1183.)* Parathyroid hyperplasia may be associated with either primary or secondary hyperparathyroidism. In contrast to primary hyperparathyroidism, secondary hyperparathyroidism results from hypocalcemia and causes secondary hypersecretion of parathyroid hormone (PTH). This results in the combination of hypocalcemia and increased PTH. This abnormality is principally found in patients with chronic renal failure, where phosphate retention is thought to cause hypocalcemia. Since the failing kidney is not able to synthesize 1,25-dihydroxycholecalciferol, the most active form of vitamin D, this deficiency leads to poor absorption of calcium from the gut and relative hypocalcemia, which stimulates excess PTH secretion. Chronic renal failure is the most important cause, but secondary hyperparathyroidism also occurs in vitamin D deficiency, malabsorption syndromes, and pseudohypoparathyroidism. In any of the causes of parathyroid hyperplasia, all four parathyroid glands are typically enlarged. Parathyroid hyperplasia can be differentiated from parathyroid adenomas by the fact that parathyroid hyperplasia, either primary or secondary, results in enlargement of all four glands, while a parathyroid adenoma or parathyroid carcinoma produces enlargement of only one gland. In most cases the other three glands are smaller than normal.

5-7. The answer is a. (*Nolte, pp 375–394, 451–467, 538–545, 548–555. Siegel and Sapru, pp 204–220, 346–348.*) This section is taken at the level of the mammillary bodies (at ventral levels) and includes parts of the anterior thalamus (at dorsal levels). The lenticular fasciculus (D), situated just below the thalamic fasciculus and immediately above the subthalamic nucleus at the level of this brain section, arises from the dorsomedial aspect of the medial pallidal segment and projects to the VL, VA, and CM nuclei of the thalamus. Damage to the neurons of the medial pallidal segment would cause degeneration of the efferent projections from this region, one pathway of which is the lenticular fasciculus. The subthalamic nucleus (F), which lies on the dorsal surface of the internal capsule, maintains reciprocal connections with the globus pallidus through a pathway called the *subthalamic fasciculus*. Damage to the subthalamic nucleus has been associated with the onset of hemiballism. The anterior nucleus of the thalamus (A), which lies at the rostral end of the thalamus in a dorsomedial position, receives a major input from the mammillary bodies via the *mammillothalamic tract*. The mammillary bodies (E), situated at the base of the posterior aspect of the hypothalamus, are the origin of the mammillothalamic (G) tract, which innervates the anterior thalamic nucleus. The region immediately below the tail and body of the caudate nucleus is occupied by a major output pathway of the medial amygdala (within the temporal lobe), the *stria terminalis* (H). It supplies the medial preoptic region, bed nucleus of the stria terminalis, and medial hypothalamus. The thalamic fasciculus can be seen in sections taken through the caudal half of the thalamus and is clearly visualized in a position dorsal to the subthalamic nucleus and lenticular fasciculus. The *thalamic fasciculus* (C) also projects to the ventral lateral and VA thalamic nuclei. While many of the fibers contained in this bundle arise from the medial pallidal segment, others arise directly from the dentate nucleus of cerebellum. A large nuclear mass situated in the medial aspect of the posterior two-thirds of the thalamus is the mediodorsal thalamic nucleus (B). This nucleus projects extensively to wide regions of the frontal lobe, including the prefrontal cortex. In turn, the prefrontal region of the cortex and adjoining regions of the frontal lobe project their axons back to the mediodorsal nucleus. Thus, there are reciprocal connections linking the mediodorsal nucleus and rostral portions of the frontal lobe. Because of the major input to the prefrontal cortex from the mediodorsal nucleus and since the prefrontal cortex plays an important role in the regulation of affective processes, damage to the mediodorsal nucleus would clearly alter emotional responses associated with the prefrontal cortex.

5-8. The answer is b. (*Moore and Dalley, pp 729–730.*) The horizontal direction of the fibers of the clavicular head of the pectoralis major muscle draws the humerus medially and causes the distal fragment of the bone to sublux. The sternal head of this muscle also has the effect of pulling the arm medially, an effect that is normally offset by the strut-like action of the clavicle. The pectoralis minor muscle **(answer c)** is a much smaller muscle and would be the second best answer. The deltoid **(answer a)** muscle would *not* cause inferior subluxation. The subclavian artery **(answer d)** and the thoracoacromial trunk **(answer e)** are blood vessels just below the broken clavicle and are at risk of being injured.

5-9. The answer is c. (*Brunton, pp 332, 624–625. Craig, pp 417–418. Katzung, pp 523–525.*) Phencyclidine (PCP; angel dust) is an hallucinogen with an amphetamine-like mechanism of action. Thus, the problems that arise are due to blockade of neuronal reuptake of such monoamines as dopamine, norepinephrine, and serotonin. The drug does not have central or peripheral muscarinic receptor antagonist activity (d), nor opioid agonist actions (b). A withdrawal syndrome (a) has not been described for this drug in human subjects. In overdose, the treatment of choice for manifestations of drug-induced psychosis is the haloperidol, although rapidly acting and highly sedating benzodiazepines may be used instead. Flumazenil (e) is a selective benzodiazepine receptor antagonist with no use in phencyclidine toxicity.

5-10. The answer is b. (*Brooks, pp 637–639. Levinson, pp 333–337. Murray PR—2005, pp 712–714. Ryan, pp 678–683.*) Endemic areas for *C. immitis* are semiarid regions, particularly the central valleys of California and southern Arizona. The infection rate is highest during the dry months of summer and autumn, when dust is prevalent. Inhalation of arthroconidia can lead to an asymptomatic infection in 60% of individuals. The other 40% may develop a self-limited influenza-like illness. Individuals with cell-mediated immunosuppression may lead to dissemination of endospores by the blood. The most frequent sites involved are skin, bones and joints, and the meninges.

Histoplasmosis is usually associated with the central river valleys of the United States, while blastomycocis is endemic primarily in the eastern United States. *M. marinum* is usually associated with fish and water, while *Mycoplasma pneumoniae* transmission is from person to person.

5-11. The answer is a. *(Brooks, pp 685–687, 688–691, 662–663, 687–690. Levinson, pp 346–347, 353–354, 367–370, 378–379, 381–382. Murray PR— 2005, pp 882–883, 907–910, 850–852, 902–905, 882–883. Ryan, pp 695–696, 723–727, 746–748, 779–784, 809–813.)* All the diseases listed in the question have significant epidemiologic and clinical features. Toxoplasmosis, for example, is generally a mild, self-limiting disease; however, severe fetal disease is possible if pregnant women ingest *Toxoplasma* oocysts. Consumption of uncooked meat may result in either an acute toxoplasmosis or a chronic toxoplasmosis that is associated with serious eye disease. Most adults have antibody titers to *Toxoplasma*, and thus would have a positive Sabin-Feldman dye test.

Trichinosis most often is caused by ingestion of contaminated pork products. However, eating undercooked bear, walrus, raccoon, or possum meat also may cause this disease. Symptoms of trichinosis include muscle soreness and swollen eyes.

Although giardiasis has been classically associated with travel in Russia, especially St. Petersburg (Leningrad), many cases of giardiasis caused by contaminated water have been reported in the United States as well. Diagnosis is made by detecting cysts in the stool. In some cases, diagnosis may be very difficult because of the relatively small number of cysts present. Alternatively, an EIA may be used to detect *Giardia* antigen in fecal samples.

Schistosomiasis is a worldwide public health problem. Control of this disease entails the elimination of the intermediate host snail and removal of streamside vegetation. Abdominal pain is a symptom of schistosomiasis.

Visceral larva migrans is an occupational disease of people who are in close contact with dogs and cats. The disease is caused by the nematodes *Toxocara canis* (dogs) and *Toxocara cati* (cats) and has been recognized in young children who have close contact with pets or who eat dirt. Symptoms include skin rash, eosinophilia, and hepatosplenomegaly.

5-12. The answer is c. *(Brunton, pp 373–374. Craig, p 331. Katzung, pp 422–423.)* For the key to the simple answer, consider the British term for local anesthetics: regional analgesics. Pain is typically the first sensation to go, the last to return. For a more detailed explanation: The primary effect of local anesthetics is intraneuronal blockade of voltage channel-gated Na channels.

Progressively increasing concentrations of local anesthetics result in an increased threshold of excitation, a slowing of impulse conduction, a decline in the rate of rise of the action potential, a decrease in the height of the action potential, and eventual obliteration of the action potential. Local anesthetics first block small unmyelinated or lightly myelinated fibers (pain), followed by heavily myelinated but small-diameter fibers, and then larger-diameter fibers (proprioception, pressure, motor). At high serum concentrations autonomic nerve function can be affected. At toxic concentrations other excitable tissues (cardiac, smooth, skeletal muscle) can be affected.

5-13. The answer is c. (*Ganong, pp 384–389. Kasper et al., pp 1700–1701.*) Vitamin D deficiency causes defective calcification of the bone matrix as a result of inadequate delivery of Ca^{2+} and PO_4^{3-} to the sites of mineralization. The disease in children is called rickets, and is characterized by growth retardation, weakness and bowing of the weight-bearing bones, dental defects, and hypocalcemia, which increases parathyroid hormone and urinary phosphate losses. Several different types of inheritance lead to the vitamin D deficiency disorders, including X-linked dominant and autosomal dominant hypophosphatemic rickets, vitamin D-dependent rickets Type I, an autosomal recessive disorder caused by inactivating mutations in the gene encoding 1α-hydroxylase enzyme, and vitamin D-dependent rickets Type II, in which there is end-organ resistance to $1,25(OH)_2D_3$, which is also usually inherited as an autosomal recessive disorder.

5-14. The answer is a. (*Young, pp 203, 207–221. Junqueira, pp 258, 268, 271, 272, 274. Kindt, pp 29–30, 494–498. Abbas, pp 211–213.*) Martin Causubon suffers from severe combined immunodeficiency (SCID) and has no T cells. The CD3 antibody recognizes a group of five proteins that are associated with the α and β chains of the T cell receptor (TCR). Recognition of antigen-MHC by the TcR-CD3 complex does not require any other molecules. Other "accessory molecules" on T cells (T_H or T_c) and their partner ligands on APCs or target cells provide a "second signal" to stimulate T cells. The region shown is a T-dependent region of the spleen. The photomicrograph shows an area of white pulp with a central artery. The sheath surrounding the central artery is known as the periarterial lymphoid sheath (PALS) and is analogous to the deep cortex (paracortex) of the lymph node or the interfollicular zone of Peyer's patches, the other T-dependent regions within lymphoid tissue.

The histologic structure of the spleen includes the presence of a connective tissue capsule with extensions into the parenchyma, forming trabeculae.

The parenchyma consists of red pulp, which represents areas of red blood cells, many of which are undergoing degradation and phagocytosis by macrophages lining the sinusoids of the red pulp, and white pulp, which represents lymphocytes involved in the filtration of the blood. The germinal centers within the white pulp are the B-dependent regions of the spleen.

(The Case of Martin Causubon is provided courtesy of the Jeffrey Modell Foundation and "The Primary Immunodeficiency Resource Center:" http://www.info4pi.org/patienttopatient/index.cfm?section=patienttopatient&c)

5-15. The answer is d. (*Murray RK, pp 335–339. Scriver, pp 677–704. Lewis, pp 234–237.*) In the classic double-helical model of DNA proposed by Watson and Crick, the purine (adenosine and guanine) and pyrimidine (cytosine and thymine) bases (see Fig. 2) attached to the sugar backbone are perpendicular to the axis and parallel to each other. They are paired (A to G or T to C) and held together by hydrogen bonds. The DNA strands (nucleotide polymers) are joined by linkages between the 3′-hydroxyl of each pentose (deoxyribose) and the 5′-phosphate of its deoxyribose neighbor. Each strand composing the double helix is different and antiparallel. The 3′ end of one strand is opposite the 5′ end of its complement and vice versa (see Fig. 2). DNA replication occurs in the 5′ to 3′ direction on both strands of DNA during the S phase of the cell cycle. It consists of five steps—unwinding by helicases, priming by short RNAs, 5′ to 3′ addition of deoxyribonucleotides via their triphosphates and DNA polymerase in elongation of the "leading" strand (discontinuously using Okazaki fragments for the "lag" strand), replacement of RNA primers with newly synthesized DNA, and sealing of gaps (on the lag strand) with DNA ligase. DNA repair occurs at all cell cycle phases, and among the types is excision repair that uses endonuclease to nick strands adjacent to thymine dimers, DNA polymerase to degrade and replace damaged nucleotides, ligase to restore integrity. All types of DNA synthesis will incorporate deoxyribonucleotide triphosphates rather than isolated bases or deoxyribose residues, and the new nucleotides are synthesized in the 5′ to 3′ direction using both strands of the DNA helix as templates.

5-16. The answer is c. (*Adams, p 1074. Kandel, pp 861–866, 1306–1309. Siegel and Sapru, pp 360–376.*) The spinocerebellar cortical (Purkinje) cells project mainly to the fastigial nucleus. The interposed nuclei receive inputs from the intermediate zone of the hemispheres; the dentate nucleus receives inputs from the lateral aspect of the hemispheres; the superior cerebellar peduncle contains the axons of the interposed and dentate nuclei.

5-17. The answer is b. (*Kumar, pp 803–805. Rubin, pp 673–676.*) The presence of columnar epithelium lining part or all of the distal esophagus is known as Barrett's esophagus. It is considered an acquired change resulting from reflux of acidic gastric contents with ulceration of the esophageal squamous epithelium and replacement by metaplastic, acid-resistant, columnar epithelium. Endoscopically it has a velvety-red appearance. Microscopically, intestinal-type epithelium is most common, but gastric-type epithelium is also seen. Varying degrees of dysplasia may be present. The risk of carcinoma is increased 30- to 40-fold. Virtually all of these tumors are of the adenocarcinoma type and they account for up to 10% of all esophageal cancers.

5-18. The answer is d. (*Kumar, pp 320–324.*) Ultraviolet rays are associated with the formation of skin cancers, including squamous cell carcinoma, basal cell carcinoma, and malignant melanoma. The ultraviolet portion of the spectrum (ultraviolet rays) is divided into three wavelength ranges: UVA (320 to 400 nm), UVB (280 to 320 nm), and UVC (200 to 280 nm). UVB is the wavelength range that is responsible for the induction of skin cancers. The carcinogenic property of UVB is related to the formation of pyrimidine dimers in DNA. UVC, although a potent mutagen, is not significant because it is filtered out by the ozone layer around the earth.

Some DNA viruses and RNA viruses are associated with the development of dysplasia and malignancy. For example, infection with human papillomavirus (HPV), especially types 16 and 18, is associated with cervical dysplasia; Epstein-Barr virus (EBV) is associated with Burkitt's lymphoma and nasopharyngeal carcinoma; hepatitis B virus (HBV) and hepatitis C virus (HCV) are associated with primary hepatocellular carcinoma; and HHV-8 is associated with Kaposi's sarcoma. HTLV-I is an RNA retrovirus that is associated with the formation of a peculiar type of hematologic malignancy called adult T-cell leukemia/lymphoma. These patients have malignant cells in their lymph nodes and blood. This malignancy is endemic in southern Japan and the Caribbean region.

5-19. The answer is a. (*Nolte, pp 225–232. Afifi, pp 59–89.*) First-order neurons that convey pain and temperature sensations to the spinal cord terminate principally in the ipsilateral laminas I and II upon dendrites of cells located in adjacent laminas.

5-20. The answer is b. (*Moore and Dalley, pp 107–109.*) The lymphatic drainage of the mammary gland, which follows the path of its blood supply, generally parallels the tributaries of the axillary, internal thoracic (mammary), thoracoacromial, and intercostal vessels. Because about 75% of the breast lies lateral to the nipple, the more significant lateral and inferior portions of the breast drain toward the axillary nodes. The smaller medial portion drains to the parasternal lymphatic chain paralleling the internal thoracic vessels (**answers c and d**), whereas the very small superior portion drains toward the nodes associated with the thoracoacromial trunk and the supra-clavicular nodes. Lymph rarely crosses the midline (**answer a**). Lymph generally reaches subscapular (apical axillary) nodes after passing through axillary nodes (**answer e**).

5-21. The answer is d. (*Kumar, pp 1353–1354. Rubin, pp 1449–1451.*) Neural tube developmental defects are caused by defective closure of the neural tube. These defects, which may occur anywhere along the extent of the neural tube, are classified as either caudal or cranial defects. Failure of development of the cranial end of the neural tube results in anencephaly, while failure of development of the caudal end of the neural tube results in spina bifida. Anencephaly, which is not compatible with life, is characterized by the absence of the forebrain. Instead, there is a mass of disorganized glial tissue with vessels in this area called a cerebrovasculosa. Ultrasound examination will reveal an abnormal shape to the head of the fetus with an absence of the skull. Note that neural tube defects are associated with increased maternal serum levels of α-fetoprotein (AFP), which is a glycoprotein synthesized by the yolk sac and the fetal liver. Increased serum levels are also associated with yolk sac tumors of the testes and liver cell carcinomas (note that decreased AFP is associated with Down syndrome). Neural tube defects are associated with maternal obesity and decreased folate during pregnancy (folate supplementation in diet decreases the incidence of these developmental defects).

5-22. The answer is e. (*Gilroy, pp 587–588. Siegel and Sapru, pp 225, 235–237.*) The cranial nerve affected by the cold was the facial nerve (cranial nerve VII). Damage to the facial nerve will produce manifestations of facial paralysis, such as failure to close an eye, loss of the eye-blink reflex, inability to whistle, and difficulty in exposure of the teeth. In this diagram, the facial nerve passes around the dorsal aspect of cranial nerve VI and exits in a lateral position at the level of the lower pons.

5-23. The answer is e. (*Brunton, pp 686–689, 691–692. Craig, pp 262–263, 312–314. Katzung, pp 581–582, 991.*) Sodium bicarbonate (IV) can be an important adjunct to managing severe salicylate poisoning for two main reasons: (1) it helps raise blood pH, which as stated earlier is profoundly reduced from metabolic plus respiratory acidosis; (2) it alkalinizes the urine, which (via a pH-dependent mechanism, *a la* Henderson-Hasselbach) converts more aspirin molecules into the ionized form in the tubules, thereby reducing tubular reabsorption of a substance we want to eliminate from the body as quickly as possible.

Acetaminophen (a), even though it is usually an effective antipyretic, is not good for managing fever of severe aspirin poisoning. It would add yet another drug that might complicate the clinical picture, and ordinary (and ordinarily safe) doses aren't likely to do much to lower temperature quickly or sufficiently. (Thus, we use physical means to lower body temperature.) N-acetylcysteine (c), the antidote for acetaminophen poisoning, does nothing for salicylate poisoning. Amphetamines (b) might seem rational for managing ventilatory depression that characterizes late stages of severe aspirin poisoning. The more likely outcome of giving an amphetamine is simply to hasten the onset of seizures. Phenobarbital (d), or other CNS depressants, would aggravate an already bad state of CNS/ventilatory depression. (However, if seizures develop they must be managed—for example, with IV lorazepam and phenytoin, even though they cause CNS depression. Without them, the patient may quickly die from status epilepticus.)

5-24. The answer is b. (*Moore and Dalley, pp 117–118.*) The fluid level in the right pleural cavity is indicative of hemothorax caused by bleeding into the pleural space. As blood collects, lung tissue is displaced and cannot expand fully, thereby impairing ventilation. However, perfusion continues so that the ventilation-perfusion ratio is altered. There would be *no* fluid line if it were a pneumothorax **(answer c)**. A puncture wound often produces a flailing chest [**(answer a)** moving inward as the rest of the thoracic cage expands during inspiration]. Paralysis of the right hemidiaphragm **(answer d)** would result in the diaphragm becoming stationary near its normal expiration height.

5-25. The answer is d. (*Moore and Dalley, pp 277– 280.*) The colon normally has two regions where it is retroperitoneal: the ascending and descending colon. There are also two normal points of flexure: the hepatic (right) and splenic (left) flexures. Therefore, the sigmoid colon, splenic flexure, and hepatic flexure are the regions where the gastroenterologist has the greatest difficulty passing the fiberoptic scope, and thus have the greatest risk of bowel perforation. This is perhaps most easily visualized by looking at Fig. 2.44 on p 278 of Moore & Dalley. Other answers **(answers a, b, c, and e)** are *not* correct.

5-26. The answer is b. (*Adams, pp 443–445, 453–459. Siegel and Sapru, pp 475–478.*) This case is an example of a lesion of the left (usually dominant) parietal lobe, most often in the angular gyrus, with some involvement of the precentral gyrus in the posterior frontal lobe. There is contralateral UMN weakness (with a positive Babinski's sign), as well as several cortical sensory defects—specifically, right-left confusion, agraphia (inability to write, independent of motor weakness), acalculia (the inability to calculate), and finger agnosia (the inability to designate the fingers). The latter four elements are sometimes referred to as the *Gerstmann's syndrome* by neurologists, and all represent spatial discriminatory functions of the parietal lobe (often the dominant parietal lobe, which is usually the left). The parietal lobe also subserves other visual-spatial functions such as construction of complex drawings. There are other locations within the CNS where UMN weakness can occur; however, the combination with parietal lobe signs can occur only in this location. If the damage was slightly more extensive, it may have involved Broca's area, causing aphasia.

5-27. The answer is b. (*Brooks, pp 637–639. Levinson, pp 333–337. Murray PR—2005, pp 712–714. Ryan, pp 680–683.*) In patients with coccidioidomycosis, a positive skin test to coccidioidin appears 2–21 days after the appearance of disease symptoms and may persist for 20 years without reexposure to the fungus. A decrease in intensity of the skin response often occurs in clinically healthy people who move away from endemic areas. A negative skin test frequently is associated with disseminated disease. CF immunoglobulin G (IgG) antibodies, which may not appear at all in mild disease, rise to a high titer in disseminated disease, a poor prognostic sign. For this reason, a persistent or rising CF titer combined with clinical symptoms indicates present or imminent dissemination. Rarely is the CF titer negative. Most persons infected with *C. immitis* are immune to reinfection.

5-28. The answer is d. (*Brunton, pp 238, 240t–241t, 250–251. Craig, pp 101–102, 112t. Katzung, pp 136–137, 212–213.*) Dobutamine behaves, for all practical purposes, as a selective β_1 agonist. Norepinephrine is a β_1 agonist that also activates α-adrenergic receptors effectively. However, when it is administered with phentolamine (prototype α blocker) its spectrum of activity is, qualitatively, identical to that of dobutamine.

High doses of dopamine (a) cause positive inotropic and chronotropic effects, but also release neuronal norepinephrine and probably activate α-adrenergic receptors directly (causing unwanted vasoconstriction). These vasoconstrictor effects would negate vasodilator effects due to stimulation of dopamine D_1 receptors found in some arterioles and of D_2 receptors found on some ganglia, and in the cardiovascular control center of the CNS. Ephedrine (b) weakly activates all adrenergic receptors and also leads to norepinephrine release. Overall, its effects are quite similar to those produced by norepinephrine itself. Regardless, if one administers ephedrine with propranolol (c), the prototypic nonselective (β_1 and β_2) beta blocker, ephedrine's remaining actions amount to selective α-adrenergic activation (i.e., phenylephrine-like)—not at all like dobutamine, and not at all what we want in this situation.

Phenylephrine (α agonist) plus atropine (muscarinic antagonist) (e) causes effects that in no way resemble those of dobutamine or the norepinephrine-phentolamine combination. From a cardiovascular perspective, this combination would give us a rise of blood pressure due to peripheral vasoconstriction. The vasoconstriction would elicit a baroreceptor reflex tantamount to withdrawing sympathetic tone and increasing opposing parasympathetic tone. However, the presence of atropine would blunt parasympathetic-mediated cardiac slowing. The overall and combined effect on heart rate of reduced sympathetic tone to the SA node, and concomitant blockade of ACh–mediated cardiac slowing (also an effect on the SA node) can vary. However, it would be reasonable to predict a slight increase of rate over predrug rates. Nonetheless, there would not be a positive inotropic response, which is what would occur with either dobutamine or a norepinephrine-phentolamine combination.

5-29. The answer is b. (*Murray RK, pp 481–497. Scriver, pp 2275–2296.*) An elevation of pyruvate and a deficiency of acetyl-CoA suggest a deficiency of pyruvate dehydrogenase (PDH). This multisubunit enzyme assembly contains pyruvate dehydrogenase, dihydrolipoyl transacetylase, dihydrolipoyl dehydrogenase, and two enzymes involved in regulation of the overall enzymatic activity of the complex. PDH requires thiamine pyrophosphate as a coenzyme, dihydrolipoyl transacetylase requires lipoic acid and CoA, and dihydrolipoyl dehydrogenase has an FAD prosthetic group that is reoxidized by NAD^+. Biotin, pyridoxine, and ascorbic acid are not coenzymes for PDH. An ATP-dependent protein kinase can phosphorylate PDH to decrease activity, and a phosphatase can activate PDH. Increases of ATP, acetyl-CoA, or NADH (increased energy charge) and of fatty acid oxidation increase phosphorylation of PDH and decrease its activity. PDH is less active during starvation, increasing pyruvate, decreasing glycolysis, and sparing carbohydrates. Free fatty acids decrease PDH activity and would not be appropriate therapy for PDH deficiency. PDH deficiency (246900, 312170) exhibits genetic heterogeneity, as would be expected from its multiple subunits, with autosomal and X-linked recessive forms. The infant also could be classified as having Leigh's disease (266150), a heterogenous group of disorders with hypotonia and lactic acidemia that can include PDH deficiency.

5-30. The answer is c. *(Brunton, p 756. Craig, p 246. Katzung, p 250.)* Thiazides and thiazide-like diuretics (e.g., chlorthalidone, metolazone) may elevate blood glucose levels, impair glucose tolerance, and cause frank hyperglycemia. The loop diuretics may do the same.

Several mechanisms have been proposed to explain the effect: decreased release of insulin from the pancreas; increased glycogenolysis and decreased glucogenesis; a reduction in the conversion of proinsulin to insulin; and a reduced responsiveness of adipocyte and skeletal myocyte insulin receptor response to the hormone.

(You might recall that diazoxide [mainly used as a parenteral drug for prompt lowering of blood pressure] can be used in its oral dosage form to raise blood glucose levels in some hypoglycemic states. It is, chemically, a thiazide, but is not used as a diuretic.)

5-31. The answer is b. *(Murray RK, pp 237–241. Scriver, pp 1667–1724.)* Phenylalanine is an essential amino acid that is converted to tyrosine by phenylalanine hydroxylase. Tyrosine is metabolized to various dopamine metabolites as well as melanin. Children with phenylketonuria (PKU-261600) have deficient phenylalanine hydroxylase and develop elevated phenylalanine with severe mental deficiency that is perhaps related to brain dopamine pathways. Dietary treatment of PKU is effective if begun before age 2–3 months (hence neonatal screening that may not be done in underdeveloped countries), but it must be monitored because phenylalanine cannot be completely excluded from the diet. Complete absence of phenylalanine will cause protein malnutrition and failure to grow. Tyrosine is a precursor to melanin, so deficient tyrosine synthesis in children with PKU often causes a lighter hair and skin color than usual for their family. Phenylalanine and tyrosine levels must be monitored every 3–4 months in children on low phenylalanine diets to ensure balance between accumulation and deficiency.

5-32. The answer is a. *(Brooks, pp 526–527. Levinson, pp 211, 297. Murray PR—2005, p 644. Ryan, p 592.)* Dengue (breakbone fever) is caused by a group B togavirus that is transmitted by mosquitoes. The clinical syndrome usually consists of a mild systemic disease characterized by severe joint and muscle pain, headache, fever, lymphadenopathy, and a maculopapular rash. Hemorrhagic dengue, a more severe syndrome, may be prominent during some epidemics; shock and, occasionally, death result.

5-33. The answer is d. (*Alberts, pp 1005, 1335–1336. Kumar p 100. Ross and Pawlina, pp 80–81, 91.*) Increased transcription of the transcription factor, E2F leads to loss of cell cycle control. E2F is regulated through phosphorylation and dephosphorylation of Retinoblastoma protein (Rb), a key "negative" regulator of the cell cycle. Cells that enter G_1 have dephosphorylated Rb protein that is subsequently phosphorylated, allowing passage of cells from G_1 to "S." Dephosphorylated Rb is inhibitory because it sequesters E2F. Upon Rb phosphorylation, E2F is released and induces the expression of various genes associated with the initiation of the cell cycle.

The phosphorylation or absence of Rb facilitates E2F binding to DNA **(answer e).** Bcl-2 is an antiapoptotic gene **(answer c).** Accumulation of bcl-2 has been associated with the increased incidence and severity of prostate carcinoma in African-American males. Cell division kinase inhibitors block activation of cyclin-CDk [cyclin dependent kinase complexes **(answer b)**] and cell cycle progression **(answer a).** p53 and Rb are tumor suppressor genes. In the absence of Rb or p53, tumor suppression and normal control are lost. p53 increases in the presence of DNA damage, resulting in the inhibition of cell division. p53 mutations inhibit cell division kinase (Cdk) inhibitors such as p21, resulting in uncontrolled cell division. The absence of p53 also permits proliferation of damaged cells. For more details on the regulation of the cell cycle, see "High-Yield Facts."

5-34. The answer is e. (*Sadler, pp 129–131.*) In achondroplasia, the common mutations cause a gain of function of the *FGFR3* gene, resulting in decreased endochondral ossification, inhibited proliferation of chondroblasts in growth plate cartilage, decreased cellular hypertrophy, and decreased cartilage matrix production **(answers b and c).** Growth in the length of long bones after birth (postnatally) occurs through cell proliferation of chondroblasts (immature chandrocytes) in the secondary ossification centers of the epiphyses. The primary ossification centers "close" soon after birth **(answer d).** Fetal development of long bones occurs by the process of endochondral ossification in which a cartilage model is replaced by bone. Before birth, growth in length of the long bone occurs primarily through the proliferation of chondroblasts within the diaphysis of the cartilage model (primary ossification center). Growth in the width of the long bone occurs by the addition of osteoblasts from the periosteum and deposition of a periosteal collar (**answer a**). This is appositional growth without a cartilage intermediate (intramembranous ossification). It is one of the best examples of intramembranous ossification, even though it occurs in the development of a long bone. The action of osteoblasts is to deposit bone matrix and secrete alkaline phosphatase; they do not proliferate in either the primary or the secondary ossification centers.

5-35. The answer is b. (*Brunton, pp 227–228, 356. Craig, pp 342, 344. Katzung, pp 410–411.*) Although a rare occurrence, halothane and other inhaled volatile liquid anesthetics may cause malignant hyperthermia, the signs and symptoms of which we have described in the question. Apparently, this occurs mainly in genetically susceptible individuals (whether a personal or familial history, as the predisposition seems to be heritable). The prevalence of the reaction is increased by concomitant use of succinylcholine. Indeed, the halothane-succinylcholine interaction is most commonly cited as the main cause of malignant hyperthermia.

5-36. The answer is c. (*Ganong, pp 706–708.*) When water is filtered across the glomerulus, the protein concentration (and thus the oncotic pressure) within the capillaries increases, which in turn increases the efficiency by which water reabsorbed from the proximal tubule is returned to the circulatory system. If GFR increases, it results in a larger increase in oncotic pressure. This in turn increases the amount of water reabsorbed from the proximal tubule.

5-37. The answer is c. (*Afifi, pp 59–83. Nolte, pp 220–235. Siegel and Sapru, pp 142–155.*) Sensory fibers that terminate in the medulla are located in the dorsal columns. Fibers mediating conscious proprioception from the upper limb are contained in the fasciculus cuneatus (A). The lateral spinothalamic tract (D) transmits pain and temperature information directly to the thalamus. The lateral corticospinal tract (B) originates in the contralateral cortex and crosses over at the level of the lower medulla. This important pathway mediates control over volitional movements. When these fibers are cut, there is a clear loss of ability to produce volitional movements. The rubrospinal tract (C), situated adjacent to the lateral corticospinal tract, originates from the red nucleus of the midbrain and facilitates the actions of flexor motor neurons. The lateral vestibulospinal tract (E) powerfully facilitates alpha motor neurons of extensor muscles. This tract is located in the ventral funiculus adjacent to the gray matter. The axons of the cells situated in this part of the gray matter (i.e., ventral horn) innervate extensor motor neurons.

The posterior (or dorsal) spinocerebellar tract (H) transmits information from muscle spindles to the cerebellum via the inferior cerebellar peduncle. This tract is located on the lateral aspect of the lateral funiculus of the cord, just above the anterior (or ventral) spinocerebellar tract. Pain and temperature fibers from the periphery terminate directly in the region of the dorsal horn, called the *substantia gelatinosa* (I). A smaller component of the corticospinal tract, the anterior corticospinal tract (F), originates from the cerebral cortex and passes ipsilaterally to the spinal cord. In its ventromedial position, the fibers are ipsilateral to their cortical origin. Just prior to their termination, many of the fibers are distributed to the contralateral side of the cord. The anterior (or ventral) spinocerebellar tract (G) arises from wide regions of the gray matter of the cord. These fibers pass contralaterally to the lateral aspect of the lateral funiculus to reach a position just below the dorsal spinocerebellar tract. These fibers then ascend to the cerebellum via the superior cerebellar peduncle, conveying information from Golgi tendon organs located in the lower limbs.

5-38. The answer is d. *(Murray RK, pp 358–373. Scriver, pp 3–45. Lewis, pp 185–204.)* The gene that produces the deadly toxin of Corynebacterium diphtheriae comes from a lysogenic phage that grows in the bacteria. Prior to immunization, diphtheria was the primary cause of death in children. The protein toxin produced by this bacterium inhibits protein synthesis by inactivating elongation factor 2 (EF-2, or translocase). Diphtheria toxin is a single protein composed of two portions (A and B). The B portion enables the A portion to translocate across a cell membrane into the cytoplasm. The A portion catalyzes the transfer of the adenosine diphosphate ribose unit of NAD_1 to a nitrogen atom of the diphthamide ring of EF-2, thereby blocking translocation. Diphthamide is an unusual amino acid residue of EF-2.

5-39. The answer is e. *(Brunton, pp 632, 1196. Craig, pp 553–554. Katzung, p 749.)* This "red man" syndrome is characteristically associated with vancomycin. It is thought to be caused by histamine release. The risk or severity can be reduced dramatically by infusing the drug more slowly, and by pretreatment with antihistamines (H_1 receptor blockers, e.g., diphenhydramine).

5-40. The answer is d. *(Brooks, p 650. Levinson, pp 338–341. Ryan, pp 678–680.)* This description is a typical picture of mucormycosis occurring in a diabetic patient. The organism is a member of *Phycomycetes*, which forms uniseptate hyphae. In candidiasis, septate hyphae and budding yeast are seen in infected tissues. Nocardiosis, erysipelas, and gas gangrene are not mycotic infections. They are caused by bacteria (*N. asteroides, Streptococcus pyogenes, and Clostridium perfringens* respectively).

5-41. The answer is b. (*Ganong, pp 317–332. Kasper et al., pp 2107–2109.*) Secretion of TSH is regulated primarily by the pituitary levels of T_3. As plasma thyroid hormone levels increase, pituitary T_3 levels rise and lead to inhibition of TSH synthesis and secretion. TSH stimulates thyroid gland function by binding to specific cell membrane receptors and increasing the intracellular levels of cAMP. The thyroid gland secretes thyroxine (T_4) and triiodothyronine (T_3); the latter is the physiologically active hormone. The majority of T_3 is formed in the peripheral tissues by deiodination of T_4.

5-42. The answer is b. (*Afifi, pp 82–85. Siegel and Sapru, pp 152–154.*) The medial vestibulospinal tract arises from the medial vestibular nucleus and descends in the MLF to cervical levels, where it controls lower motor neurons (LMNs), which innervate (flexor) muscles controlling the position of the head. The lateral vestibulospinal tract facilitates extensor motor neurons of the limbs, the rubrospinal tract facilitates flexor motor neurons of the limbs, and the reticulospinal tracts modulate muscle tone of the limbs.

5-43. The answer is d. (*Favus, pp 58–59, 150–152, 277–282. Kierszenbaum, pp 126–128. Reszka, pp 45–52.*) The woman in the vignette is diagnosed with osteoporosis. The DXA "T" score of -2 indicates that she is four times more likely to have a spine fracture than a person with a normal bone mineral density (BMD). The -2.5 "T" score indicates she is five times more likely to have a hip fracture than a person with a normal BMD. Bisphosphonate treatment is the most effective current treatment for osteoporosis. Bisphosphonates are analogues of the pyrophosphates and suppress bone resorption by osteoclasts. Inhibition of osteoblastic activity **(answer a)** would inhibit new bone deposition but also inhibit the production of RANK-L (receptor for activation of nuclear factor kappa beta-ligand) and M-CSF (macrophage colony-stimulating factor) by osteoblasts. RANK-L binds to RANK on the osteoclast and stimulates osteoclastic activity. M-CSF stimulates the differentiation of monocytes into osteoclasts. Increased RANK-L **(answer b)** and M-CSF **(answer c)** secretion by osteoblasts and upregulation of RANK **(answer e)** on the surface of osteoclasts will all increase osteoclastic activity. Some of the bisphosphonates are metabolized to a toxic analogue that targets mitochondria and apoptosis of the osteoclasts. Others interfere with cholesterol-dependent pathways in the osteoclast. The interactions of RANK, RANK-L, and osteo-protegerin (OPG) are shown in the following figure.

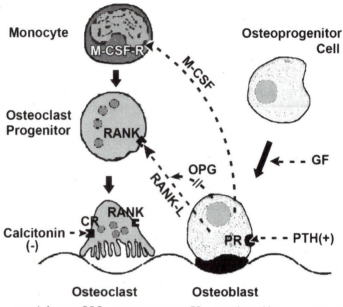

GF = growth factors, OPG = osteoprotegerin, PR = parathyroid hormone receptor,
PTH = parathyroid hormone, RANK = receptor for activation of nuclear factor
kappa B, RANK-L = ligand for RANK, M-CSF = macrophage colony-stimulating factor,
M-CSF-R = MCSF receptor.

5-44. The answer is e. (*Ross, p 254. Junqueira, p 238. Kumar, p 620.*) The bone marrow begins to function in the second month and becomes the pre-dominant hematopoietic site during months 5 to 9 of gestation, The first site of blood cell development (hematopoiesis) is extraembryonic, in the yolk sac (**answer b**), which produces hematocytoblasts and primitive ery-throblasts from the third week through the second month of gestation. Hepatic erythropoiesis (**answer a**) begins during the sixth week, reaches its maximum in the third month, and then ceases about the seventh month. Whereas, the spleen (**answer c**) is involved specifically in the production of red blood cells (erythropoiesis) from months 2 to 5 of gestation with some activity continuing postnatally. The spleen continues to produce monocytes and lymphocytes throughout life. From the second month of gestation, the lymph nodes produce lymphocytes, and the thymus (**answer d**) is responsible for the education of T cells. Those T lymphocytes are seeded to T-dependent areas, such as the deep cortex of the lymph node and periarteriolar lymphoid sheath (PALS) of the spleen.

5-45. The answer is a. (*Kierszenbaum, pp 427–429. Kumar, pp 844–845. Kasper, pp 222–223.*) The area shown in the photomicrograph is the glycocalyx (brush border consisting of microvilli) of the small intestinal epithelium. It is the location of the brush border enzymes including lactase. The patient in the scenario is suffering from lactase deficiency which often has an adult onset since lactase activity decreases after childhood. The absence of lactase or reduced lactase activity results in passage of undigested lactose into the colon. Colonic bacteria carry out fermentation of the lactose to organic acids and hydrogen. The bloating, cramping, and abdominal pain are due to the breakdown of lactose and production of the hydrogen gas. The microvilli are also the site of the glucose/galactose transporter (**answers b and c**). However, the glucose/galactose transporter is *not* the site of the deficiency in lactose intolerance. Other brush border enzymes include the other monosaccharidases and enterokinase, which is important for cleavage of pancreatic zymogens (e.g., trypsinogen) to their active form.

Digestion of lipids occurs through the action of bile (from the liver and bile duct) and lipase (from the pancreas). Bile serves to emulsify the lipid to form micelles, whereas lipase breaks down the lipid from triglycerides to fatty acids, glycerol, and monoglycerides (**answers d and e**). Those three breakdown products diffuse freely across the microvilli to enter the apical portion of the enterocyte by passive diffusion. Triglycerides are resynthesized in the smooth endoplasmic reticulum. Proteins are synthesized in the RER and are combined with sugar and lipid portions in the Golgi to form glycoproteins and lipoproteins. Those two types of molecules form the coverings of the triglyceride cores of the chylomicra. The chylomicra are released at the basolateral membranes by exocytosis into the lacteals. From the lacteals, the chylomicra travel into the cisterna chyli and eventually into the venous system by way of the thoracic duct. Digestion of fat occurs to a greater extent in the duodenum and jejunum than in the ileum.

Sugars are broken down by amylase in the oral cavity, with continued digestion by brush border monosaccharidases. Proteins are broken down by pepsinogen in the stomach with continued breakdown in the small intestine by the enzymes of the pancreatic juice (e.g., trypsin, chymotrypsin, and carboxypeptidases). The products of protein digestion are amino acids that are actively transported by transporters also located in the brush border.

5-46. The answer is e. *(Alberts, pp 720–722, 724, 729–730, 744–745. Junqueira, pp 39, 50.)* The child is suffering from inclusion (I)–cell disease. There is an absence or deficiency of N-acetylglucosamine phosphotransferase and an absence of mannose-6-phosphate (M6P) on the lysosomal enzymes. The failure to add M6P in the cis-Golgi results in inappropriate vesicular segregation by M6P receptors in the trans–Golgi network (TGN). The default pathway is transport to the cell membrane and secretion from the cell by exocytosis for proteins lacking M6P. Lysosomal enzymes are secreted into the bloodstream, and undigested substrates build up within the cells. There is no missorting back to the Golgi **(answer a)**. Peroxisomal enzymes, which are sorted by the presence of three specific amino acids located at the C-terminus: Ser–Lys–Leu–COO⁻, are not affected **(answer b)**. KDEL **(answer c)** is the signal used for retrieval of proteins from the Golgi back to the endoplasmic reticulum. SNAREs [soluble-N-ethylemalemide sensitive factor (NSF) attachment protein receptors] are the receptors for SNAPs [soluble-N-ethylemalemide sensitive factor (NSF) attachment proteins] and bind vesicles to membranes **(answer d)**. Trafficking to other structures, such as the nucleus and mitochondria, is regulated by nuclear localization signals (NLSs) or an N-terminal signal peptide, respectively.

5-47. The answer is c. *(Moore and Dalley, p 304.)* Obstruction of any portion of the biliary tree will produce symptoms of gallbladder obstruction. If the common hepatic duct **(answer b)** or bile duct **(answer a)** is occluded by stone or tumor, biliary stasis with accompanying jaundice occurs. In addition, blockage of the duodenal papilla (of Vater), distal to the juncture of the bile duct with the pancreatic duct **(answer e)**, can lead to complicating pancreatitis. If only the cystic duct is obstructed, jaundice will not occur because bile may flow freely from the liver to the duodenum. Bile duct obstruction also may arise as a result of pressure exerted on the duct by an external mass, such as a tumor in the head of the pancreas. **Answser d** is not anatomically correct.

5-48. The answer is c. *(Kumar, pp 673–674. Rubin, pp 1122–1126.)* Chronic lymphocytic leukemia (CLL) is the most common leukemia and is similar in many aspects to small lymphocytic lymphoma (SLL). It is typically found in patients older than 60 years of age. Histological examination of the peripheral smear reveals a marked increase in the number of mature-appearing lymphocytes. These neoplastic lymphocytes are fragile and easily damaged. This fragility produces the characteristic finding of numerous smudge cells in the peripheral smears of patients with CLL. About 95% of the cases of CLL are of B-cell origin (B-CLL) and are characterized by having pan–B-cell markers, such as CD19. These malignant cells characteristically also have the T-cell marker CD5. The remaining 5% of cases of CLL are mainly of T-cell origin. Patients with CLL tend to have an indolent course and the disease is associated with long survival in many cases. The few symptoms that may develop are related to anemia and the absolute lymphocytosis of small, mature cells. Splenomegaly may be noted. In a minority of patients, however, the disease may transform into prolymphocytic leukemia or a large cell immunoblastic lymphoma (Richter's syndrome). Prolymphocytic leukemia is characterized by massive splenomegaly and a markedly increased leukocyte count consisting of enlarged lymphocytes having nuclei with mature chromatin and nucleoli.

5-49. The answer is d. (*Kumar, pp 695–696. Henry, pp 605–606.*) The myelodysplastic syndromes (MDS) are a group of disorders characterized by defective hematopoietic maturation and an increased risk of developing acute leukemia. These disorders characteristically have hypercellular bone marrows but pancytopenia in the peripheral blood. The two basic types of MDS are an idiopathic (primary) form and a therapy-related (secondary) form. Both have numerous dysplastic features affecting all blood cell lines. Red cell dysplastic features include the presence of ringed sideroblasts, megaloblastoid erythroid precursors, and misshapen erythroid precursors. A dimorphic population of red cells may be seen in the peripheral blood of some patients with some types of MDS. White cell dysplastic features include hypogranular cells or Pelger-Huët white blood cells, which are abnormal appearing neutrophils having only two nuclear lobes. Megakaryocytes may be abnormal and have only a single nuclear lobe or multiple separate nuclei, so-called "pawn ball" megakaryocytes. Chromosomal abnormalities are commonly associated with the MDSs, especially 5q_ and trisomy 8.

Except for chronic myelomonocytic leukemia (CMML), which is characterized by a marked increase in the number of monocytes, the MDSs are subclassified by the number of blasts present within the bone marrow. The FAB classification of MDS is as follows: if there are less than 5% blasts present, the MDS is either refractory anemia (RA) or RA with ring sideroblasts (RARS). RA with excess blasts (RAEB, pronounced "rab") has between 5 and 20% blasts, while refractory anemia with excess blasts in transformation (RAEBIT, pronounced "rabbit") has between 20 and 30% blasts in the marrow. Acute leukemia is defined as the presence of more than 30% blasts in the marrow. The WHO (World Health Organization) has a similar classification of the MDS except that in their classification the number of blasts in the bone marrow needed for the diagnosis of acute leukemia is only 20%.

5-50. The answer is e. (*Goldman, pp 1093–1095. Kumar, pp 156–158.*) Lipids are transported in the blood complexed to proteins called apo-lipoproteins. Abnormalities of this lipid transport or metabolism result in hyperlipoproteinemias, which are responsible for most syndromes of premature atherosclerosis. The primary hyperlipidemias are divided into five distinct electrophoretic patterns. Type I hyperlipoproteinemia, caused by a mutation in the lipoprotein lipase gene, results in increased chylomicrons and triglycerides. Type II hyperlipoproteinemia, perhaps the most frequent Mendelian disorder, is caused by a mutation in the low-density lipoprotein (LDL) receptor gene. This results in increased LDL and cholesterol. Homozygotes for this gene defect have markedly increased plasma cholesterol levels and develop severe atherosclerosis at an early age. Xanthomas of the Achilles tendon are somewhat specific for this disorder. Mutations in the apolipoprotein E gene result in type III hyperlipoproteinemia, which is characterized by increased intermediate-density lipoproteins (IDLs), triglycerides, and cholesterol. Type IV hyperlipoproteinemia causes increased very-low-density lipoproteins (VLDLs) and triglycerides. The genetic defect causing this abnormality is a mutation in the lipoprotein lipase gene. Type V hyperlipoproteinemia, caused by a mutation in apolipoprotein CII, results in increased VLDLs, chylomicrons, triglycerides, and cholesterol.

Block 6

Answers

6-1. The answer is a. (*Ganong, p 688. Kasper et al., p 1568. Levitzky, pp 12, 116–117. Stead et al., pp 273–274.*) When air enters the pleural space due to interruption of the pleural surface through either the rupture of the lung or a hole in the chest wall, the pressure in the pleural space becomes atmospheric, the lung on the affected side collapses because of the lung's tendency to recoil inward, and the chest wall on the affected side recoils outward. Because the intrapleural pressure is atmospheric, the mediastinum shifts farther to the normal side with each inspiration. With collapse of the lung, the $\dot{V}/\dot{Q}$ ratio on the affected side decreases.

6-2. The answer is b. (*Murray RK, pp 314–357. Scriver, pp 4571–4636. Lewis, pp 205–240.*) The offspring of a woman with sickle cell anemia must receive one of her abnormal β-globin alleles and be a heterozygote or carrier known as sickle cell trait. Approximately 1 in 12 African Americans will have sickle trait, justifying its inclusion in American neonatal screening protocols. Caucasians, especially those of Mediterranean origin, can also be affected. Individuals with sickle trait will be asymptomatic under normal conditions, but may show symptoms under conditions of low oxygen tension (high altitudes, diving, etc.) due to the lower oxygen-binding capacity of their red blood cells (half normal, half sickle cell hemoglobin). Those with sickle trait will have one β-globin gene with a sickle mutation that ablates the sixth codon MstII site, yielding a 680 bp fragment by Southern blot in addition to the 515 and 165 bp fragments yielded by the normal β-globin gene. RNA transcription and processing willl not be affected, yielding a β-globin mRNA of about 700 bp. The sickle hemoglobin will have a different charge and conformation due to its glutamic acid to valine substitution, migrating differently by electrophoresis and yielding a second, abnormal hemoglobin band in addition to that of normal hemoglobin.

6-3. The answer is e. (*Alberts, pp 584–592, 608–612.*) The patient in the scenario is suffering from cirrhosis in which there are alterations in plasma lipoproteins. Binding of an antibody to a cell surface receptor results in lateral diffusion of protein in the lipid bilayer, resulting in increased membrane fluidity—patching and capping. Rotational and lateral movements of both proteins and lipids contribute to membrane fluidity. Restriction reduces membrane fluidity (**answer a**). Phospholipids are capable of lateral diffusion, rapid rotation around their long axis, and flexion of their hydrocarbon (fatty acyl) tails. They undergo transbilayer movement (**answer b**), known as "flip-flop," between bilayers in the endoplasmic reticulum; however, in general this does not occur in the plasma membrane. Other factors reduce membrane fluidity. An increase in the amount of cholesterol relative to phospholipid (**answer c**) has been shown by a variety of physicochemical techniques to decrease fluidity in both biological and artificial membranes by interacting with the hydrophobic regions near the polar head groups and stiffening this region of the membrane. Association or binding of integral membrane proteins with cytoskeletal elements (**answer d**) on the interior of the cell and peripheral membrane proteins on the extracellular surface limit membrane mobility and fluidity.

6-4. The answer is c. (*Damjanov, pp 1006–1008. Kumar, pp 753–756.*) Infection by the protozoan *P. carinii* is characterized by the presence of oval and helmet-shaped organisms whose capsules are made more visible by use of Gomori's methenamine-silver staining technique. This organism, although it has low virulence, is opportunistic; it is often seen to attack severely ill, immunologically depressed patients. It is frequently the first opportunistic infection to be diagnosed in HIV-1-positive patients, and it is a leading cause of death in patients with AIDS.

6-5. The answer is c. (*Murray RK, pp 374–395. Scriver, pp 525–537. Lewis, pp 205–216.*) Southern analysis using methylation-sensitive or insensitive endonuclease restriction in the first two panels of the figure suggests both p57 alleles in the tumor are methylated. Only the larger fragment is detected in the patient sample when restricted with methylation-sensitive endonuclease (second panel). The accompanying Northern blot shows markedly decreased amounts of p57 mRNA, supporting a connection between p57 allele methylation and silencing of expression. The maternal allele of p57 is undermethylated and expressed in normal tissues, and its loss of imprinting (methylation) is one of the few situations where epigenetic silencing appears to be the sole carcinogenic event.

6-6. The answer is d. (*Martin, pp 42–49. Afifi, pp 194–195. Siegel and Sapru, pp 240–242.*) The trochlear nerve controls downward movement of the eyes when it is situated in a medial position. After exiting the brain, this cranial nerve enters the cavernous sinus (along with cranial nerves III, V, and VI) and enters the orbit through the superior orbital fissure. Therefore, pressure exerted on the cavernous sinus could easily affect the function of this nerve.

6-7. The answer is a. *(Alberts, pp 742–743, Fig. 13-35. Rubin, pp 785–787. Kumar, pp 910–911. Kasper, pp 409–410.)* The patient in the scenario suffers from Wilson's disease in which copper accumulates in the tissues. For example, in the liver the mutation in ATP7B prevents translocation of copper from the cytosol to the late endosome blocking biliary copper excretion via lysosomes and resulting in accumulation of copper in the liver. The late endosome is part of the endocytic pathway. Cargo proteins from the late endosome reach the lysosome by development into lysosomes, transport to lysosomes via vesicles, or fusion with lysosomes. Clathrin-coated pits and vesicles **(answer b)** endocytose and subsequently deliver proteins to the early endosome in the first stages of the endocytic process. Multivesicular bodies (MVBs) are the means of transport from early to late endosomes **(answer c)**. The CGN *(cis-Golgi network)* receives transitional elements in the form of coatomer-coated vesicles carrying proteins and lipids from the rough endoplasmic reticulum and participates in phosphorylation. The remaining Golgi stacks are the *cis*, medial, *trans*, and TGN (trans-Golgi network). The medial compartment is responsible for the removal of mannose and the addition of N-acetylglucosamine. The *trans* face is responsible for the addition of sialic acid and galactose. The TGN serves as a sorting station for proteins destined for various organelles (e.g., lyosomes), the plasma membrane, and protein for export from the cell **(answer e)**. Golgi-derived transport and secretory vesicles bud off from the TGN. Recycling of receptors occurs from early endosomes to the plasma membrane **(answer d)**.

6-8. The answer is e. *(Junqueira, pp 423–428. Kumar, pp 1172–1173. Moore and Persaud, Developing, pp 215–217.)* The patient is suffering from Graves' disease, an autoimmune disease that occurs much more frequently in women than in men. Graves' disease accounts for approximately 85% of diagnosed hyperthyroidism. Patients with Graves' disease produce autoantibodies to TSH receptors. $CD8^+$-T cells are also generated against the TSH receptors, leading to their destruction. The result is an increase in TSH produced by the anterior pituitary with a concomitant increase in thyroid hormone production [T4 (tetraiodothyronine, thyroxine) and T3 (tetraiodothyronine)] from the thyroid. The elevated thyroid hormone secretion leads to the nervousness, weight loss, and extreme mood changes experienced by the patient.

The thyroid gland is shown in the photomicrograph and is most often confused histologically with lactating mammary gland, which differs from the thyroid in the presence of an elaborate duct system. The thyroid is composed of follicles filled with colloidal material and surrounded by follicular cells with a cuboidal-to-columnar epithelium. The C cells are found outside the follicular cells and produce calcitonin, synthesized by the interfollicular "C" (parafollicular) cells derived embryologically from the ultimobranchial bodies (fourth and possibly fifth pair of branchial pouches). Calcitonin decreases elevated serum calcium levels by transiently inhibiting osteoclastic activity through receptors on osteoclasts. In Graves' disease there are no autoantibodies to the C cells (answer a). Destruction of C cells would lead to an absence of calcitonin and high serum calcium levels. Autoantibodies to principal cells of the parathyroid (answer b) would lead to decreased serum calcium levels as parathyroid hormone (PTH) synthesis and secretion would be reduced. PTH increases osteoclastic resorption and also stimulates Ca^{2+} uptake from the gut and Ca^{2+} reabsorption by the kidneys. The thyroid gland is under the direct regulation of TSH (thyrotropin) production by the anterior pituitary, which in turn is regulated by TSH-releasing factor (TSH-RF) released from the hypothalamus. TSH-RF is transported by the hypothalamic-hypophyseal (pituitary)-portal system to the anterior pituitary. Autoantibodies to TSH-RF (answer c) would result in elevated TSH and T3 and T4, but the receptors would be located in the anterior pituitary on thyrotrophs. Autoantibodies to thyroglobulin and thyroid peroxidase result in Hashimoto's thyroiditis (answer d).

Asthenia is loss of strength and tachycardia is accelerated heart rate. Pretibial myxedema presents as an orange-peel-like rash on the shins in some patients with Graves' disease.

The thyroid follicular epithelial cells import iodide and amino acids from the capillary lumen. The follicular cells synthesize thyroglobulin from amino acids. When iodide enters the follicular cells, it undergoes oxidation. Thyroglobulin is iodinated while in the colloid, and iodinated thyroglobulin (not the thyroid hormones) is the storage product in the thyroid colloid. The thyroid follicular cells process iodinated thyroglobulin, and the activity of lysosomes breaks down the colloid to form thyroxine (T4), triiodothyronine (T3), diiodotyrosine (DIT), and monoiodotyrosine (MIT). Most of the secretion of the human thyroid gland is composed of thyroxine, although triiodothyronine is more potent.

6-9. The answer is d. *(Kandel, pp 282–284. Siegel and Sapru, pp 115–118. Siegel et al., pp 244–246.)* The biosynthesis of catecholamines includes the following steps: Tyrosine is converted into L-DOPA by tyrosine hydroxylase. L-DOPA is then decarboxylated by a decarboxylase to form dopamine (and CO_2). The conversion of dopamine to norepinephrine comes about by the action of the enzyme dopamine β-hydroxylase. The rate-limiting enzyme in the biosynthesis of serotonin is tryptophan hydroxylase. In this process, tryptophan is converted to 5-hydroxytryptophan by tryptophan hydroxylase and by 5-hydroxytryptophan decarboxylase into serotonin.

6-10. The answer is b. *(Brooks, pp 216–218, 220, 640–642, 7. Levinson, pp 164, 481s–482s, 333–337. Murray PR—2005, pp 417–418, 289–292, 714–715. Ryan, pp 649–650, 676–683.)* Actinomycosis is a chronic suppurative and granulomatous infection that produces pyogenic lesions with interconnecting sinus tracts that contain granules composed of microcolonies of bacteria embedded in tissue components. The etiologic agents are closely related to normal oral flora with most cases being due to *Actinomyces israelii*, a facultative anaerobe. The three most common forms are cervicofacial, thoracic, and abdominal, with trauma being the mechanism that introduces these organisms into the mucosa tissues. The bacteria bridge the mucosal surfaces of the mouth, respiratory tract, and lower GI tract. Infection is associated with dental caries, gingivitis, surgical complication, or trauma, as mentioned above. Aspiration may lead to pulmonary infection. Cervicofacial disease presents as a swollen, erythematous process in the jaw area, producing draining fistulas. *A. bovis* seldom causes human disease. Nocardia infection is usually caused by inhalation of the organism and relate to pulmonary infections. *H. capsulatum* could be identified by microscopic examination of exudate, showing large, spherical thick-walled macroconidia with peripheral projections of cell wall materials.

6-11. The answer is c. *(Brooks, pp 438–440, 420–428, 599–601, 562–566, 442–446. Levinson, pp 248–249, 249–250, 255–256, 256–257, 281. Murray PR—2005, pp 550–553, 533–539, 523–524, 597, 559–561. Ryan, pp 509–510, 564–565, 568, 579, 619.)* Varicella- zoster virus is a herpesvirus. Chickenpox is a highly contagious disease of childhood that occurs in the late winter and early spring. It is characterized by a generalized vesicular eruption with relatively insignificant systemic manifestations.

Adenovirus has been associated with adult respiratory disease among newly enlisted military troops. Crowded conditions and strenuous exercise may account for the severe infections seen in this otherwise healthy group.

Papillomavirus is one of two members of the family Papovaviridae, which includes viruses that produce human warts. These viruses are host-specific and produce benign epithelial tumors that vary in location and clinical appearance. The warts usually occur in children and young adults and are limited to the skin and mucous membranes. Rubeola (measles) virus produces a maculopapular rash. No vesicles or pustule forms are developed and no successive crops of lesions are formed. Infectious mononucleosis caused by CMV is clinically difficult to distinguish from that caused by EBV. Lymphocytosis is usually present, with an abundance of atypical lymphocytes. CMV-induced mononucleosis should be considered in any case of mononucleosis that is heterophil-negative and in patients with fever of unknown origin.

6-12. The answer is f. *(Katzung, p 333.)* You should know N-acetylcysteine as an antidote for acetaminophen poisoning. When used for that purpose, it is given orally or intravenously. The sulfhydryl groups that are part of the molecule are important, as they react with the toxic acetaminophen metabolite and spare glutathione-depleted hepatocytes from oxidative attack. N-acetylcysteine is also a mucolytic (mucus-thinning) drug, given by inhalation in a nebulized solution or by intratracheal instillation, to reduce the viscosity of airway mucus that can then be removed easier by coughing, postural drainage and chest percussion, or by airway suctioning. Here, too, the mechanism is based on its—SH rich composition. N-acetylcysteine lacks other airway effects such as bronchodilation or suppression or inflammation.

6-13. The answer is d. *(Kandel, pp 1213–1216. Siegel et al., pp 1080–1082.)* Lithium has been used for a number of years as an effective drug for the treatment of bipolar disorders. It has been shown to decrease the length, severity, and recurrence of manic states as well as the depressive components of this disorder. The mechanism of action of lithium in effectively combating bipolar disorder is not absolutely clear, since it has a wide variety of biological effects. In part, these include changes in the expression of some G-proteins and subtypes of adenyl cyclase, alteration of the coupling of G-proteins to neurotransmitter receptors, alterations of monoamine levels and receptors, and effects upon ion channels. Monoaminergic drugs are generally used for the treatment of panic disorders and, to some extent, to treat anxiety. Anxiety attacks are also treated with benzodiazepine drugs. For schizophrenia, a wide range of drugs have been used; these include those that affect monoaminergic, cholinergic, and GABAergic systems.

6-14. The answer is b. (*Moore and Dalley, pp 359–360.*) The sacrococcygeal joint. The indicated line represents the sacroiliac joint. These structures are seen bilaterally between the alae of the sacrum and the ilia. The body of the sacrum (**answer a**) is in the midline and normal. The sacroiliac ligaments might have been sprained by the trauma of the fall. The pathway for spinal nerves (**answer c**) is through foramina of the sacrum, *not* through long bony canals. Similarly, the pathway for the gluteal arteries (**answers d and e**) is through the greater sciatic foramen between the ilium and the sacrum.

6-15. The answer is d. (*Murray RK, pp 205–218. Scriver, pp 2863–2914.*) The shell of apoproteins coating blood transport lipoproteins is important in the physiologic function of the lipoproteins. Some of the apoproteins contain signals that target the movement of the lipoproteins in and out of specific tissues. B48 and E seem to be important in targeting chylomicron remnants to be taken up by liver. B100 is synthesized as the coat protein of VLDLs and marks their end product, LDLs, for uptake by peripheral tissues. Other apoproteins are important for the solubilization and movement of lipids and cholesterol in and out of the particles. CII is a lipoprotein lipase activator that VLDLs and chylomicrons receive from HDLs. The A apoproteins are found in HDLs and are involved in lecithin–cholesterol acyl transferase (LCAT) regulation. Familial hypercholesterolemia (144010) causes early heart attacks in heterozygotes, particularly in males, and childhood disease in rare homozygotes. The daughter's chest pain was likely angina due to coronary artery occlusion and her skin patches were fatty deposits known as xanthomata.

6-16. The answer is b. (*Ganong, pp 484, 496, 504–505. Stead et al., pp 149–154.*) Inflammation of the duodenum may lead to increased acid output, hypocalcemia, and microcytic anemia. Increased basal and maximal acid outputs may result from excessive stimulation of the parietal cell (e.g., hypergastrinemia) or reduced inhibitory feedback (i.e., reduced effect of enterogastrone and the enterogastric reflex). The latter may occur when the proximal small intestine is inflamed. Although calcium is absorbed along the entire length of the small intestine, it is absorbed primarily in the duodenum. Similarly, iron is absorbed primarily in the duodenum. Microcytic anemia is the result of reduced stores of iron, the most common anemia. Glucose-6-phosphatase deficiency is the most common metabolic disorder of red blood cells, and is also associated with a microcytic anemia, as is α-thalassemia.

6-17. The answer is c. (*Ganong, p 81. Kasper et al., pp 261–265, 1375. Stead et al., pp 231–232.*) An increase in extracellular K^+ makes the membrane potential more positive. Depolarizing the membrane opens K^+ channels causing an increase in membrane conductance. Prolonged depolarization, whether caused by an increase in extracellular K^+ or by an action potential, inactivates Na^+ channels, which decreases the excitability of the nerve membrane. The activity of the Na^+-K^+ pump is reduced in hypokalemia, not hyperkalemia.

6-18. The answer is c. (*Murray RK, pp 5–13. Scriver, pp 3–45. Lewis, pp 185–204.*) The amino acid cystine, essentially a dimer of cysteine, accumulates in the lysosomes of patients with cystinosis (219800). It has a sulfhydryl side group with a pKa of 8.3 that is different from the amino side groups of lysine, arginine, and glutamine (pKas 9–12). These patients exhibit progressive vision problems and renal failure, but these problems can be forestalled by cysteamine treatment, which complexes with cystine and allows egress from lysosomes.

6-19. The answer is a. (*Brunton, pp 538, 1256–1258. Craig, p 370. Katzung, p 454.*) This cutaneous response, called *livedo reticularis*, is characteristically associated with amantadine. Recall that this seldom-used antiparkinson drug probably works by releasing endogenous dopamine and blocking its neuronal reuptake. Livedo reticularis is not associated with levodopa (used alone or with carbidopa; c or d), nor with the dopamine agonists bromocriptine (d) or pramipexole (e; a newer and generally preferred drug for starting treatment of mild parkinsonian signs and symptoms). (You might also recall that amantadine is also used for prophylaxis of some strains of influenza virus infections.)

6-20. The answer is D. (*Siegel and Sapru, pp 225, 240–243.*) The inability to move the right eye to the right (i.e., in a lateral direction) is the result of damage to the right abducens nerve (cranial nerve VI). Normally, activation of the right abducens nerve causes the right eye to be moved laterally to the right. This cranial nerve exits the brain at the level of the lower pons just above the medulla at a position medial to the exit of the facial nerve. The cell bodies of origin of this nerve lie in the caudal aspect of the dorsomedial pons at a position just below where the facial nerve arches over and around cranial nerve VI before it exits the brainstem.

21. The answer is d. (*Brooks, pp 316, 645–647. Levinson, pp 25, 182, 484s. Murray PR—2005, p 397. Ryan, p 904.*) Microscopic examination can readily demonstrate clue cells (epithelial cells with *Gardnerella* bacteria attached) or pseudohyphae (*Candida*). A wet mount will be needed to demonstrate motile *Trichomonas* cells. *Candida, Trichomonas,* and bacterial vaginitis are seen most often. *Staphylococcus aureus* is involved much less frequently. While *E. coli* may be a common cause of genitourinary infection, clue cells are usually absent. See the table below for a comparison of these bacteria.

6-22. The answer is c. (*Murray RK, pp 173–179. Scriver, pp 3181–3218.*) Triacylglycerols are assembled from glycerol and saturated fatty acids that are synthesized from condensation of malonyl and acetyl CoA through the fatty acyl synthase complex. Plasmalogens and certain signaling agents like platelet activating factor are ether lipids, distinguished by an ether (C-O-C) bond at carbon 1 of glycerol. Ether lipid synthesis is initiated by placing an acyl group on carbon 1 of dihydroxyacetone phosphate (DHAP) using DHAP acyltransferase. The acyl side chain is then exchanged with an alcohol to form an ether linkage by an acylDHAP synthase—the acyltransferase and synthase plus other enzymes of ether lipid synthesis are localized in peroxisomes. Subsequent additions of phosphocholine yield ether/acyl glycerols analogous to lecithins (including platelet activating factor), and addition of a phosphoethanolamine to carbon 3 of ether (alkyl) glycerols forms plasmalogens. Acetyl and palmitoyl CoA can contribute to these ether lipid modifications after the core carbon 1 ether linkage has produced an alkylglycerol. Disruption of peroxisome structure by mutations in various peroxisomal membrane proteins ablates DHAP acyltransferase and other enzymes for ether lipid/plasmalogen synthesis, causing deficienty of brain lipids, severe neurologic disease, hypotonia, and liver failure—the most severe phenotype of which is Zellweger syndrome (214100).

6-23. The answer is e. (*Goldman, pp 560, 566. Ayala, pp 121, 125.*) Respiratory alkalosis results from an increase in the respiratory rate that decreases blood CO_2 (hypocapnia) and results in decreased arterial [H^+] and [HCO_3^-]. The body tries to compensate for the increased pH through renal mechanisms, namely, decreased H^+ excretion and decreased reabsorption of HCO_3^-. Note that there is also no respiratory compensation for respiratory alkalosis. Causes of respiratory alkalosis include diseases or states that cause hypoxemia (such as living at high altitude), psychogenic causes, and ingestion of salicylates (which can cause a mixed respiratory alkalosis and metabolic acidosis).

Respiratory acidosis is caused by a decrease in the respiratory rate, which increases blood CO_2 (hypercapnia) and results in increased arterial [H^+] and [HCO_3^-]. The body tries to compensate for the decreased pH through renal mechanisms, namely, increased H^+ excretion (through titratable H^+) and increased reabsorption of HCO_3^-. Note that there is no respiratory compensation for respiratory acidosis. Causes of respiratory acidosis include substances that inhibit the medullary respiratory center (such as opiates, sedatives, and anesthetics), impairment of the respiratory muscles (due to neurologic diseases such as multiple sclerosis), airway obstruction, and other pulmonary diseases, such as ARDS and COPD.

6-24. The answer is b. *(Moore and Dalley, pp 778, 819–822.)* The patient has a classic case of carpal tunnel syndrome, in which the median nerve is compressed as it passes through the carpal tunnel formed by the flexor retinaculum in the wrist. Evidence for involvement of the median nerve is weakness and atrophy of the thenar muscles (abductor pollicis brevis, opponens pollicis) and lumbricals 1 to 3. Sensory deficits also follow the distribution of the median nerve. The median nerve enters the hand, along with the tendons of the superficial and deep digital flexors, through a tunnel framed by the carpal bones and the overlying flexor retinaculum. Symptoms are worse in the early morning and in pregnancy because of fluid retention, resulting in swelling that entraps the median nerve. Flexing the wrist for an extended period exaggerates the paresthesia ("Phelan's" sign) by increasing pressure on the median nerve.

Neither the ulnar nerve **(answer c)**, radial nerve **(answer e)**, *nor* radial artery **(answer a)** passes through the carpal tunnel. The ulnar nerve supplies the third and fourth lumbricals and only the short adductor of the thumb. The radial nerve innervates mostly long and short extensors of the digits and the dorsal aspect of the hand. Proper digital nerves **(answer a)** lie distal to the carpal tunnel but are only sensory.

6-25. The answer is a. *(Murray RK, pp 434–473. Scriver, pp 4029–4240.)* The β-adrenergic catecholamines like epinephrine are type II hormones that act at cell membranes, stimulating second messengers including cAMP and protein kinases. These hormones are secreted by the adrenal medulla in keeping with its neural crest derivation and response to neural stimulation (e.g., anxiety, fight or flight response). The actions of epinephrine (adrenaline) and norepinephrine are catabolic; that is, these catecholamines are antagonistic to the anabolic functions of insulin and, like glucagon, are secreted in response to low blood glucose or during "fight or flight" stress. Glycolysis is an anabolic process that is decreased in the presence of elevated catecholamines. Unlike glucagon, which only acts on the liver, the catecholamines affect most tissues, including liver and muscle. The catabolic processes increased by secretion of epinephrine and norepinephrine include glycogenolysis, gluconeogenesis, lipolysis, and ketogenesis. Thus, products that increase blood sugar or spare it, such as ketone bodies and fatty acids, are increased. Prolonged synthesis of adrenergic hormones causes a "hypermetabolic" or catabolic state, inhibiting anabolism and favoring energy expenditure/depletion (fatigue) and weight loss rather than inactivity and weight gain.

6-26. The answer is e. (*Kumar, pp 846–851. Rubin, pp 727–734.*) The two inflammatory bowel diseases (IBDs), Crohn's disease (CD) and ulcerative colitis (UC), are both chronic, relapsing inflammatory disorders of unknown etiology. They both may show very similar morphologic features and associations, such as mucosal inflammation, malignant transformation, and extragastrointestinal manifestations that include erythema nodosum (especially ulcerative colitis), arthritis, uveitis, pericholangitis (especially with ulcerative colitis, in which sclerosing pericholangitis may produce obstructive jaundice), and ankylosing spondylitis. CD is classically described as being a granulomatous disease, but granulomas are present in only 25 to 75% of cases. Therefore, the absence of granulomas does not rule out the diagnosis of CD. CD may involve any portion of the gastrointestinal tract and is characterized by focal (segmental) involvement with "skip lesions." Involvement of the intestines by CD is typically transmural inflammation, which leads to the formation of fistulas and sinuses. The deep inflammation produces deep longitudinal, serpiginous ulcers, which impart a "cobblestone" appearance to the mucosal surface of the colon. Additionally in Crohn's disease, the mesenteric fat wraps around the bowel surface, producing what is called "creeping fat," and the thickened wall narrows the lumen, producing a characteristic "string sign" on x-ray. This narrowing of the colon, which may produce intestinal obstruction, is grossly described as a "lead pipe" or "garden hose" colon. In contrast to CD, UC affects only the colon, and the disease involvement is continuous. The rectum is involved in all cases, and the inflammation extends proximally. Because UC involves the mucosa and submucosa, but not the wall, fistula formation and wall thickening are absent (but toxic megacolon may occur). Grossly, the mucosa displays diffuse hyperemia with numerous superficial ulcerations. The regenerating, nonulcerated mucosa appears as "pseudopolyps."

6-27. The answer is b. (*Ganong, pp 684–686. Levitzky, pp 234–239.*) Hypoxemia at high altitude stimulates the peripheral chemoreceptors to increase ventilation, causing arterial Pco_2 to decrease and arterial pH to rise (respiratory alkalosis). Tissue hypoxia also stimulates erythropoietin production, which increases the number of red blood cells and the hemoglobin concentration, which increases arterial oxygen content, and thus tissue oxygen delivery. Hypoxia also increases the concentration of 2,3-bisphosphoglycerate, which decreases hemoglobin's affinity for oxygen, thereby increasing oxygen release to the tissues. Alveolar hypoxia constricts the pulmonary vessels at high altitude causing an increase in pulmonary vascular resistance and pulmonary artery pressure (pulmonary hypertension).

6-28. The answer is b. *(Brooks, pp 242–244, 218–220. Levinson, pp 27, 83, 470s–471s. Murray PR—2005, pp 260–262, 417–418. Ryan, pp 294, 457–459, 870–871.)* The patient probably has actinomycosis. These laboratory data are not uncommon. There is no reason to work up all the contaminating bacteria. A fluorescent microscopy test for *A. israelii* is available. If positive, the FA provides a rapid diagnosis. In any event, it may be impossible to recover *A. israelii* from such a specimen. High-dose penicillin has been used to treat actinomycosis.

6-29. The answer is b. *(Brooks, pp 677–682. Levinson, pp 349–353. Murray PR—2005, pp 861–865. Ryan, pp 711–722.)* The case history presented in the question is characteristic of infection with *P. falciparum,* the causative agent of malignant tertian malaria. The long duration of the febrile stage rules out other forms of malaria. The presence of ringlike young trophozoites and crescent-like mature gametocytes—as represented in the illustration below— as well as the absence of schizonts is diagnostic of *P. falciparum* malaria.

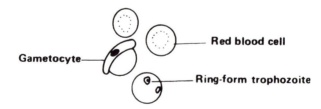

6-30. The answer is e. *(Ganong, pp 246–247, 378–379, 729–730. Kasper et al., pp 213–214. Stead et al., pp 77–78, 226–228.)* An increase in antidiuretic hormone is associated with isovolemic, hypotonic hyponatremia, and an increase in both urine osmolarity and urine sodium. The etiology of syndrome of inappropriate antidiuretic hormone secretion (SIADH) includes idiopathic overproduction of ADH that is often associated with disorders of the CNS (encephalitis, stroke, head trauma) and pulmonary disease (TB, pneumonia). Hyperaldosteronism leads to decreased sodium (and water) excretion and thus hypernatremia and an increase in extracellular fluid volume. A decrease in aldosterone would be associated with hypovolemic hyponatremia. A decrease in ANP would lead to decreased sodium and water excretion.

6-31. The answer is e. (*Ganong, p 684. Kasper et al., pp 210–211. Levitzky, p 156. Stead et al., pp 262–263.*) Cyanosis is the blue color of the skin produced by desaturated hemoglobin. Cyanosis appears when 5 g of hemoglobin per 100 mL of blood are desaturated. For a person with a normal hemoglobin concentration of 15 g/100 mL, cyanosis appears when one-third of the blood is desaturated. For a person with polycythemia (a higher-than-normal concentration of hemoglobin), cyanosis may appear when only one-fourth of the hemoglobin is desaturated (e.g., if hemoglobin concentration is 20 g/100 mL). This individual may not be hypoxic because of the high concentration of saturated hemoglobin. On the other hand, a person with anemia (a lower than normal concentration of hemoglobin) may have a significant portion of the hemoglobin desaturated without displaying cyanosis. This individual will not appear cyanotic but may be hypoxic.

6-32. The answer is b. (*Kumar, p 752. Damjanov, pp 886–887, 928–930. Duchin, pp 949–955.*) Severe acute respiratory distress syndrome (SARS) is a highly contagious and very severe atypical pneumonia that was first described in the fall of 2002. The illness was particularly prevalent among the young and health care workers. In March of 2003, investigators identified the cause of SARS as a novel coronavirus (SARS-CoV). Note that the two main strains of human coronaviruses, types 229E and OC43, are major causes of the common cold. It appears that the SARS-CoV may be the first coronavirus to cause severe disease in otherwise healthy individuals as it differs from previous coronaviruses because it can infect the lower respiratory tract and spread throughout the body. Patients develop a dry cough with fever, chills, and malaise after an incubation of up to 10 days. In contrast to atypical pneumonia caused by Mycoplasma, SARS is not usually associated with a sore throat. Up to one-third of the patients improve, but the majority of patients progress to severe respiratory distress and almost 10% die from the disease.

   The diagnosis of SARS relies on the presence of fever and respiratory symptoms. Interestingly, the most consistent laboratory finding occurring early in the disease is peripheral lymphopenia. Examination of lung tissue from confirmed cases has revealed the presence of hyaline membrane formation, interstitial mononuclear inflammation, and desquamation of pneumocytes into the alveoli. The Center for Disease Control (CDC) has defined several criteria to be used in the diagnosis of SARS. One of the epidemiologic criteria is: "travel (including transit in an airport) within 10 days of symptom onset to an area with current, recently documented, or suspected community transmission of SARS", such as China or Hong Kong.

In contrast to Coronavirus, the Hantavirus genus belongs to the Bunyaviridae family and includes the causative agent of a group of diseases that occur throughout Europe and Asia and are referred to as hemorrhagic fever with renal syndrome. The characteristic features of this syndrome are hematologic abnormalities, renal involvement, and increased vascular permeability. Respiratory involvement is generally minimal in these diseases. Although several species of rodents in the United States are known to be infected with Hantavirus, no human cases were reported until an outbreak of severe, often fatal respiratory illness occurred in the United States in May 1993 in the Four Corners area of New Mexico, Arizona, Colorado, and Utah. This illness resulted from a new member of the genus Hantavirus that caused a severe disease characterized by a prodromal fever, myalgia, pulmonary edema, and hypotension. The main distinguishing feature of this illness, which is called Hantavirus pulmonary syndrome, is noncardiogenic pulmonary edema resulting from increased permeability of the pulmonary capillaries. Laboratory features common to both Hantavirus pulmonary syndrome and hemorrhagic fever with renal syndrome include leukocytosis, atypical lymphocytes, thrombocytopenia, coagulopathy, and decreased serum protein concentrations. Abdominal pain, which can mimic an acute abdomen, may be found in both Hantavirus pulmonary syndrome and hemorrhagic fever with renal syndrome.

Dengue fever virus is a type of flavivirus, and flaviviruses are similar to alphaviruses. Dengue fever (breakbone fever) is initially similar to influenza but then progresses to a rash, muscle pain, joint pain, and bone pain. It can produce a potentially fatal hemorrhagic disorder. Ebola virus is a member of the Filoviridae family, which causes a severe hemorrhagic fever. Outbreaks occur in Africa and typically make the national news.

6-33. The answer is b. (*Young, p 91. Junqueira, pp 68–70, 72.*) The child in the vignette suffers from microvillous inclusion disease (MID) which results in the absence of microvilli in the small intestinal absorptive cell (enterocyte) brush border (apical structure labeled between the arrows in the photomicrograph). MID is associated with an inability to absorb even simple nutrients; the disease presents as refractory diarrhea in the newborn period with chronic dependency on total parenteral nutrition. In MID, microvilli are found as inclusions in the apical enterocyte. Microvilli increase surface area for specialized uptake of molecules by pinocytosis, receptor-mediated endocytosis, and phagocytosis. The microvilli also contain the brush border enzymes such as lactase and alkaline phosphatase. Microvilli are supported by a core of microfilaments and are capable of movement; however, cilia (**answer a**) function in the movement of substances, such as mucus and foreign material, over the surface. Cell movement is controlled by interactions between the cytoskeleton and the extracellular matrix (**answer c**), while microtubules facilitate organellar movement within the cytoplasm (**answer d**). Transitional epithelium characteristic of the urinary system facilitates distensibility and stretch (**answer e**). A table listing functions and locations of epithelia is provided below.

EPITHELIAL TYPES, LOCATION, AND FUNCTION

Epithelial Type	Location	Function
Simple		
Simple squamous	Endothelium of blood vessels	Transport, absorption, secretion
Simple cuboidal	Collecting ducts of kidneys	Transport, reabsorption, secretion
Simple columnar	Epithelium of the gut: stomach, intestines	Absorption, protection, lubrication (mucus)
Stratified		
Stratified cuboidal	Sweat ducts	Transport
Stratified columnar	Excretory ducts of salivary glands	Transport
Stratified squamous (keratinized)	Epidermis	Protection, water conservation
Stratified squamous (nonkeratinized)	Esophagus, anus, vagina	Protection, lubrication, secretion
Pseudostratified	Respiratory system (trachea with cilia), male reproductive system (no cilia)	Movement of material across epithelial surface
Transitional	Urinary system: ureter, bladder	Stretch, protection

6-34. The answer is c. (*Murray RK, pp 580–597. Scriver, pp 645–664. Lewis, pp 331–454.*) This case is an example of Burkitt lymphoma, which may affect the tonsils or other lymphoid tissues. The translocation places the myc oncogene on chromosome 8 downstream of the very active heavy-chain locus on chromosome 14, activating myc gene expression in B-cells and their derivatives. The translocation is likely an aberrant form of the normal DNA rearrangements that generate unique heavy-chain genes in each B-cell. The translocation joins one chromosome 8 to one chromosome 14, leaving their homologues unaffected. The cause for the phenotype must therefore be transacting, since cis-acting effects would pertain only to the translocated loci and not affect the homologous untranslocated loci. Activation of a tumor-promoting gene (oncogene) on chromosome 8 could produce an enlarged tonsil, while underactivity of immunoglobulin production due to one-half expression could decrease immune function but would not completely ablate the processes in choices a, b, d, and e. At the genetic level, transacting events are autosomal dominant in that one of the two homologous loci is abnormal and produces a phenotype. Mutations of cis-acting events must disrupt both homologous loci to produce phenotypes, making them autosomal recessive at the genetic level.

6-35. The answer is c. (*Murray RK, pp 30–39. Scriver, pp 3–45. Lewis, pp 185–204.*) The carbon next to a carboxyl (C = O) group may be designated as the α carbon, with subsequent carbons as β, γ, δ, etc. α-Amino acids contain an amino group on their α-carbon, as distinguished from compounds like γ-aminobutyric acid, in which the amino group is two carbons down (γ-carbon). In α-amino acids the amino acid, carboxylic acid, and the side chain or R group are all bound to the central α-carbon, which is thus asymmetric (except when R is hydrogen, as for glycine). Amino acids are classified as acidic, neutral hydrophobic, neutral hydrophilic, or basic, depending on the charge or partial charge on the R group at pH 7. Hydrophobic (water-hating) groups are carbon-hydrogen chains like those of leucine, isoleucine, glycine, or valine. Basic R groups, such as those of lysine and arginine, carry a positive charge at physiologic pH owing to protonated amide groups, whereas acidic R groups, such as glutamic acid, carry a negative charge owing to ionized carboxyl groups. Threonine with its hydroxyl side chain is neutral at physiologic pH.

Leucine, isoleucine, and valine are amino acids with branched side groups, and they share a pathway for degradation that is deficient in children with maple syrup urine disease (248600). Their amino groups can be removed, but the resulting carboxy-acids accumulate with resulting acidosis, coma, and death unless a diet free of branch-chained amino acids is instituted.

6-36. The answer is b. (*Kumar, pp 205, 1309.*) A variety of different diseases have an association with certain human leukocyte antigen (HLA) types.

The exact mechanism of this association is unknown. These diseases can be grouped into three broad categories: inflammatory diseases, inherited errors of metabolism, and autoimmune diseases. The classic example of an inflammatory disease associated with a certain HLA is the association of ankylosing spondylitis with HLA-B27. Ankylosing spondylitis is one type of spondyloarthropathy that lacks the rheumatoid factor found in rheumatoid arthritis. Other seronegative spondyloarthropathies include Reiter syndrome, psoriatic arthritis, and enteropathic arthritis. All of these are associated with an increased incidence of HLA-B27. Ankylosing spondylitis, also known as rheumatoid spondylitis or Marie-Strümpell disease, is a chronic inflammatory disease that primarily affects the sacroiliac joints of adult males. Calcification of the vertebral and paravertebral ligaments produce low back pain and stiffness and are seen radiographically as a "bamboo spine."

HLA types are also associated with inherited errors of metabolism and autoimmune diseases. An example of an inherited error of metabolism being associated with a certain HLA type is the association of hemochromatosis with HLA-A3, while autoimmune diseases can be associated with the DR locus. Two examples of this are the associations of rheumatoid arthritis with DR4 and of insulin-dependent diabetes with DR3/DR4.

6-37. The answer is e. (*Brooks, pp 469–470. Levinson, pp 289–291. Murray PR—2005, pp 685–687. Ryan, pp 551–552.*) HCV is a positive-stranded RNA virus, classified as a flavivirus. About half of HCV patients develop chronic hepatitis. A large number of infections appear among IV drug abusers. About 90% of the cases of transfusion-associated hepatitis are thought to be caused by HCV.

6-38. The answer is b. (*Brunton, pp 351–353. Craig, pp 292t, 297. Katzung, pp 411–412, 415–416.*) The scenario describes most of the classic responses to ketamine, a "dissociative anesthetic": analgesia; an ostensibly light sleep-like state; a trance-like and cataplectic state (including increased muscle tone); and activation of most cardiovascular parameters (in patients with normal cardiovascular status to begin with). The various psychosis-like emergence reactions are the main disadvantages to using a drug that, otherwise, causes many of the desired elements of balanced anesthesia, usually without the need for complicated and expensive anesthesia administration devices or personnel. Ketamine undergoes significant metabolism in humans, with about 20% of the absorbed dose recovered as metabolites. The only other drug listed that provides adequate analgesia is fentanyl (a). Midazolam (c; benzodiazepine), succinylcholine (d; depolarizing neuromuscular blocker), and thiopental (e; thiobarbiturate) lack analgesic activity; moreover, if any cardiovascular or autonomic changes were to occur in response to any of those drugs, they would be better characterized as depression, not activation.

6-39. The answer is b. (*Ganong, pp 657–658. Levitzky, pp 49–51.*) Respiratory muscles consume oxygen in proportion to the work of breathing. The work of breathing is equal to the product of the change in volume for each breath and the change in pressure necessary to overcome the resistive work of breathing and the elastic work of breathing. Resistive work includes work to overcome tissue as well as airway resistance; thus a decreased airway resistance will decrease the work of breathing and the oxygen consumption of the respiratory muscles. A decreased lung compliance would increase the elastic work of breathing. An increase in respiratory rate or tidal volume increases the work of breathing.

6-40. The answer is e. (*Junqueira, pp 206–209. Moore and Dalley, p 160. Kierszenbaum, pp 335–336.*) The site at which coronary arteries become occluded are: first, at the left anterior descending (thus affecting both ventricles anteriorly); second, at the origin of the right coronary artery affecting both the right atrium and ventricle and disrupting cardiac rhythm; and third, the circumflex branch (affecting both left atria and ventricle). Atherosclerosis is initiated by damage to the endothelial cells, which exposes the subjacent connective tissue (subendothelium). The loss of the antithrombogenic endothelium results in aggregation of platelets. Atherosclerosis is one form of arteriosclerosis (hardening of the arteries) that involves deposition of fatty material primarily in the walls of the conducting arteries. The intima and media become infiltrated with lipid. Intimal thickening occurs through the addition of collagen and elastin with an abnormal pattern of elastin cross-linking. Platelets release mitogenic substances that stimulate proliferation of smooth muscle cells. The thickening of the intima is also called an atheromatous plaque and worsens with repeated damage to the endothelium. It is most dangerous in small vessels, particularly the coronary arteries, where occlusion can result in a myocardial infarction. Atherosclerotic plaques also lead to thrombi and aneurysms.

6-41. The answer is e. (*Kumar, pp 649, 699–700. Ravel, pp 76–77.*) Polycythemia refers to an increased concentration of red blood cells (RBCs) in the peripheral blood. This is manifested by an increase in the red blood cell count, hemoglobin concentration, or hematocrit. The differential diagnosis of polycythemia includes primary polycythemia, which is due to a defect in myeloid stem cells (polycythemia rubra vera), and secondary polycythemia, which is caused by an increase in the production of erythropoietin (EPO). In patients with primary polycythemia, a myeloproliferative disorder, the red cell mass is increased but the levels of EPO are normal or decreased. That is, the abnormality is a primary defect in the red blood cells themselves. In contrast, with secondary polycythemia, the polycythemia is secondary to the increased EPO. This secondary increase in the EPO may be appropriate or inappropriate. Appropriate causes of increased EPO, in which the oxygen saturation of hemoglobin will be abnormal, include lung disease, cyanotic heart disease, living at high altitudes, or abnormal hemoglobins with increased oxygen affinity. Inappropriate causes of increased EPO include EPO-secreting tumors, such as renal cell carcinomas, hepatomas, or cerebellar hemangioblastomas. In contrast, pancreatic adenocarcinoma may be associated with migratory thrombophlebitis (Trousseau's sign).

It is important to understand that an increase in red blood cell count, reported clinically as number of cells per microliter, is not the same thing as the RBC mass, which is a radioactive test that is reported in mL/kg. The RBC count and the RBC mass do not necessarily parallel each other. For example, a decreased plasma volume increases the RBC count but does not affect the RBC mass. An increased red blood cell concentration may be a relative polycythemia or an absolute polycythemia. A relative polycythemia is due to a decrease in the plasma volume (hemoconcentration), causes of which include prolonged vomiting or diarrhea (as seen with acute gastroenteritis), or the excessive use of diuretics.

To summarize these clinical findings, an increased total red cell mass indicates an absolute polycythemia, increased serum EPO indicates a secondary polycythemia, and a normal oxygen saturation of hemoglobin suggests an inappropriate secretion of EPO, such as seen with renal cell carcinoma.

6-42. The answer is b. (*Afifi, p 250. Siegel and Sapru, p 484.*) The superior temporal gyrus is the primary auditory receiving area in the cerebral cortex. Accordingly, the primary afferent source to this region arises from the medial geniculate nucleus, which constitutes a specific thalamic relay for processing of auditory information.

6-43. The answer is c. (*Afifi, pp 187–213. Nolte, pp 266–277. Siegel and Sapru, pp 198–200, 206. Waxman, p 94.*) The superior colliculus (E), situated at a more rostral level of the tectum, plays an important role in tracking or pursuit of moving stimuli as well as movements of the eyes up and down. Damage to this region would clearly affect the ability to produce these movements. The medial geniculate nucleus (D), which is part of the forebrain, actually sits over the lateral aspect of the midbrain and can be seen at rostral levels of the midbrain. It is part of an auditory relay system and receives its inputs from the inferior colliculus via fibers of the brachium of the inferior colliculus. Damage to this relay nucleus would affect auditory acuity and one's ability to localize and discriminate sound. The pars compacta is situated in the medial aspect of the substantia nigra (A) and contains dopamine neurons whose axons innervate the striatum. Damage to these dopamine neurons produces Parkinson's disease, which is characterized by rigidity, tremor, and akinesia. The red nucleus (C), a structure associated with motor functions, receives direct inputs from both the cerebral cortex and the cerebellum. The contralateral limb ataxia could be accounted for by the loss of inputs from the red nucleus to the cerebellum via the inferior olivary nucleus. The loss of pupillary constriction and ability to move the eye medially could be accounted for by the fact that the fibers of the oculomotor nerve pass ventrally in proximity to the red nucleus. Thus, damage to the red nucleus would also affect the oculomotor nerve. The oculomotor nerve (cranial nerve III) (F), located at the level of the superior colliculus, contains general somatic efferent components that innervate extraocular eye muscles and general visceral efferent components whose postganglionic fibers innervate smooth muscles associated with pupillary constriction and bulging of the lens. As just noted, damage to the oculomotor nerve would produce impairment of vertical and medial movements of the eyes as well as loss of the pupillary light reflex.

6-44. The answer is h. (*Afifi, pp 47–58, 422–424, 426–430, 476–477. Siegel and Sapru, pp 8–13, 287–289, 312–315.*) This figure is a midsagittal section of the brain. A major portion of the anterior commissure (E) contains fibers mediating olfactory signals that arise from the olfactory bulb and decussate to the contralateral olfactory bulb. The septum pellucidum (G) forms the medial wall of the lateral ventricle, which in fact separates the lateral ventricle on one side from that on the opposite side. The cingulate gyrus (H) is a prominent structure on the medial aspect of the cerebral cortex and constitutes a component of the limbic lobe. As part of the limbic system, its functions relate in part to the regulation of emotional behavior. Accordingly, tumors of this region have resulted in marked changes in emotionality. The primary visual cortex lies on both banks of the calcarine fissure. Cells located on the upper bank of this fissure (B) receive inputs from the lateral geniculate nucleus that relate to the lower visual field. Therefore, a lesion of this region would result in a lower visual field deficit. The major output pathway of the hippocampal formation is the fornix system of fibers (A), which arises from cells in its subicular cortex and adjoining regions of the hippocampus. These fibers are then distributed to the anterior thalamic nucleus, mammillary bodies, and septal area. Accordingly, the most effective way of activating the output pathways of the hippocampal formation would be to stimulate these fibers of the fornix. The basilar portion of the pons (D) lies in the ventral half of this region of the brainstem. It receives inputs from each of the lobes of the cerebral cortex, which it then relays to the cerebellar cortex. As noted in the answer to Question 2, this circuit mediates functions associated with the regulation of voluntary movements of the limbs. Disruption of any part of this circuit, whether at the level of the internal capsule or basilar pons, would affect inputs from the cerebral cortex to the hemispheres of the cerebellar cortex, thus eliminating key inputs necessary for the expression of smooth, coordinated movements. With respect to the neurons located on the lower bank of the calcarine fissure (C), they receive inputs from the lateral geniculate nucleus that relate to the upper retinal (or temporal) visual fields. Therefore, a lesion of this region would produce an upper quadrantanopia (i.e., loss of one-quarter of the visual field). The corpus callosum (F) constitutes the major channel by which the cerebral cortex on one side can communicate with the cortex of the opposite side. In order to stop the spread of seizures from one hemisphere to the other (when the seizures are severe), cutting of the corpus callosum is carried out.

6-45. The answer is a. (*Afifi, pp 171–177. Nolte, pp 294–301. Siegel and Sapru, pp 237–240.*) The spinal trigeminal nucleus receives its sensory inputs from first-order neurons contained in the ipsilateral descending tract of cranial nerve V. A central property of the spinal trigeminal nucleus is that it is uniquely associated with pain inputs (to the exclusion of the main sensory nucleus and mesencephalic nucleus). Fibers from this nucleus mainly project contralaterally to the ventral posteromedial nucleus of the thalamus. Surgical interruption of these descending first-order pain fibers is a practical approach and one that has been carried out by neurosurgeons. Destruction of the ventral posterolateral nucleus would not necessarily destroy the major pain inputs to the cerebral cortex and would additionally be a more difficult structure to destroy surgically. The main sensory nucleus of the trigeminal nerve is not known to convey pain inputs to thalamus and cortex. The substantia gelatinosa conveys pain and temperature sensation from the body and not the head. The midbrain periaqueductal gray constitutes part of a pain-inhibitory system, not one that transmits pain sensations to the cerebral cortex.

6-46. The answer is d. (*Kumar, pp 79–83, 381–386.*) Granulomatous inflammation is characterized by the presence of granulomas, which by definition are aggregates of activated macrophages (epithelioid cells, not epithelial cells). These cells may be surrounded by mononuclear cells, mainly lymphocytes, and multinucleated giant cells. These cells result from the fusion of several epithelioid cells together. The source of macrophages (histiocytes) are monocytes from the peripheral blood.

Granulomatous inflammation is a type of chronic inflammation initiated by a variety of infectious and noninfectious agents. Indigestible organisms or particles, or T cell–mediated immunity to the inciting agent, or both, appear essential for formation of granulomas. Tuberculosis is the classic infectious granulomatous disease and is characterized by finding rare acid-fast bacilli within areas of caseous necrosis. In addition to tuberculosis, several other infectious disorders are characterized by formation of granulomas, including deep fungal infections (coccidioidomycosis and histoplasmosis), schistosomiasis, syphilis, brucellosis, lymphogranuloma venereum, and cat-scratch disease. In sarcoidosis, a disease of unknown cause, the granulomas are noncaseating, which may assist in histologic differentiation from tuberculosis. No organisms are found in the noncaseating granulomas of sarcoidosis.

6-47. The answer is c. (*Kumar, pp 107, 110, 112–113.*) Tissue repair occurs through the regeneration of damaged cells and the replacement of tissue by connective tissue. Tissue repair involves the formation of granulation tissue, which histologically is characterized by a combination of proliferating fibroblasts and proliferating blood vessels. Proliferating cells are cells that are rapidly dividing and usually have prominent nucleoli. This histologic feature should not be taken as a sign of dysplasia or malignancy. It is important not to confuse the term granulation tissue with the similar-sounding term granuloma. The latter refers to a special type of inflammation that is characterized by the presence of activated macrophages (epithelioid cells).

6-48. The answer is b. (*Kumar, pp 103–105. Rubin, pp 78–84.*) The extracellular matrix (ECM) is composed of fibrous structural proteins and interstitial matrix, the latter being composed of adhesive glycoproteins embedded within a ground substance. The structural proteins of the ECM include collagen fibers, reticular fibers, and elastic fibers. Collagen is a triple helix of three polypeptide α-chains that is secreted by fibroblasts and has a high content of glycine and hydroxyproline. Collagens may be either fibrillar or nonfibrillar. The fibrillar (interstitial) types of collagen (types I, III, and V) are found within the ECM (interstitial tissue), while the nonfibrillar type IV collagen is found within the basement membranes, which are special organizations of the interstitial matrix found around epithelial, endothelial, and smooth-muscle cells. Type I collagen is found in skin, tendon, bone, dentin, and fascia; type II collagen is found only in cartilage; and type III collagen (reticulin) appears in the skin, blood vessels, uterus, and embryonic dermis.

The adhesive glycoproteins include fibronectin and laminin. Laminin, the most abundant glycoprotein in basement membranes, is a cross-shaped glycoprotein that is capable of binding multiple matrix components, such as type IV collagen and heparan sulfate. It also binds to specific receptors on the surface of some cells. Fibronectin, secreted by fibroblasts, monocytes, and endothelial cells, is also capable of binding many substances, such as collagen, fibrin, proteoglycans, and integrins. Basically, fibronectin links the ECM component and macromolecules to integrins and is chemotactic for fibroblasts and endothelial cells. Instead of being cross-shaped like laminin, fibronectin is a large glycoprotein composed of two chains held together by disulfide bonds. Albumin is secreted by hepatocytes and is mainly responsible for intravascular oncotic pressure, while immunoglobulins are secreted by plasma cells and are important in mediating humoral immunity.

6-49. The answer is d. (*Kumar, pp 104, 154–155. Ayala, p 179.*) Several diseases result from abnormalities involving defects in structural proteins. Marfan's syndrome is an autosomal dominant disorder that results from defective synthesis of fibrillin causing connective tissue abnormalities. It is characterized by specific changes involving the skeleton, the eyes, and the cardiovascular system. Skeletal changes seen in individuals with Marfan's syndrome include arachnodactyly (spider fingers) and a large skeleton causing increase in height. Eyes in patients with Marfan's syndrome typically have a subluxed lens (ectopia lentis) in which the lens is found in the anterior chamber. The lens dislocation in Marfan's syndrome is usually upward, in contrast to the downward dislocation seen with homocystinuria. Cardiovascular lesions associated with Marfan's syndrome include MV prolapse and cystic medial necrosis of the aorta.

Abnormalities of copper metabolism is seen with Wilson's disease, which is characterized by varying liver disease and neurologic symptoms due to excess copper deposition within the liver and basal ganglia of the brain. Decreased levels of vitamin D can produce rickets in children or osteomalacia in adults. Type VI Ehlers-Danlos syndrome is characterized by decreased lysyl hydroxylation of collagen, which causes decreased cross-linking of collagen. These individuals have eye problems along with hyper-extensible skin and joint hypermobility. Finally, osteogenesis imperfecta (OI) results from defective synthesis of type I collagen. These patients have "brittle bones" and also typically develop blue scleras and hearing loss.

6-50. The answer is e. (*Kumar, pp 1352–1353.*) Increased intracranial pressure can result from mass lesions in the brain, cerebral edema, or hydrocephalus. Increased intracranial pressure can cause swelling of the optic nerve (papilledema), headaches, vomiting, or herniation of part of the brain into the foramen magnum or under a free part of the dura.

Brain herniations are classified according to the area of the brain that is herniated. Subfalcine herniations are caused by herniation of the medial aspect of the cerebral hemisphere (cingulate gyrus) under the falx, which may compress the anterior cerebral artery. Transtentorial herniation, which occurs when the medial part of the temporal lobe (uncus) herniates over the free edge of the tentorium, may result in compression of the oculomotor nerve, which results in pupillary dilation and ophthalmoplegia (the affected eye points "down and out"). Tentorial herniation may also compress the cerebral peduncles, within which are the pyramidal tracts. Ipsilateral compression produces contralateral motor paralysis (hemiparesis), while compression of the contralateral cerebral peduncle against Kernohan's notch causes ipsilateral hemiparesis. Further caudal displacement of the entire brainstem may cause tearing of the penetrating arteries of the midbrain (Duret hemorrhages). This caudal displacement may also stretch the trochlear nerve (cranial nerve VI), causing paralysis of the lateral rectus muscle (the abnormal eye turns inward). Masses in the cerebellum may cause tonsillar herniation, in which the cerebellar tonsils are herniated into the foramen magnum. This may compress the medulla and respiratory centers, causing death. Tonsillar herniation may also occur if a lumbar puncture (LP) is performed in a patient with increased intracranial pressure. Therefore, before performing an LP, check the patient for the presence of papilledema.

Block 7

Answers

7-1. The answer is c. (*Siegel and Sapru, pp 331–336, 338–339*). The deficits observed in this patient were due to damage to the left internal capsule. The tumor impinged upon both genu and posterior limbs of the internal capsule, thus affecting corticospinal and some corticobulbar fibers. Such damage would account for both the contralateral limb paresis (due to damage to the corticospinal tract) and the loss of expression of the contralateral lower jaw (due to damage to corticobulbar fibers that supply the ventral aspect of the facial nucleus, whose axons innervate the lower jaw).

7-2. The answer is a. (*Avery, pp 306–310. Guyton, pp 740–741.*) The woman in the scenario suffers from Sjögren's syndrome, which like other autoimmune diseases (presence of ANA and RF), is much more common in women than men. The striated ducts resorb Na^+ and secrete K^+ **(answer b)** from the isotonic saliva converting it to a hypotonic state. Na^+-independent chloride-bicarbonate anion exchangers appear to be involved in these processes by generating ion fluxes into the salivary secretion. The striated duct is the primary region for electrolyte transport in the salivary gland duct system. The primary secretion produced by the acinar cells is comprised of amylase, mucus, and ions in the same concentrations as those of the extracellular fluid. In the duct system, Na^+ is actively absorbed from the lumen of the ducts, Cl^- is passively absorbed [although the tight junctions between striated duct cells inhibit Cl^- from following Na^+ **(answer c)**]. HCO_3^- is secreted **(answer d)**; Ca^{2+} transport is not a factor **(e)**. The result is a hypotonic sodium and chloride concentration and a hypertonic potassium concentration.

7-3. The answer is d. (*Kasper et al., pp 164–165.*) The optical field defect is produced by an enlarged pituitary gland, which impinges on the optic chiasm. Compression of the optic chiasm by the pituitary gland damages the nasal portion of each optic nerve, which produces a loss of vision in the temporal visual field of both eyes. This defect is referred to as a bitemporal hemianopia.

7-4. The answer is e. *(Brunton, p 957. Craig, pp 273–275. Katzung, pp 571–573.)* Gemfibrozil mainly lowers triglycerides and is used specifically for that purpose. This fibric acid derivative is sometimes classified as a peroxisomal proliferator-receptor activator (PPAR). It stimulates lipoprotein lipase synthesis and hydrolysis of triglycerides in chylomicrons and VLDL. The net effect is increased clearance of triglycerides. Clofibrate is a related (but lesser used) fibrate. As you should recall, atorvastatin (a; and other statins) inhibits cholesterol synthesis by inhibiting HMG CoA reductase, and depending on a host of factors they may or may not lower triglycerides; cholestyramine (b) and colestipol (c) are bile acid sequestrants; ezetimibe (d), a relatively new drug, inhibits uptake of dietary cholesterol from the gut. Those other drugs may have beneficial effects on serum triglyceride levels, but they are not first-line drugs for managing hypertriglyceridemia with or without concomitant hypercholesterolemia.

7-5. The answer is d. *(Siegel and Sapru, pp 240–242.)* The patient was suffering from a lateral gaze paralysis resulting from an infarction of the dorsomedial pons, thus affecting the abducens nerve (cranial nerve VI), whose nucleus is located in the region of the infarction. The fibers of the abducens nerve pass ventrally, exiting the brain in a relatively medial position at the level of the lower pons.

7-6. The answer is h. *(Parslow, pp 128–129, 401–405, 426–430. Levinson, pp 423–428, 453–462. Kasper, pp 1960–1967.)* Loss of tolerance by the immune system to certain self-components can lead to the formation of antibodies, causing tissue and organ damage. Such diseases are referred to as *autoimmune diseases.* There are a host of autoimmune diseases characterized by the autoantibodies. The presence of a "butterfly" rash is a classic cutaneous sign of SLE and is characterized by a rash over the bridge of the nose and on the cheeks.

7-7. The answer is c. *(Brunton, pp 242, 254, 263–264. Craig, pp 100–102. Katzung, pp 133–134, 136–138, 148.)* Phenylephrine is the prototypic α-adrenergic agonist. It terminated the arrhythmia reflexly, via the baroreceptors, in response to a vasopressor effect. (Raising blood pressure quickly and markedly is a risky way of terminating this tachycardia, of course, due to such risks as causing a hemorrhagic stroke.) All the other drugs would also terminate the arrhythmia, but by actions in the heart. Edrophonium (a) is an ACh esterase inhibitor with a fast onset of action and a brief duration. It would slow heart rate by increasing the effects of ACh on the SA node, slowing the spontaneous rate of phase 4 depolarization. Esmolol is a β blocker (nonselective) that also has a fast onset and short duration of action. It and propranolol (d) would slow heart rate via the direct β-blocking effects on the SA node. Verapamil (e) will do the same by blocking AV nodal calcium channels.

7-8. The answer is e. *(Afifi, pp 104–117. Siegel and Sapru, pp 142–149, 237–239.)* The nucleus gracilis (A) contains cells that respond to movement of the lower limb as a result of joint capsule activation. Damage to this region will result in loss of conscious proprioception associated with the leg, and, additionally, the loss of conscious proprioception will result in ataxia because this input is essential for normal ambulation to occur. The nucleus cuneatus (B) contains cells that respond to a variety of stimuli applied to the upper limb, including vibratory stimuli. One component of the descending MLF (E) contains fibers that arise from the medial vestibular nucleus that project to cervical levels and contribute to reflex activity associated with the position of the head. The descending track of the trigeminal nerve (C) contains first-order fibers mediating pain and temperature information from the head region. Because of its lateral position in the brainstem, a surgical procedure is sometimes carried out to cut these fibers as a means of alleviating excruciating pain. Fibers of the medial lemniscus (D) arise from the contralateral dorsal column nuclei and ascend to the ventral posterolateral nucleus of the thalamus. These fibers transmit the same information noted earlier for the dorsal column nuclei, which includes two-point discrimination and conscious proprioception from the opposite side of the body.

7-9. The answer is e. *(Lewis, pp 75–94. Scriver, pp 5903–5934.)* The presence of consanguinity (double line in the figure) is a red flag for autosomal recessive inheritance because, although disease-causing alleles are rare, the probability of a homozygous individual escalates dramatically when the same rare allele descends through two branches of a family. Using a lowercase r to denote the retinitis pigmentosa allele, the affected male (individual II-2 in the figure accompanying the question) has a genotype of rr. His prospective mate has a very low risk to be a carrier for this rare disease, making her genotype RR. Their children will all have genotypes Rr, making them carriers but not affected. Retinitis pigmentosa is another disease manifesting genetic heterogeneity, with autosomal dominant (180100), autosomal recessive (268000), and X-linked recessive (312650) forms. Carriers of autosomal recessive diseases are heterozygotes with one normal and one abnormal allele. Many autosomal recessive diseases involve enzyme deficiencies, indicating that 50% levels of enzymes found in heterozygotes are sufficient for normal function. The probability that an affected individual will encounter a mate who is a carrier is approximately twice the square root of the disease incidence. This figure derives from the Hardy-Weinberg law. Since most recessive diseases have incidences lower than 1 in 10,000, the risk for unrelated mates to be carriers is less than 1 in 50, and the chance of having an affected child is less than $\frac{1}{50} \times \frac{1}{4}$ = less than 1 in 200. Disorders that are fairly common in certain ethnic groups, such as cystic fibrosis, are exceptions to this very low risk.

7-10. The answer is d. (*Simon, pp 138–145.*) A neuritis involving the optic disk would affect the size of the visual field loss around the optic disk, which corresponds to the blind spot. In general, this kind of neuritis would expand somewhat the size of the blind spot but would cause no further visual loss.

7-11. The answer is a. (*Junqueira, pp 51–54. Ross and Pawlina, p 78.*) Triple A syndrome is an autosomal recessive neuroendocrinological disease caused by mutations in a gene that encodes the nucleoporin ALADIN, a component of the nuclear pore complex labeled with the arrows in the electron micrograph. The immediate effect of mutations in the nucleoporins is decreased import of macromolecules from the cytoplasm. Patients with triple A syndrome have adrenocorticotrophic (ACTH)-resistant adrenal failure, achalasia (abnormal esophageal motility most often due to inability of the esophageal sphincter to relax), and alacramia (reduced ability to produce tears). They also demonstrate neurological symptoms affecting the cranial nerves, autonomic nervous system (Horner's syndrome and orthostatic hypotension). Phosphorylation (breakdown) and dephosphorylation (reconstitution) of the lamins regulates nuclear envelope stability during the cell cycle **(answers b and c)**. Condensation of chromosomes would not be directly affected **(answer d)** and the nucleus is the site of RNA synthesis **(answer e)**.

7-12. The answer is c. (*Lewis, pp 75–94, 267–282. Scriver, pp 3827–3876.*) The probability that any one sibling is homozygous normal is one-third. The human leukocyte antigen (HLA) cluster on chromosome 6 consists of several loci that are each highly polymorphic. Because the loci are clustered together, their polymorphic products form haplotypes (i.e., A1-B8-DR2 on one chromosome and A9-B5-DR3 on another chromosome). Since recombination among HLA loci is unlikely, the chances of two siblings being HLA-identical are essentially those of inheriting the same parental chromosomes, that is, $^1/_4$. The chance for a sibling to be both homozygous normal for Tay-Sachs disease and HLA-compatible is $^1/_3 \times \, ^1/_4 = \, ^1/_{12}$. Since there are three siblings, the total chance is $^1/_{12} \times 3 = \, ^1/_4$.

7-13. The answer is a. *(Parslow, pp 117, 302–305. Levinson, pp 431, 432, 463–465.)* Bruton's agammaglobulinemia is a congenital defect that becomes apparent at approximately 6 months of age, when maternal IgG is diminished. It occurs in males and is characterized by a defective *btk* gene, very small tonsils, low levels of all five classes of immunoglobulins, and no mature B cells. Thus, the child is unable to produce immunoglobulins and develops a series of bacterial infections characterized by recurrences and progression to more serious infections such as septicemia. The most common organisms responsible for infection are *H. influenzae* and *S. pneumoniae*. Cell-mediated immunity is not affected, and the child is able to respond normally to diseases that require this immune response for resolution. Treatment consists of pooled IgG.

Note: Immunodeficiency is characterized by unusual and recurrent infections:

- B cell (antibody) deficiency—bacterial infections
- T cell deficiency—viral, fungal, and protozoal infections
- Phagocytic cell deficiency—pyogenic infections (bacterial), skin infections, systemic bacterial opportunistic infections
- Complement deficiencies—pyogenic infections (bacterial)

7-14. The answer is e. *(Brunton, pp 1064–1066. Craig, p 609. Katzung, pp 879–881.)* Both trimethoprim-sulfamethoxazole (not listed) and pentamidine are effective in pneumonia caused by *P. carinii*. This protozoal disease usually occurs in immunodeficient patients, such as those with AIDS. Nifurtimox is effective in trypanosomiasis and metronidazole in amebiasis and leishmaniasis, as well as in anaerobic bacterial infections. Penicillins are not considered drugs of choice for this particular disease.

7-15. The answer is d. *(Brunton, pp 14–22. Craig, pp 52–53. Katzung, pp 45–46.)* Here is how you solve the problem.

Note: It's easy to be misled by inconsistent use of units of measurement (mcg vs. mg, mL vs. L), so be sure you convert units as necessary.

First calculate the drug's elimination rate constant:

$$k_e = 0.693/t_{1/2} \quad \text{or}$$

$$k_e = 0.693/0.5 \text{ h} = 1.386/\text{h}$$

Then calculate the clearance:

$$Cl = k_e \times V_d, \quad \text{or} \dots.$$

$Cl = 1.386/\text{h} \times 45 \text{ L}$, which equals 62.37 L/h, or 62,370 mL/h

Recall that $C_{ave} = (F/Cl) \times (\text{Dose}/t)$, where t represents the dosing interval (time; given as 4 h).
Rearrange to solve for the dose.

$$\text{Dose} = (C_{ave} \times Cl \times t)/F, \quad \text{or}$$
$$\text{Dose} = [(2 \text{ mcg/mL}) \times (62,370 \text{ mL/h}) \times 4 \text{ h}]/1.0$$

Thus, Dose = 499,000 mcg, or 499 mg (close enough to 500 mg).

7-16. The answer is b. (*Brunton, pp 509–510, 1860t. Craig, pp 53, 377–378. Katzung, pp 380–382.*) The hepatic enzymes responsible for phenytoin metabolism (mainly CYP 2C9) become saturated at plasma drug concentrations above approximately 10–15 mcg/mL, which are clearly within the typical therapeutic range yet well below maximum or peak therapeutic levels. At daily dosages associated with or below those 10–15 mcg/mL values, dose increases give relatively proportional increases in plasma drug concentrations, and phenytoin elimination follows usual first-order kinetics (a constant fraction of drug is eliminated with the passing of each half-life). Once the metabolic capacity is exceeded (as it has in our patient, which may arise with intentional or inadvertent increases in the daily dose), small increases in dosage lead to disproportionately large increases of serum concentrations (and effects) because, in essence, "drug in greatly exceeds drug out": zero-order kinetics now describes the drug's elimination, such that a constant amount (not fraction) of drug is eliminated per unit time. Therefore, the first-order half-life does not apply; elimination is slower, and the plasma concentration will be much greater than 15 mcg/mL (half of 30 mcg/mL; ans. e) 24 h after the initial blood sample is taken.

The figure shows an *approximation* of the relationship between plasma phenytoin levels and daily doses (the placement of the curve can vary from patient to patient along the x-axis). From the rapid rise in the curve at dosages above about 300 mg/day you can deduce a significant reduction of clearance rates owing to slowed metabolism (since metabolism is the main pathway for phenytoin's elimination).

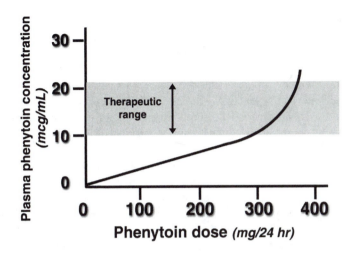

Answer (a) is incorrect; flumazenil is a benzodiazepine receptor antagonist (competitive blocker) that has no effects (beneficially or not; pharmacokinetic or otherwise) on the elimination or effects of phenytoin. It would be inappropriate—and dangerous—to give an amphetamine or any other CNS stimulant to counteract the excess CNS depression. Titrating upwards the dose of a CNS stimulant to combat CNS depression (whether caused by a drug or from another cause) is a risky endeavor, due to the chance of inducing seizures from excessive CNS stimulation, and the risks are far greater in a person with a history of seizure disorders.

Phenobarbital (d) is a classic example of a P450 inducer, and indeed it is metabolized mainly by CYP2C9, on which phenytoin's elimination is mainly dependent. In theory, giving phenobarbital might increase phenytoin's metabolism *via* P450 induction. In reality, the pharmacokinetic outcomes of a phenobarbital-phenytoin interaction are quite variable (and dependent on blood levels of each drug), but the more likely consequence is inhibited phenytoin elimination as the barbiturate competes with it for conversion by the same cytochromes. Regardless, adding phenobarbital is likely to add to the generalized CNS depression caused by the phenytoin, and complicate both the clinical picture and its management. Therefore, this approach, too, would be inappropriate.

7-17. The answer is a. (*Favus, pp 321–323. Kumar, pp 1284–1286. Greenspan, pp 326–329. Kasper, pp 2279–2281.*) The correct diagnosis is Paget's disease, also known as osteitis deformans because of its deforming capabilities (e.g., skull or femoral head enlargement). In this disease the serum calcium is normal, but there is an increase in osteoclastic activity (osteolytic lesions and elevated 24-hour urine hydroxyproline) and an increase in osteoblastic activity (elevated osteocalcin and alkaline phosphatase). Patients with Paget's disease exhibit a marked increase in osteoid, and the bone actually enlarges. The osteoid is never normally mineralized in this disease. In this patient, the bone scan shows significant uptake of labeled bisphosphonates, which are incorporated into newly formed osteoid during bone formation. Her proximal femur is enlarged and no longer fits properly into the acetabulum, which results in the hip pain.

There are a number of useful biochemical markers of bone metabolism. Osteoclasts synthesize tartrate-resistant acid phosphatase so that increased osteoclastic activity is reflected in increased serum levels of tartrate-resistant acid phosphatase. Bone resorption fragments of type I collagen and noncollagenous proteins increase as bone matrix is resorbed. Hydroxyproline is a good urinary marker of bone metabolism because hydroxyproline is released and excreted in the urine as collagen is broken down. The presence of pyridinoline cross-links, which are involved in the bundling of type I collagen, is used for measurement of bone resorption. Those cross-links are released only during degradation of mineralized collagen fibrils as occurs in bone resorption. Usually, pyridinoline cross-links are measured by immunoassay over a 24-hour period to detect excess bone resorption and collagen breakdown in disorders such as Paget's disease.

Markers of bone formation include osteocalcin, alkaline phosphatase, and the extension peptides of type I collagen. Osteocalcin is a vitamin K–dependent γ-carboxyglutamic acid protein, that is, synthesized by osteoblasts and secreted into the serum in an unchanged state. Serum concentrations of osteocalcin are, therefore, directly related to osteoblastic activity. It is a more specific marker than alkaline phosphatase, because other organs, such as the liver and kidney, produce that enzyme.

Radiologic methods such as conventional x-ray can be used to detect osteoporosis, but only after patients have lost 30–50% of their bone mass. Dual-beam photon absorptiometry allows a much more accurate diagnosis of loss of bone mass.

7-18. The answer is c. (*Lewis, pp 95–112. Scriver, pp 3–45.*) Anticipation refers to the worsening of the symptoms of disease in succeeding generations. The famous geneticist L.S. Penrose dismissed anticipation as an artifact, but the phenomenon has been validated by the discovery of expanding trinucleotide repeats. Steinert myotonic dystrophy is caused by unstable trinucleotide repeats near a muscle protein kinase gene on chromosome 19; the repeats are particularly unstable during female meiosis and may cause a severe syndrome of fetal muscle weakness and joint contractures. Variable expressivity could also be used to describe the family in the question, but the concept implies random variation in severity rather than progression with succeeding generations. Diseases that involve triplet repeat instability exhibit a bias for exaggerated repeat amplification during meiosis (e.g., women with the fragile X syndrome or myotonic dystrophy and men with Huntington chorea). The explanation for this bias is unknown.

7-19. The answer is b. *(Kasper et al., pp 1748–1759.)* Withdrawal from long-term use of proton pump inhibitors prescribed for peptic ulcer disease may be associated with rebound gastric hypersecretion. Pharmacological suppression of gastric acid secretion can occur when the administered drug binds to a receptor present on the parietal cell or when it antagonizes the hydrogen-potassium-ATPase pump responsible for the active secretion of hydrogen ion into the gastric lumen. At the present time, the most effective antisecretory compounds work by blocking the histamine type-2 (H_2) receptor present on the parietal cell or by inhibition of the hydrogen pumps. The latter are the most potent and long-acting, thus increasing the probability of increasing serum gastrin.

7-20. The answer is b. *(Gilroy, pp 201–215, 357–362. Siegel and Sapru, p 156. Simon, pp 170–171, 179.)* ALS is characterized by a progressive loss of motor functions, first seen as weakness in limb muscles, especially those of the fingers, and later of the other limbs. Sensory functions are not affected. Over time, there is wasting, atrophy, and fasciculations of limb muscles, followed by UMN signs and the patients ultimately die because of respiratory failure or complications of pneumonia. Electromyogram abnormalities can also be observed of the upper and lower extremities. In MS, there is also sensory loss, such as loss or blurring of vision, as well as bladder problems. Poliomyelitis and myasthenia gravis involve LMN symptoms, while a cerebral cortical stroke would result in a UMN disorder without LMN signs.

7-21. The answer is a. *(Murray, pp 60–71. Scriver, pp 4571–4636.)* Many enzymes that catalyze initial or rate-limiting reactions in metabolic pathways are subject to allosteric effects, where cofactors or substrates (effectors) activate the enzyme and end-products of the pathway inhibit the enzyme (feedback inhibition). The binding of an effector to the regulatory subunit of an allosteric enzyme causes a conformational change that either increases or decreases the activity of the enzyme's separate catalytic site. There are also cascades of regulation illustrated by the glycogen phosphorylases of liver and muscle. Each are responsive to cAMP through inhibitor proteins, phosphorylation of phosphorylase kinase, and phosphorylation of phosphorylase kinase that then acts on phosphorylase. Several types of mutations that alter activity or allosteric regulation of glycogen phosphorylase or its kinase have been characterized (e.g., glycogen storage disease type IV, 232700).

7-22. The answer is d. (*Brooks, pp 338–340. Levinson, pp 99, 100, 172, 483s. Murray PR—2005, pp 438–441. Ryan, pp 430–431.*) Leptospirosis is a zoonosis of worldwide distribution. Human infection results from ingestion of water or food contaminated with leptospirae. Rats, mice, wild rodents, dogs, swine, and cattle excrete the organisms in urine and feces during active illness and during an asymptomatic carrier state. Drinking, swimming, bathing, or food consumption may lead to human infection. Children acquire the disease from dogs more often than do adults. Treatment can include doxycycline, ampicillin, or amoxicillin. Symptoms in humans range from fever and rash to jaundice through aseptic meningitis.

7-23. The answer is d. (*Junqueira, pp 45, 47, 153–154, 160–163.*) The cells labeled with GFAP are activated astrocytes. Astrocytes are the most abundant cell type in the human brain. Astrocytes are activated following CNS damage and form the glial scar. These glial cells interact with neurons, blood vessels and the *pia mater* by their stellate processes. Regulation of the microenvironment including the concentrations of ions, metabolites and neurotransmitters (e.g., glutamate) is an important function of astrocytes. Astrocytes are also the source of the most common glioma, astrocytoma. The barrier function of the blood-brain-barrier is established by tight junctions (*zonula occludentes*) between endothelial cells in the blood vessels of the brain. However, astrocytes establish and maintain the blood-brain barrier and thus control the entry of compounds into the brain parenchyma. During development the astrocytes are critical to normal migration of developing neurons. The patient in the vignette suffers from NeuroAIDS. In that disease, astrocytes are believed to be infected with the AIDS virus. Astrocytes can be infected with HIV-1, however, there appears to be only limited replication. Infection can lead to changes in gene expression (of the cell) and some of the released products can have deleterious effects on neurons. Astrocytes integrate neuronal inputs, exhibit calcium excitability, and communicate bidirectionally with neighboring neurons and synapses, but do not synapse with neurons **(answer a)**. Microglia present antigen and phagocytose dying neurons **(answers b and c)**. Oligodendrocytes myelinate axons in the CNS **(answer e)**.

7-24. The answer is c. *(Brunton, pp 1521–1524. Craig, pp 749–750. Katzung, p 656.)* Cardiovascular and related hemodynamic changes, mostly arising from or related to tachycardia, increased ventricular contractility, and potentially leading to acute myocardial ischemia, are among the hallmarks of thyroid hormone excess, whether drug-induced or idiopathic (e.g., thyrotoxicosis of other causes). Increased thyroid hormone levels "up-regulate" the β-adrenergic receptors, leading to heightened and potentially lethal responses that involve overactivation of those receptors. β–Blockade provides important and prompt symptom relief, and may be lifesaving in situations such as this. Other interventions aimed at lowering thyroid hormone synthesis or release ultimately will be important, but saving the patient's life with administration of propranolol or a suitable alternative is the most important first step.

7-25. The answer is a. *(Murray, pp 163–172. Scriver, pp 1489–1520.)* Hereditary fructose intolerance (229600) is a defect in aldolase B, causing accumulation of fructose-1-phosphate and other hexose phosphates. The accumulated hexose phosphates deplete cellular phosphate pools, inhibiting generation of ATP through glycolysis or oxidative-phosphorylation (with increased lactate). Altered AMP/ATP ratios cause increased uric acid formation, and inhibition of glycogen phosphorylase by fructose phosphates produces hypoglycemia. Once recognized, hereditary fructose intolerance can be treated by elimination of fructose and sucrose from the diet.

7-26. The answer is c. *(Brooks, pp 554–558. Levinson, p 268. Murray PR—2005, pp 603–604. Ryan, pp 506–507.)* Parainfluenza viruses are important causes of respiratory diseases in infants and young children. The spectrum of disease caused by these viruses ranges from a mild febrile cold to croup, bronchiolitis, and pneumonia. Parainfluenza viruses contain RNA in a nucleocapsid encased within an envelope derived from the host cell membrane. Infected mammalian cell culture will hemabsorb red blood cells owing to viral hemagglutinin on the surface of the cell.

7-27. The answer is d. *(Kandel, pp 853–864. Siegel and Sapru, pp 343–351.)* The major transmitter released at terminals of neostriatal and paleostriatal fibers is GABA. Thus, the output of the basal ganglia is mainly inhibitory. This suggests that thalamic influences upon the cortex are generated through the process of disinhibition, whereby neurons of the basal ganglia are inhibited. The presence of glycine in striatal neurons has yet to be demonstrated. Enkephalins are released from terminals of neostriatal-pallidal fibers but not from other efferent neurons of the striatum. Dopamine is released from the brainstem and some adjoining hypothalamic neurons but certainly not from striatal neurons. The neostriatum receives cortical inputs that utilize glutamate, but the release of GABA from terminals of neostriatal efferent fibers has not been demonstrated.

7-28. The answer is d. (*Murray, pp 481–497. Scriver, pp 4223–4240.*) People with bowed legs and other bone malformations were quite common in the northeastern United States following the industrial revolution. This was caused by childhood diets lacking foods with vitamin D and by minimal exposure to sunlight due to the dawn-to-dusk working conditions of the textile mills. Vitamin D is essential for the metabolism of calcium and phosphorus. Soft and malformed bones result from its absence. Liver, fish oil, and egg yolks contain vitamin D, and milk is supplemented with vitamin D by law. In adults, lack of sunlight and a diet poor in vitamin D lead to osteomalacia (soft bones). Dark-skinned peoples are more susceptible to vitamin D deficiency.

Biotin deficiency can be caused by diets with excess egg white, leading to dehydration and acidosis from accumulation of carboxylic and lactic acids. Retinoic acid is a vitamin A derivative that can be helpful in treating acne but not vitamin D deficiency. Leafy vegetables are a source of B vitamins such as niacin and cobalamin.

7-29. The answer is d. (*Mandell, pp 2888–2892. Damjanov, pp 987–988.*) *G. lamblia*, a flagellate protozoan, is the most common cause of outbreaks of waterborne diarrheal disease in the United States and is seen frequently in Rocky Mountain areas. Ingestion of cysts from contaminated water results in trophozoites in the duodenum and jejunum. Identification of the trophozoite stage is done by duodenal aspiration or small-bowel biopsy; identification of the cyst stage (intermittent) is done by examination of stool. The trophozoite may appear as a pear-shaped, binucleate organism ("two eyes"). Giardiasis may cause malabsorption but is often asymptomatic. Duodenal aspiration, immunofluorescence, and ELISA testing for *Giardia* antigens are diagnostic and therapy with metronidazole or quinacrine is effective.

7-30. The answer is d. *(Brunton, pp 1478, 1485. Craig, pp 66t, 261, 781–782. Katzung, pp 552, 556.)* Phytonadione (vitamin K_1) is the antidote. It overcomes (reverses, antagonizes) warfarin's hepatic anticoagulant effects, which involve inhibited synthesis of clotting factors (VII, IX, X, and prothrombin). Aminocaproic acid is a backup (to whole blood, packed red cells, or fresh-frozen plasma) for managing bleeding in response to excessive effects of thrombolytic drugs (e.g., alteplase [tPA], streptokinase, tenecteplase). It is not indicated for warfarin-related bleeding. Epoetin alfa is a hematopoietic growth factor that stimulates erythrocyte production in peritubular cells in the proximal tubules of the kidney. Its uses include management of anemias associated with chronic renal failure, chemotherapy (of nonmyeloid malignancies), or zidovudine therapy in patients with acquired immunodeficiency syndrome. It is inappropriate for this patient. Ferrous sulfate (or fumarate or gluconate) is indicated for prevention or treatment of iron-deficiency anemias. It will do nothing to lower the patient's INR or alleviate related symptoms. Protamine sulfate is the antidote for heparin overdoses. It acts electrostatically with heparin, in the blood, to form a complex that lacks anticoagulant activity. It does nothing to the hepatic vitamin K–related problems that are at the root of excessive warfarin effects.

7-31. The answer is c. *(Levinson, pp 6–7, 133–134. Ryan, p 19.)* The periplasm is the space between the outer membrane and the plasma membrane of bacteria. The periplasmic space in *E. coli* has been shown to contain a number of proteins, sugars, amino acids, and inorganic ions. Ethylenediaminetetraacetic acid (EDTA) is a chelating agent that disrupts the cell walls of gram-negative bacteria.

7-32. The answer is b. *(Kumar, pp 701–702. Rubin, pp 1364–1365.)* Langerhans cell histiocytosis, previously known as histiocytosis X, refers to a spectrum of clinical diseases that are associated with the proliferation of Langerhans cells. These cells, not to be confused with the Langerhans-type giant cells found in caseating granulomas of tuberculosis, have Fc receptors and HLA-D/DR antigens and react with CD1 antibodies. These cells contain distinctive granules, seen by electron microscopy, that are rod-shaped organelles resembling tennis rackets. They are called LC (Langerhans cell) granules, pentilaminar bodies, or Birbeck granules. There are three general clinical forms of Langerhans histiocytosis. Acute disseminated LC histiocytosis (Letterer-Siwe disease) affects children before the age of 3 years. These children have cutaneous lesions that resemble seborrhea, hepatosplenomegaly, and lymphadenopathy. The LCs infiltrate the marrow, which leads to anemia, thrombocytopenia, and recurrent infections. The clinical course is usually rapidly fatal; however, with intensive chemotherapy 50% of patients may survive 5 years. Multifocal LC histiocytosis (Hand-Schüller-Christian disease) usually begins between the second and sixth years of life. The characteristic triad consists of bone lesions, particularly in the calvarium and the base of the skull; diabetes insipidus; and exophthalmos. These lesions are the result of proliferations of LCs. Lesions around the hypothalamus lead to decreased ADH production and signs of diabetes insipidus. Unifocal LC histiocytosis (eosinophilic granuloma), seen in older patients, is usually a unifocal disease, most often affecting the skeletal system. The lesions are granulomas that contain a mixture of lipid-laden Langerhans cells, macrophages, lymphocytes, and eosinophils.

In contrast, sarcoidosis is characterized by a proliferation of activated macrophages that form granulomas. It is not a proliferation of LCs. Dermatopathic lymphadenitis refers to a chronic lymphadenitis that affects the lymph nodes draining the sites of chronic dermatologic diseases. The lymph nodes undergo hyperplasia of the germinal follicles and accumulation of melanin and hemosiderin pigment by the phagocytic cells.

7-33. The answer is a. (*Lewis, pp 75–94. Scriver, pp 2537–2570. Murray RK, pp 293–302.*) The child has Lesch-Nyhan syndrome (308000), an X-linked recessive disorder that is caused by HGPRT enzyme deficiency. HGPRT is responsible for the salvage of purines from nucleotide degradation, and its deficiency elevates levels of PRPP, purine synthesis, and uric acid. PRPP is also elevated in glycogen storage diseases due to increased amounts of carbohydrate precursors.

7-34. The answer is a. (*Ganong, p 555. Stead et al., pp 6–8, 44–45.*) The PR interval represents the time it takes for the cardiac action potential to propagate from the SA node to the ventricular muscle. A delay in this interval, normally produced by a slowing in the conduction velocity through the AV node, is called a first-degree heart block. A second-degree heart block occurs when the action potential does not always propagate through the SA node. This produces an uneven heart beat. A third-degree block occurs when the action potential never reaches the ventricle. Under these conditions, pacemakers within the ventricle produce ventricular contraction but the rate is very slow. Inversion of the T wave and elevation of the ECG are indicators of membrane potential defects within the ventricular muscle.

7-35. The answer is d. *(Brunton, pp 886–887. Craig, p 154. Katzung, pp 205–207.)* Digoxin inhibits the sarcolemmal Na^+, K^+-ATPase ("sodium pump"). This reduces the active (ATP–dependent) extrusion of intracellular Na^+. The relative excess of intracellular Na^+ competes with intracellular Ca^{2+} for sites on a sarcolemmal 2Na–Ca exchange diffusion carrier, such that less Ca^{2+} is extruded from the cells. The net result is a rise of free $[Ca^{2+}]_i$ and greater actin-myosin interactions (i.e., a positive inotropic effect that increases cardiac output through an increase of stroke volume).

7-36. The answer is e. *(Afifi, pp 64–66. Nolte, pp 221–224. Siegel and Sapru, pp 141–142.)* The section depicted in the diagram is taken from the lower cervical cord. The cervical level of the spinal cord can be distinguished from other levels of the cord by the following characteristics: the presence of a well-defined fasciculus cuneatus, situated immediately lateral to the fasciculus gracilis; the presence of well-defined motor nuclei that are clumped into six different groups, three of which can be distinguished; an absence of an intermediolateral cell column; and relatively extensive quantities of both white and gray matter. Thus, a knife wound that destroyed the right half of the spinal cord results in a Brown-Séquard syndrome. The knife wound would cause loss of sensory and motor functions of both upper and lower limbs. The sensory loss of lower limbs would occur because of the damage to ascending fibers from spinothalamic and the fasciculus gracilis (causing loss of pain and temperature of the contralateral side of the body and conscious proprioception of the ipsilateral side), which would also include some loss of these sensations from the upper limb. At the lesion, there is additional loss of these sensations from the upper limb, which enter the cord at this level of spinal cord. Here, there would also be some bilateral pain and temperature loss at the level of the lesion because of the presence of crossing fibers. Because the lesion occurred at the cervical level, it would result in an LMN paralysis of the upper limb and a UMN paralysis involving the lower limb. Klumpke's palsy, a form of brachial plexus palsy, is characterized by weakness of the wrist and finger flexors and of small muscles of the hand, as well as loss of sensation along the medial aspect of the arm.

7-37. The answer is b. *(Damjanov, pp 2205–2206, 2363–2364. Kumar, pp 1149–1151.)* Neoplastic proliferations of the stroma of the breast may lead to the formation of either fibroadenomas or phyllodes tumors. Fibroadenomas are characterized histologically by a mixture of fibrous tissue and ducts, with no increase in cellularity or mitoses. Only the stromal cells, not the glandular cells, are clonal proliferations. Another neoplastic tumor that arises from the stromal cells is the phyllodes tumor. It is distinguished from fibroadenomas by a more cellular stroma and the presence of stromal mitoses. The phyllodes tumor, which has been called a cystosarcoma phyllodes, may either be benign or malignant. A benign phyllodes tumor is characterized by increased stromal cells with few mitoses, while a malignant phyllodes tumor has increased numbers of stromal cells that are atypical along with numerous mitoses.

7-38. The answer is b. (*Young, pp 147, 149. Junqueira, pp 208, 211, 215. Ross, p 371.*) The blood vessel in the electron micrograph is an arteriole (small artery) involved in intraorgan blood flow. There is only one layer of smooth muscle, but a distinct internal elastic membrane is present.

There is no visible internal elastic membrane in a venule. A capillary lacks smooth muscle and is composed only of a single layer of endothelial cells.

The aorta and large arteries (**answer a**) contain extensive elastic fibers that permit rapid arterial wall stretch in response to the force of ventricular contraction during systole (120 to 160 mm Hg) followed by sudden relaxation (60 to 90 mm Hg) during diastole. Blood is ejected from the left ventricle into the large arteries only during systole; however, blood flow is uniform because of the elasticity of the large, conducting arteries.

The muscular (distributing) arteries regulate blood flow to organs (**answer c**). Muscular (medium) arteries contain more smooth muscle than the arteriole (**answer b**) in the figure and distribute blood to organs. Contraction of muscular arteries is regulated by local factors as well as sympathetic innervation. The degree of contraction regulates blood flow between organs. When the tunica media of the muscular artery is contracted, less blood flow occurs to the organ. In a more relaxed state, there is increased blood flow to the same organ.

The thoracic duct (**answer d**) returns lymphocytes from the lymphoid compartment to the circulation. The thoracic duct shows complete disorganization in the wall with no distinct media or adventitia. The large veins (**answer e**), such as the vena cava, that return blood to the heart contain smooth muscle bundles in the adventitia and are also the only vessel in which one sees both cross sections and longitudinal sections of smooth muscle in the same vessel.

7-39. The answer is a. (*Brunton, pp 203–204, 211–213, 1724. Craig, pp 126–130, 347. Katzung, pp 101–104.*) Although several of the listed drugs inhibit the activity of AChE, only edrophonium is used in the diagnosis of myasthenia gravis. The drug has a more rapid onset of action (1 to 3 min following intravenous administration) and a shorter duration of action (approximately 5 to 10 min) than pyridostigmine. This fast acting/short duration profile is precisely what we want in this situation. We can quickly get our diagnostic answer, yet not have to deal too long with adverse responses (such as ventilatory paralysis) if the patient was experiencing a cholinergic crisis (excessive doses of their oral cholinesterase inhibitor); and we've now worsened the situation by inhibiting the metabolic inactivation of ACh even more with our diagnostic medication. (The short duration and the need for parenteral administration preclude use of edrophonium as a practical drug for long-term treatment of myasthenia gravis.)

Malathion (b) is used topically to treat head lice and is never used internally (intentionally). Pyridostigmine (e) is used orally for maintenance therapy of myasthenia gravis. Physostigmine (c) is indicated for treatment of glaucoma (given topically), and is also a valuable parenteral drug for treating toxicity of anticholinergic drugs such as atropine. They are all cholinesterase inhibitors. Pralidoxime (d) is a "cholinesterase reactivator" and is used adjunctively (with atropine) in the treatment of poisonings caused by "irreversible" cholinesterase inhibitors, such as the "nerve gases" used as bioweapons and some commercial insecticides.

7-40. The answer is a. (*Lewis, pp 377–496. Scriver, pp 4077–5016. Murray RK pp 434–455.*) Sex steroids are synthesized from cholesterol by side-chain cleavage (employing a P450 enzyme) to produce pregnenolone. Pregnenolone is then converted to testosterone in the testis, to estrogen in the ovary, and to corticosterone and aldosterone in the adrenal gland. The enzymes 3β-hydroxysteroid dehydrogenase, 21-hydroxylase, 11β-hydroxylase, and 18-hydroxylase modify pregnenolone to produce other sex and adrenal steroids. Deficiencies in adrenal 21-hydroxylase can thus lead to inadequate testosterone production in males and produce ambiguous external genitalia. Such children can also exhibit low sodium and high potassium due to deficiency of the more distal steroids corticol and aldosterone. 5β-reductase converts testosterone to dihydrotestosterone, and its deficiency produces milder degrees of hypogenitalism without salt wasting. Deficiency of the androgen receptor is called testicular feminization, producing normal looking females who may not seek medical attention until they present with infertility.

7-41. The answer is d. (*Levinson, pp 135–137, 475s. Ryan, pp 353, 362–363.*) Region 1 (the Oantigenic side chain of LPS is responsible for the many serotypes of *Salmonella*. A mutant of *Salmonella* deficient in region 1 is not identified as a "newport," at least by virtue of its somatic antigen; biochemical identification of this mutant would be *S. enteritidis*. Loss of region 1 does not affect genus and species classification of *Salmonella*. Recently, however, it has been recommended that *Salmonella* be referred to by genus and serovar, that is, *Salmonella newport* or *Salmonella* serovar *newport*.

7-42. The answer is d. (*Greenberg, pp 167–170.*) Multiple sclerosis is a demyelinating disease. The lesions may also involve some reactive gliosis and axonal degeneration as well. It occurs mainly in the white matter of the spinal cord and brain as well as in the optic nerve.

7-43. The answer is d. (*Stead et al., pp 237–238.*) The fractional excretion (FE) is the fraction of the filtered load that is excreted. It is calculated using the formula

$$FE = \text{Amount Excreted/Amount Filtered} = (U_{Na} \times \dot{V})/(P_{Na} \times GFR)$$

Because $GFR = (U_{creatinine} \times \dot{V}/P_{creatinine})$,

$$FE = (U_{Na} \times \dot{V})/[P_{Na} \times (U_{creatinine} \times \dot{V}/P_{creatinine})]$$

$$= (U_{Na} \times P_{creatinine})/(P_{Na} \times U_{creatinine})$$

$$= 33 \text{ mM} \times 7.5 \text{ mg/dL}/135 \text{ mM} \times 90 \text{ mg/dL} = 0.02$$

Fractional excretion is used to distinguish between a prerenal state, such as volume depletion, and intrinsic renal failure, such as acute tubular necrosis. A fractional excretion of less than 1% is consistent with volume depletion, whereas a fractional excretion of 2% or greater is consistent with acute renal failure. This patient, with a fraction excretion of 2%, was diagnosed with acute renal failure caused by excessive intake of Motrin.

7-44. The answer is c. (*Fawcett, pp 657–660. Kumar, pp 882–883. Rubin, pp 796–798.*) Cirrhosis refers to fibrosis of the liver that involves both central veins and portal triads. This fibrosis is the result of liver cell necrosis and regenerative hepatic nodules. These nodules consist of hyperplastic hepatocytes with enlarged, atypical nuclei, irregular hepatic plates, and distorted vasculature. There is distortion of the normal lobular architecture. These changes diffusely involve the entire liver; they are not focal. It is thought that the fibrosis is the result of fibril-forming collagens that are released by Ito cells, which are fat-containing lipocytes found within the space of Disse of the liver. They normally participate in the metabolism and storage of vitamin A, but they can secrete collagen in the fibrotic (cirrhotic) liver. Normally types I and III collagens (interstitial types) are found in the portal areas and occasionally in the space of Disse or around central veins. In cirrhosis, types I and III collagens are deposited throughout the hepatic lobule. These Ito cells are initiated by unknown factors and then are further stimulated by such factors as platelet-derived growth factor and transforming growth factor-beta to secrete collagen.

In contrast to Ito cells, endothelial cells normally line the sinusoids and demarcate the extrasinusoidal space of Disse. Attached to the endothelial cells are the phagocytic Kupffer cells, which are part of the monocyte-phagocyte system. Bile ducts, and thus the epithelial cells that form them, are found in the portal triads of the liver.

7-45. The answer is d. (*Ganong, pp 571–574.*) Preload is the degree to which the myocardium is stretched before it contracts, i.e., the length of the sarcomere at the end of diastole. In vivo, the variable most directly related to sarcomere length during end-diastole is left ventricular end-diastolic volume. Although blood volume, central venous pressure, pulmonary capillary wedge pressure, and left ventricular end-diastolic pressure can all influence preload, they all exert their influence through changes in end-diastolic volume.

7-46. The answer is b. (*Ganong, pp 571–576.*) Afterload is the tension at which the load is lifted during the contraction of a sarcomere. According to the law of Laplace ($T = P \times r/w$), the tension (T) is proportional to the pressure (P) and radius (r) and inversely proportional to the thickness of the ventricle wall (w) during systole. The mean left ventricular systolic pressure would therefore be the best index of afterload in vivo. Mean arterial blood pressure (MAP) is normally the same as ventricular pressure and therefore a good index of afterload. However, in a patient with aortic stenosis, the ventricular pressure is higher than the aortic pressure. Although the total peripheral resistance (TPR) can influence afterload by causing changes in mean arterial blood pressure, changes in TPR do not always cause corresponding changes in afterload. For example, during aerobic exercise, afterload (MAP) is often increased, whereas TPR is reduced and following a hemorrhage, TPR is high, whereas afterload (MAP) is low. Pulmonary capillary wedge pressure and left ventricular end-diastolic pressure are estimates of the volume of blood in the ventricle during diastole and are indices of preload.

7-47. The answer is d. (*Ganong, pp 554–556, 640. Kasper et al., pp 126–130. Stead et al., pp 44–46.*) Syncope (fainting) is a transient loss of consciousness caused by an inadequate blood flow to the brain. Transient decreases in cerebral blood flow are usually due to one of three general mechanisms: disorders of vascular tone or blood volume, cardiovascular disorders, or cerebrovascular disease. Approximately one-fourth of syncopal episodes are of cardiac origin and are due to either transient obstruction of blood flow through the heart or sudden decreases in cardiac output due to cardiac arrhythmias, such as bradycardia, heart block, or sinus arrest (neurocardiogenic syncope). Third-degree (complete) heart block results when conduction of the action potential from the atria to the ventricles is completely interrupted. Under these conditions, pacemaker cells within the His-Purkinje system or the ventricular muscle cause the ventricles to beat at a low rate (idioventricular rhythm) independently of the atria. Although the heart rate may be high enough to adequately perfuse the brain under resting conditions, Third-degree heart block is caused by conduction system disturbances, inferior wall MI, and digitalis toxicity. When the conduction disturbance is due to disease in the AV node, the idioventricular rhythm is normally about 45 beats/min. When the conduction disturbance is below the AV node (infranodal block) due to disease in the bundle of His, firing of more peripheral ventricular pacemakers can decrease heart rate to below 30 beats/min with periods of asystole that may last a minute or more. The resultant cerebral ischemia causes dizziness and fainting (Stokes-Adams syndrome). Sinus arrhythmia is a change of the heart rate produced by the normal variation in the rate of phase 4 depolarization of the SA nodal pacemaker cells between inspiration and expiration. First-degree heart block is defined as a higher-than-normal PR interval (greater than 0.2 seconds). Second-degree heart block occurs when the action potential fails to reach the ventricles some, but not all, of the time. Tachycardia is a heart rate above 100 beats per minute.

7-48. The answer is c. (*Ganong, pp 554–556. Stead et al., pp 6–8, 44–45.*) Conduction abnormalities can produce first-degree, second-degree, or third-degree heart block. In a second-degree heart block, a P wave is not always followed by a QRS complex as in trace C, where the second P wave is not followed by a QRS complex. In a first-degree heart block, trace D, the interval between the beginning of the P wave and the beginning of the QRS complex (the PR interval) is longer than normal (greater than 0.2 seconds). In a third-degree heart block, conduction between the atria and ventricles is completely blocked so the atrial beats (represented by the P waves) and the ventricular beats (represented by the QRS complex) are completely dissociated.

7-49. The answer is e. (*Ganong, pp 561–563. Kasper et al., pp 1316–1318.*) Abnormalities in coronary blood flow resulting in ischemia of the ventricular muscle will lead to a current of injury, which is reflected as an upward or downward shift in the ST segment of the ECG recording. The electrical activity of the heart does not reflect changes in ventricular contractility, blood pressure, ejection fraction, or total peripheral resistance, although all of these can be altered by changes in coronary blood flow.

7-50. The answer is c. *(Ganong, pp 565–568.)* The pressure gradient between regions of the cardiovascular system is directly proportional to the resistance of the intervening structures. During ventricular ejection, the aortic valves are open and do not offer any significant resistance to blood flow. Therefore, there is very little, if any, pressure difference between the left ventricle and the aorta. Because the tricuspid valve is closed during ventricular ejection, there is an appreciable pressure difference between the right ventricle and the left atrium, although this pressure difference is opposite in direction to the flow of blood through the circulatory system. Although pulmonary vascular resistance is relatively small compared with systemic vascular resistance, it nonetheless produces a pressure drop between the right ventricle and the left atrium. Because most of the resistance in the systemic vasculature occurs at the level of the arterioles, there is a large pressure gradient between the aorta and the capillaries.

Bibliography

Abbas AK, Lichtman AH: *Basic Immunology: Functions and Disorders of the Immune System,* 2/e. Philadelphia, Saunders/Elsevier, 2006.

Adams RD, Victor M, Ropper AW: *Principles of Neurology,* 6/e. New York, McGraw-Hill, 1997.

Afifi AK, Bergman RA: *Functional Neuroanatomy.* New York, McGraw-Hill, 1998.

Alberts B, et al: *Molecular Biology of the Cell,* 4/e. New York, Garland, 2002.

Avery JK (ed): *Oral Development and Histology,* 3/e. New York, Thieme, 2002.

Ayala C, Spellberg B: *Pathophysiology for the Boards and Wards,* 4/e. Malden, MA, Blackwell, 2003.

Behrman RE, Kliegman RM, Jenson HB: *Nelson's Textbook of Pediatrics,* 17/e. Philadelphia, Saunders, 2004.

Brooks GF et al (ed). *Jawetz's Medical Microbiology,* 23/e. New York: McGraw-Hill, 2004.

Brunton L, Lazo J, Parker K (eds). Goodman & Gilman's *The Pharmacological Basis of Therapeutics,* 11th ed.

Casals T, Bassas L, et al: Extensive analysis of 40 infertile patients with congenital absence of the vas deferens: in 50% of cases only one CFTR allele could be detected. *Hum Genet* 95(2): 205–211,1995.

Center for Disease Control Treatment Guidelines 2006, Sexually Transmitted Diseases.

Chandrasoma P, Taylor CR: *Concise Pathology,* 3/e. Stamford, CT, Appleton & Lange, 1998.

Craig CR, Stitzel RE (eds). *Modern Pharmacology with Clinical Applications,* 6/e. Lippincott Williams & Wilkins, 2004.

Damjanov I, Linder J (eds): *Anderson's Pathology,* 10/e. St. Louis, Mosby, 1996.

Duchin JS, et al: Hantavirus pulmonary syndrome: a clinical description of 17 patients with a newly recognized disease. *N Engl J Med* 330:949–955, 1994.

Favus MJ (ed): *Disorders of Bone and Mineral Metabolism,* 6/e. Washington, D.C., American Society for Bone and Mineral Research, 2006.

Flake AW, Roncarolo MG, et al: Brief report: treatment of x-linked severe combined immunodeficiency by in utero transplantation of paternal bone marrow. *N Engl J Med* 335(24):1806–1810, 1996.

Ganong WF: *Review of Medical Physiology,* 22/e. New York, The McGraw-Hill Companies, Inc., 2005.

Gilroy J: *Basic Neurology*, 3/e. New York, McGraw-Hill, 2000.

Goldman L, Ausiello D. *Cecil Textbook of Medicine*. 22nd ed. Philadelphia, PA, Saunders; 2004.

Greenberg DA, Aminoff MJ, Simon RP. *Clinical Neurology*, 5/e. New York, McGraw-Hill, 2002.

Greenspan FS, Gardner DG: *Basic and Clinical Endocrinology*, 7/e. New York, Lange Medical Books/McGraw-Hill, 2004.

Guyton AC, Hall JE: *Textbook of Medical Physiology*, 10/e. Philadelphia, W.B. Saunders, 2000.

Henry JB, et al (eds): *Clinical Diagnosis and Management by Laboratory Methods*, 20/e. Philadelphia, Saunders, 2001.

Junqueira LC, Carneiro J: *Basic Histology: Text and Atlas*, 11/e. New York, McGraw-Hill, 2005.

Kandel ER, Schwartz JH, Jessell TM: *Principles of Neural Science*, 4/e. New York, McGraw-Hill, 2000.

Kasper DL et al (eds). *Harrison's Principles of Internal Medicine*, 16/e. New York: McGraw-Hill, 2005.

Katzung BG (ed): *Basic and Clinical Pharmacology*, 9/e. New York: McGraw-Hill, 2004.

Kierszenbaum AL: *Histology and Cell Biology*. St. Louis, Mosby, 2002.

Kindt TJ, Goldsby RA, Osborne BA: *Immunology*, 6/e. New York, W.H. Freeman and Company, 2007.

Kumar V, Abbas AK, Fausto N: *Robbins and Cotran Pathologic Basis of Disease*, 7/e. Philadelphia, Saunders, 2004.

Levinson W et al. *Medical Microbiology and Immunology*, 8/e. New York: McGraw-Hill, 2004.

Levitzky MG: *Pulmonary Physiology*, 6/e. New York, The McGraw-Hill Companies, Inc., 2003.

Lewis R: *Human Genetics: Concepts and Applications*. 5/e. New York, McGraw-Hill, 2003.

Lobov IB, Brooks PC, Lang RA: Angiopoietin-2 displays VEGF-dependent modulation of capillary structure and endothelial cell survival in vivo, Proc. Natl. Acad. Science (USA) 99:11205–11210, 2002.

Mandell GL, et al (eds): *Principles and Practice of Infectious Diseases*, 5/e. New York, Churchill Livingstone, 1998.

Martin JH: *Neuroanatomy*, 2/e. Stamford, CT, Appleton & Lange, 1996.

McPhee SJ, et al: *Pathophysiology of Disease*, 4/e. Stamford, CT, Appleton & Lange, 2002.

Moore KL and Dalley AF: *Clinically Oriented Anatomy*, 5/e Philadelphia, Lippincott Williams & Wilkins, 2006.

Moore KL and Persaud TVN: *Before We Are Born: Essentials of Embryology and Birth Defects*, 6/e. Philadelphia, W.B. Saunders, 2003.

Murray PR et al. *Medical Microbiology*, 5/e. St. Louis, MO: Mosby; 2005.

Murray RK, Granner DK, Mayes PA, Rodwell VW. *Harper's Illustrated Biochemistry*. 26/e. New York, McGraw-Hill, 2003.

Nolte J: *The Human Brain: An Introduction to Its Functional Anatomy*, 4/e. St. Louis, MO, Mosby, 1999.

Paller AS, Mancini AJ. *Hurwitz Clinical Pediatric Dermatology e-dition: Text with Continually Updated Online Reference*. 3rd ed. Philadelphia, PA, Saunders; 2003.

Parslow TG et al. *Medical Immunology*, 10/e. New York: McGraw-Hill, 2001.

Ravel R: *Clinical Laboratory Medicine*, 6/e. St. Louis, Mosby-Year Book, 1995.

Reszka AA, Rodan GA: Mechanism of action of bisphosphonates. *Curr. Osteoporosis Rep.* 1:45–52, 2003.

Ross MH, Pawlina W: *Histology: A Text and Atlas*, 5/e. Baltimore, Lippincott Williams & Wilkins, 2006.

Rubin E, Farber JL: *Pathology*, 3/e. Philadelphia, Lippincott, 1999.

Ryan KJ et al (ed). *Sherris Medical Microbiology*, 4/e. New York: McGraw-Hill, 2001.

Sadler TW: *Langman's Medical Embryology*, 10/e. Baltimore, Williams & Wilkins, 2006.

Scriver CR, Beaudet AL, Sly WS, Valle D: *The Metabolic and Molecular Bases of Inherited Disease*. 8/e. New York, McGraw-Hill, 2001.

Siegel GJ, Agranoff BW, Albers RW, Fisher SK, Uhler MD: *Basic Neurochemistry*, 6/e. Philadelphia, PA, Lippincott, Williams & Wilkins, 1999.

Siegel A, Sapru HN: *Essential Neuroscience*. Philadelphia, PA, Lippincott, Williams & Wilkins, 2006.

Simon RP, Aminoff MJ, Greenberg DA: *Clinical Neurology*, 4/e. New York, McGraw-Hill, 1999.

Stead LG, Stead SM, Kaufman MS, McFarlane SI: *First Aid for the Medicine Clerkship*, 2/e. New York, The McGraw-Hill Companies, Inc., 2006.

Waxman SG: *Correlative Neuroanatomy*, 24/e. New York, McGraw-Hill, 2000.

Widmaier E, Hershel R, Strang K: *Vander's Human Physiology*, 10/e. New York, The McGraw-Hill Companies, Inc., 2006.

Young B, Heath JW: *Wheater's Functional Histology*, 4/e. New York, Churchill Livingstone, 2000.